ADVANCES IN NEPHROLOGY

From The Necker Hospital

VOLUME 8

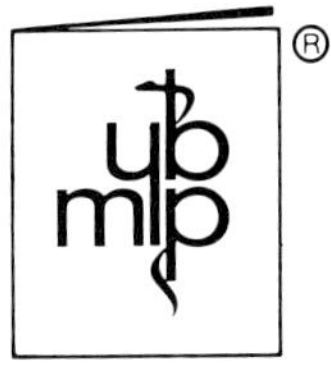

ADVANCES IN NEPHROLOGY

VOLUMES 1 through 3 (out of print)

VOLUME 4

VOLUME 5

VOLUME 6

VOLUME 7

ADVANCES IN NEPHROLOGY

From the Necker Hospital

FRENCH EDITORS

JEAN HAMBURGER, M.D.

JEAN CROSNIER, M.D.

JEAN-PIERRE GRÜNFELD, M.D.

Department of Nephrology, Necker Hospital, Paris, France

AMERICAN EDITOR

MORTON H. MAXWELL, M.D.

Clinical Professor of Medicine, University of California (Los Angeles) Medical Center

VOLUME 8 • 1979

YEAR BOOK MEDICAL PUBLISHERS · INC.

CHICAGO • LONDON

Library of Congress Catalog Card Number: 73-154325

International Standard Serial Number: 0084-5957

International Standard Book Number: 0-8151-4117-3

Contributors

ASSAN, R., M.D., *Professeur Agrégé, Hôpital Necker, Paris, France*

AYED, K., M.D., *Hôpital Broussais, Paris, France*

BAGDADE, J. D., M.D., *Department of Medicine, School of Medicine, University of Washington and the Providence Medical Center, Seattle, Washington*

BARBANEL, C., M.D., *Ancien Chef de Clinique, Hôpital Necker, Paris, France*

BARIETY, J., M.D., *Hôpital Broussais, Paris, France*

BERNAUDIN, J. F., M.D., *Hôpital Henri Mondor, Créteil, France*

BRAUTBAR, N., M.D., *Assistant Professor of Medicine, Division of Nephrology, University of California, Los Angeles, School of Medicine, Los Angeles, California*

BROWN, D. M., M.D., *Professor of Pediatrics and Laboratory Medicine and Pathology, University of Minnesota School of Medicine, Minneapolis, Minnesota*

CAPPEL, J., M.D., *Assistant, Service de Virologie, Brugmann University Hospital, Brussels, Belgium*

CROSNIER, J., M.D., *Professeur and Chef de Service, Hôpital Necker, Paris, France*

DE ROY, G., M.D., *Adjoint, Service d'Anatomie Pathologique, Brugmann University Hospital, Brussels, Belgium*

DROZ, D., M.D., *Chef de Clinique, Hôpital Necker, Paris, France*

DRUET, E., M.D., *Attachée-assistant, Faculté de Médecine, Université Paris VI, Paris, France*

DRUET, P., M.D., *Hôpital Broussais, Paris, France*

DUBERNARD, J. M., M.D., *Cliniques Universitaires de Néphrologie et d'Urologie and Unité INSERM U 80, Hôpital Edouard Herriot, Lyon, France*

DUPONT, E., M.D., *Premier Assistant, Département de Néphrologie, Brugmann University Hospital, Brussels, Belgium*

FINCH, T. W., M.D., *Hôpital Necker, Paris, France*

FRANTZ, P., M.D., *Unité de Transplantation de la Clinique Urologique, Groupe Hospitalier Pitié-Salpétrière, Paris, France*

GARABEDIAN, M., M.D., *Chargée de Recherches au C.N.R.S., Hôpital Necker-Enfants Malades, Paris, France*

GIRARD, J. F., M.D., *Hôpital Broussais, Paris, France*

GUNDERSEN, H. J. G., M.D., *Lecturer in Stereology, Kommunehospitalet, Aarhus, Denmark*

HINGLAIS, N., M.D., *Chargée de Recherches, INSERM U 28, Hôpital Broussais, Paris, France*

JACOBS, C., M.D., *Service de Néphrologie, Groupe Hospitalier Pitié-Salpétrière, Paris, France*

JONES, M. R., PH.D., *Medical and Research Services, Veterans Administration, Wadsworth Medical Center and Schools of Medicine and Public Health, University of California, Los Angeles, Los Angeles, California*

KINNAERT, P., M.D., *Adjoint Principal, Service de Chirurgie, Brugmann University Hospital, Brussels, Belgium*

KLEEMAN, C. R., M.D., *Professor of Medicine, Chief, Division of Nephrology, University of California, Los Angeles, School of Medicine, Los Angeles, California*

KOPPLE, J. D., M.D., *Medical and Research Services, Veterans Administration, Wadsworth Medical Center and Schools of Medicine and Public Health, University of California, Los Angeles, Los Angeles, California*

KREIS, H., M.D., *Professeur Agrégé, Hôpital Necker, Paris, France*

LACOMBE, M., M.D., *Professeur, Hôpital Necker, Paris, France*

LEGRAIN, M., M.D., *Service de Néphrologie, Groupe Hospitalier Pitié-Salpétrière, Paris, France*

LIEBOWITCH, M., M.D., *Ancienne Chef de Clinique, Hôpital Necker, Paris, France*

LOCKWOOD, C. M., M.B.B.C.H., M.R.C.P., *Research Fellow and Honorary Senior Registrar, Renal Unit, Department of Medicine, Royal Postgraduate Medical School, London, England*

LUNDBAEK, K., M.D., *Professor of Medicine, Kommunehospitalet, Aarhus, Denmark*

MACINTYRE, I. M. B., CH.B., PH.D., D.SC., *Professor of Endocrine Chemistry and Director, Endocrine Unit, Royal Postgraduate Medical School, University of London, London, England*

MALIK, M. C., M.D., *Cliniques Universitaires de Néphrologie et d'Urologie and Unité INSERM U 80, Hôpital Edouard Herriot, Lyon, France*

MAUER, S. M., M.D., *Associate Professor of Pediatrics, Director, Pediatric Hemodialysis Program, University of Minnesota School of Medicine, Minneapolis, Minnesota*

MAXWELL, M. H., M.D., *Clinical Professor of Medicine, University of California and Director of Hypertension Division, Cedars-Sinai Medical Center, Los Angeles, California*

MOGENSEN, C. E., M.D., *Lecturer in Medicine, Kommunehospitalet, Aarhus, Denmark*

MOREAU, J. F., M.D., *Professeur Agrégé, Hôpital Necker, Paris, France*

NEYRA, P., M.D., *Cliniques Universitaires de Néphrologie et d'Urologie and Unité INSERM U 80, Hôpital Edouard Herriot, Lyon, France*

NOEL, L. H., M.D., *Hôpital Necker, Paris, France*

ØSTERBY, R., M.D., *Director of Electron Microscopic Laboratory for Diabetes Research, Kommunehospitalet, Aarhus, Denmark*

PETERS, D. K., M.B., B.CH., F.R.C.P., *Professor of Medicine and Consultant Physician, Royal Postgraduate Medical School, London, England*

PUSSEL, B., F.R.A.C.P., *Royal Postgraduate Medical School, London, England*

RÉACH, G., M.D., *Chef de Clinique, Hôpital Necker, Paris, France*

REVILLARD, J.-P., M.D., *Maitre de Conférences Agrégé d'Immunologie, Clinique de Néphrologie et des Maladies Métaboliques et Rénales, Université Claude Bernard, Lyon, France*

ROTTEMBOURG, J., M.D., *Service de Néphrologie, Groupe Hospitalier Pitié-Salpétrière, Paris, France*

SAPIN, C., *Attachée de Recherches au CNRS, INSERM U 8, Hôpital Broussais, Paris, France*

SEYER-HANSEN, K., M.D., *Kommunehospitalet, Aarhus, Denmark*

SLAMA, G., M.D., *Service de Diabétologie, Hôpital Hôtel-Dieu, Paris, France*

STEFFES, M. W., M.D., *Associate Professor, Laboratory of Medicine and Pathology and Director of Clinical Chemistry, University of Minnesota School of Medicine, Minneapolis, Minnesota*

TCHOBROUTSKY, G., M.D., *Associate Professor of Endocrinology and Metabolism, Université Pierre et Marie Curie and Head, Department of Diabetology, Hôpital Hôtel-Dieu, Paris, France*

THIRY, L., M.D., *Professeur, Service de Virologie, Brugmann University Hospital, Brussels, Belgium*

TOURAINE, J. L., M.D., *Cliniques Universitaires de Néphrologie et d'Urologie and Unité INSERM U 80, Hôpital Edouard Herriot, Lyon, France*

TOUSSAINT, C., M.D., *Professeur de Clinique Médicale, Département de Néphrologie, Brugmann University Hospital, Brussels, Belgium*

TRAEGER, J., M.D., *Cliniques Universitaires de Néphrologie et d'Urologie and Unité INSERM U 80, Hôpital Edouard Herriot, Lyon, France*

TRANCHANT, D., M.D., *Cliniques Universitaires de Néphrologie et d'Urologie and Unité INSERM U 80, Hôpital Edouard Herriot, Lyon, France*

ULMANN, A., M.D., *Chef de Clinique Assistant, Hôpital Necker-Enfants Malades, Paris, France*

VAN GEERTRUYDEN, J., M.D., *Professeur de Clinique Chirurgicale, Brugmann University Hospital, Brussels, Belgium*

VANHERWEGHEM, J. L., M.D., *Premier Assistant, Département de Néphrologie, Brugmann University Hospital, Brussels, Belgium*

VEREERSTRAETEN, P., M.D., *Adjoint Principal, Département de Néphrologie, Brugmann University Hospital, Brussels, Belgium*

WILSON, C. B., M.D., *Scripps Clinic, La Jolla, California*

Table of Contents

PART I

Diabetic Nephropathy

Preface

What is happening in nephrology is exciting, and so is this volume of ADVANCES IN NEPHROLOGY .

The main subject of the volume, diabetic nephropathy, is treated in depth. After a general review of diabetes mellitus by Doctor Assan of Paris, Doctor Mauer and his colleagues (Minnesota) show from experimental diabetes in animals that diabetic nephropathy is a consequence of the diabetic state, rather than a separately inherited genetic disorder. Insulin therapy retards diabetic nephropathy in animals. New information indicates that alterations in glomerular hemodynamics (increased glomerular filtration rate) apparently can influence the rate of development of experimental diabetic glomerulopathy. Professor Gundersen and his colleagues from Denmark reach almost identical conclusions from long-term serial studies in patients with both early and late diabetic nephropathy. Doctor Mauer's thesis regarding alterations in glomerular hemodynamics is strengthened by the demonstration by Gundersen et al. that antihypertensive therapy reduces the fall in the glomerular filtration rate and postpones the onset of uremia in diabetes.

Professor Tchobroutsky of Paris presents a detailed analysis of the medical literature and concludes that the microangiopathic and neuropathic complications of diabetes mellitus are secondary to insulin deficiency and hyperglycemia. Doctor Bagdade of Seattle then reviews the various mechanisms related to abnormal glucose metabolism in uremia. This symposium is concluded with two clinical articles. In the first, Doctor Jacobs and his colleagues (Paris) formulate a reasonable approach to the treatment of end-stage renal failure in insulin-dependent diabetes, based upon 32 patients who were treated by dialysis and/or renal transplantation. They state that the exclusion of insulin-dependent diabetics with end-stage renal failure from dialysis therapy and/or renal transplantation is not acceptable, but caution that these modes of therapy should be instituted when creatinine clearance is above 10 ml/minute, i.e., before irreversible complications occur. In the second article, Professor Traeger of Lyon describes his experience with pancreatic transplantation in patients with renal insufficiency. Most fascinating is his detailed report of a patient who first received a pancreas, which then permitted kidney transplantation.

A smaller symposium on the kidney, vitamin D and renal osteodystrophy is presented next. Based upon his own experiments and others, Professor MacIntyre (London), demonstrates that the kidney is the organ of central importance in the regulation of calcium metabolism. He emphasizes the roles of growth hormone and prolactin. Doctors Garabedian and Ulmann from Paris review the effect of various vitamin D metabolites on target organs and explain their cellular mechanisms of action. These two basic introductory reviews are followed by a summary of the causes, sequence of events and proper therapy in human renal osteodystrophy by Brautbar and Kleeman of Los Angeles.

The rest of this volume contains articles of both basic and clinical interest in important areas in nephrology. Several large clinical studies include a report of 267 patients undergoing hemodialysis, of whom 33% showed evidence of liver disease (Toussaint et al., Brussels), and an analysis of early renal failure following cadaver kidney transplantation among 172 patients (Kreis et al., Paris). Lockwood et al. from London demonstrate the unquestioned value of intensive plasma exchange therapy in fulminating nephritis in a prospective study of 44 patients.

Other areas treated in Volume 8 include necrotizing angiitis, experimental immune glomerulonephritis, the use of angiotensin antagonists in renovascular hypertension and amino acid metabolism in uremia.

As in past volumes of ADVANCES IN NEPHROLOGY, two important subjects are treated in depth, and individual contributions reflect advances in other areas.

MORTON H. MAXWELL, M.D.

Part I

DIABETIC NEPHROPATHY

1

Present Concepts in Diabetology

R. ASSAN, M.D., G. RÉACH, M.D., AND
C. BARBANEL, M.D.

Hôpital Necker, Paris, France

Is it legitimate to study the problems posed by diabetes mellitus in a book for nephrologists? Diabetes mellitus is directly related to nephrology only through diabetic nephropathy, which is a fairly infrequent cause of chronic renal insufficiency, and through the impairment of glucoregulation, which complicates diuretic and immunosuppressive therapy. Diabetes mellitus, however, is now a focus of attention for all physicians. This severe, incapacitating and common disease, the treatment of which was for a long time empirical and at best palliative, has become in the past few years an area for the application of molecular biology and genetic studies utilizing histocompatibility markers and immunopathologic techniques. The pathophysiology of diabetes is being partially, if not fully, clarified. Diabetes is also the object of renewed therapeutic approaches by better use of conventional means, as well as by new techniques.

Diabetes mellitus affects 5% of the population in the United States, that is, 10 million people.[61, 62, 67] It is the third most frequent cause of death. The incidence of the disease increased by 50% between 1965 and 1973. In France, a similar frequency has been documented: diabetes is the fourth most frequent listed disease.[22] The diagnosis of diabetes appears on 2.9% of all death

3

0084-5957/79/080003-19$3.75

certificates. Diabetes is an incapacitating disease because of its complications: it is the most frequent cause of acquired adult blindness in Western countries. Renal damage is 17 times more frequent, and coronary artery disease 2.5 times more frequent in diabetics than in nondiabetics. Life expectancy for diabetics is reduced by one third.[61, 62, 67]

Today, there is neither a definite cure for diabetes nor a means of systematic prevention. More than 50 years after the discovery of insulin, the control of diabetes remains in most cases a daily symptomatic treatment. The efficacy of this treatment for the chronic complications is still a matter of controversy.[16, 36, 72] The use of sulfonylureas and biguanides only adds to the debate.

Considerable progress has been made in the past few years in the understanding and treatment of diabetes. The respective roles of genome, viruses and environment in triggering the disease and its complications are beginning to be clarified. The artificial pancreas, the graft or implantation of islets of Langerhans and the industrial production of insulin by biologic procedures (genetic manipulation of bacteria and yeast) have introduced into the field of diabetology the techniques of biomedical engineering.

At the level of health policy, because diabetes demonstrates the need for early detection, a teaching program for patients and an evaluation of the economics, it is a research model for other chronic diseases.

What Is Diabetes Mellitus?

The definition of diabetes mellitus is essentially biologic: permanent or intermittent hyperglycemia secondary to insulin deficiency. There is no strict enzymatic, bacteriologic or anatomical definition. The genetic definition remains unclear. The characterization by other metabolic or hormonal abnormalities is more complex and does not improve the sensitivity or specificity of the definition.

EMPIRICAL DEFINITION OF DIABETES BY HYPERGLYCEMIA

Hyperglycemia, as a consequence of decreased glucose uptake by the tissues and increased output by the liver, can be permanent or intermittent. Fasting hyperglycemia is not constant in insulin-independent diabetics in whom severe postprandial hyperglycemia can occur. The measurement of fasting blood glucose levels is an insensitive diagnostic parameter.

The oral glucose tolerance test (OGTT) is well codified, sensitive, specific and simple to perform. It is relatively physiologic, involving the complex process of digestion, the enteroportal absorption of glucose, the release of the insulin-stimulating enterohormones, the release of gastric and pancreatic somatostatin and, finally, the glucose uptake by the liver. Because it is a pragmatic test for diabetes, OGTT must be performed under strict guidelines regarding the methodology (e.g., sampling, glucose assay, amount of glucose administered) and the physiologic preparation of the subject (e.g., overnight fast after several days of carbohydrate-rich diet, interruption of interfering drugs). Finally, the results must be interpreted taking into account the age, anamnestics and general pathophysiologic status of the subject.[26] The need for a specific glucose assay must be stressed among nephrologists, because other reducing substances (uric acid, creatinine) may interfere with the less-specific assay systems: an overestimation of the blood glucose level may lead to severe drug-induced hypoglycemia in uremic patients.

A firm diagnosis, or at least a strong presumption, can be made most of the time in clinical practice from the results of OGTT. However, the absence of clear-cut discontinuity between the normal and pathologic states, some time-related variations and the operational character of the definition of diabetes by OGTT make the genetic and physiologic analyses of diabetes more difficult.

CAN DIABETES BE DEFINED BY ABNORMAL INSULIN SECRETION?

The lack of insulin is almost complete in patients with ketotic, insulin-dependent juvenile diabetes. A residual endogenous insulin secretion is still present for several years, however, as demonstrated by the C-peptide assay.[70] In patients with nonketotic, maturity onset diabetes, the fasting insulin level in plasma is normal (or elevated in the case of overweight patients), but the glucose-induced release is delayed. Since the early phase of insulin release is needed for an appropriate uptake of glucose by the liver, a major part of the glucose ingested escapes the liver in these patients. The same defect in early insulin release has been observed in subjects who are still normal but liable to develop diabetes: identical twins of diabetics and subjects whose parents are both diabetic.[17] The same problem occurs in some laboratory rodents whose diabetes appears very similar to human nonketotic diabetes.[65] In these rodents, the release of cyclic adenosine monophosphate (AMP) by islets, which is associated with the insulin secretory process, is also delayed.[64] This kinetic abnormality of insulin release, which is present even before the appearance of overt diabetes, might be an early clue or possibly a genetic marker of maturity-onset diabetes.

CAN DIABETES BE DEFINED BY OTHER HORMONAL, METABOLIC OR ANATOMICAL ANOMALIES?

Hypersecretion of glucagon occurs in all types of human diabetes mellitus[79] except when the patient has undergone total pancreatectomy.[76] This hyperglucagonemia contributes to hyperglycemia and ketosis.[79] In diabetics, the glucagon secretion is neither inhibited by the administration of glucose nor stimulated by hypoglycemia.[32] The hypothesis of a primitive A-cell anomaly has been proposed, suggesting that diabetes mellitus could be a bihormonal disease, at least certain types of diabetes.[79] But glucagon concentration is very often normal in genetically prediabetic subjects.[21] Diabetic hyperglucagonemia is corrected by strict control of hyperglycemia.[8] The hypothesis of a primary bihormonal disturbance in patients with diabetes appears improbable to date.[24]

An abnormal elevation of somatostatin concentration has been recently observed in the islets of Langerhans in human and experimental diabetes. The significance of this needs to be clarified. The excessive secretion of somatotropin often encountered in patients with poorly treated juvenile diabetes is normalized, as with glucagon, by strict control of blood glucose levels.[39] A normal secretion of somatotropin has been observed in identical twins of juvenile diabetics.[40] The characterization in the plasma of synalbumin, a genetically transmitted inhibitor of insulin, remains controversial.[81]

The early occurrence of specific vascular lesions (microangiopathy) preceding the detectable metabolic abnormalities (hyperglycemia in particular) has been the subject of strong controversy. This hypothesis of anatomical, genetically transmitted criteria for diabetes cannot be supported today in the light of experimental,[54] biochemical[73, 74] and epidemiologic[63] studies, which are discussed in other parts of this book.

Summary

The impairment of glucose metabolism is only part of the diabetic metabolic disturbances; however, the common features of all diabetic syndromes are permanent or intermittent hyperglycemia and a partial or complete insulin deficiency. The diabetic syndrome thus defined can appear in two forms: ketotic diabetes in which a profound lack of insulin appears most often in juvenile subjects, and diabetes without spontaneous ketosis appearing most often in adults. All the diabetic syndromes have in common the late appearance of anatomical vascular lesions, particularly retinal and renal. The common denominator of hyperglycemia plus insulin deficiency plus microangiopathy might be secondary to several diseases that differ in their genetic and environmental causes.

Why Do People Become Diabetic?

The simple scheme of the lack of insulin causing hyperglycemia, suggested by the experimental diabetes that follows pancreatectomy, has been difficult to extend to human diabetics, first because minute lesions were seen in the pancreas of patients, and also because nonnegligible amounts of insulin were measured in the plasma of most nonketotic diabetics. For these reasons, insulin resistance rather than insulin lack has been hypothesized by many workers. An absolute or relative deficiency in B cells is found in all cases of human diabetes; some factors of insulin resistance can possibly be added. The causes of insulin lack and resistance appear to be multiple.

Causes of Insulin Deficiency

Genetic *and* acquired factors can cause insulin deficiency in pancreatic B cells.

The Role of the Genome

Diabetes mellitus remains "the geneticist's nightmare"[56] because of its variable clinical appearance, the absence of a reliable genetic marker and the influence of environmental factors. Several studies on diabetic laboratory rodents suggest an intervention of multiple alleles. In humans, several well-conducted studies suggest heterogeneity in the transmission of different diabetic syndromes. Differences appear between the genetic transmission of the juvenile type and maturity-onset diabetes.[60]

MONOZYGOTIC TWINS. — Twins are convenient human models for discriminating between the roles of genetic and environmental factors. Near 100% of monozygotic twins are concordant for diabetes when the disease appears after 40 years of age; the concordance is less than 50% when diabetes appears before age 40 (Table 1–1). Discordant twins of diabetics display no metabolic or hormonal abnormalities evocative of prediabetes. Thus, maturity-onset rather than juvenile diabetes seems to be genetically transmitted.[76]

THE CHILDREN OF TWO DIABETIC PARENTS. — These subjects are another means for studying diabetes. The parents are usually maturity onset, nonketotic diabetics. Only 6–10% of these children present with frank diabetes. The proportion increases to 25–40% if OGTT is used for diagnosis. Impairment of glucoregulation increases with increasing age.[76]

PARENTS OF JUVENILE KETOTIC DIABETICS. — The incidence of nonketotic diabetes is not increased.[50] In the twin studies, when both twins present with maturity-onset diabetes, one of the two parents is diabetic in 50% of cases; diabetes is rare in parents of twins when one of these is a ketotic diabetic. This also emphasizes the possibility of a clear-cut genetic factor in maturity-onset diabetes and of an important environmental role in ketotic diabetes.

TABLE 1–1. — DIABETES AND MONOZYGOTOUS TWINS

AUTHORS	NO. OF PAIRS	CONCORDANT	DIABETES DIAGNOSED BEFORE 40 YR OF AGE		DIABETES DIAGNOSED AFTER 40 YR OF AGE	
			CONCORDANT	DISCORDANT	CONCORDANT	DISCORDANT
Gottlieb	30	15	5	15	10	0
Tattersall	96	65	31	28	34	3

HISTOCOMPATIBILITY MARKERS AND DIABETES MELLITUS. — The risk of juvenile diabetes is two to four times higher than normal in individuals with HLA-B8 and BW15 antigens.[20, 49, 57] A stronger association has recently been found with DW3 and DW4 antigens, the risk increasing to 6.4 and 3.7, respectively, times the control population. The HLA-B7 antigen, on the contrary, seems to be associated with protection from diabetes.[46]

An association between maturity-onset diabetes and the HL-A system has not been found. This is surprising, since a genetic transmission seems to be manifest in maturity-onset diabetes, whereas ketotic diabetes appears more likely to be transmitted genetically. To explain this contradiction, it has been suggested that HL-A antigens favor a viral infection or an immunologic disorder that leads to an autoimmune attack on the islet.

From a practical standpoint, the association between the HL-A markers and diabetes mellitus is less definitive than in other diseases (ankylosing spondylitis, for instance); HL-A typing cannot serve as a diagnostic tool for diabetes but may be used to characterize the high-risk subjects.

OTHER DISEASES. — Another approach to the localization of the gene(s) favoring diabetes consists of searching for associations between diabetes mellitus and other hereditary diseases[68]: 34 genetic syndromes are often associated with diabetes, including in particular Friedreich's ataxia, Huntington's chorea and gonadal dysgenesis. The multiplicity of chromosomes involved is compatible with the hypothesis of a polygenetic transmission.[23]

ANTI-ISLET ANTIBODIES. — Diabetes mellitus can be associated with autoimmune diseases such as thyroid diseases, adrenal insufficiency, Schmidt's syndrome, Biermer's anemia, myasthenia gravis and vitiligo. Autoantibodies directed against the corresponding tissues (endocrine, gastric, muscular and cutaneous) have been detected in juvenile diabetics.[16] Anti-islet autoantibodies, as well as cellular autoimmune processes,[35-38] have been demonstrated recently in the plasma of juvenile diabetics. The incidence of HLA-B8 marker in most patients with autoimmune processes seems to be increased.

NO INBORN ERROR OF INSULINOGENESIS CAN BE SAID TO CAUSE DIABETES. — An immunoassayable but biologically inactive insulin in diabetics has never been verified. The genetic absence of cliving enzyme causes the secretion of proinsulin alone.[29] Although proinsulin is much less active, biologically, than insulin, glucose tolerance is normal in subjects affected by this abnormality, owing to the increased secretory response of the islets. The hypothesis of a bound, biologically inactive, circulating insulin has never been confirmed.[4]

Acquired Lesions of the Islets

CONVENTIONAL ACQUIRED PANCREATOPATHIES. — Pancreatectomy in humans suppresses insulin secretion but does not cause an increased release of extrapancreatic glucagon, in contrast to what occurs in dogs. The same seems to happen in hemochromatosis, calcifying pancreatitis and other diseases. However, the incidence of diabetes in patients with hemochromatosis or calcifying pancreatitis is higher in cases of familial antecedents of diabetes, suggesting that a genetic factor of diabetes aggravates the hormonal consequences of the acquired pancreatopathy.[47]

INSULITIS AND JUVENILE DIABETES. — Inflammatory lesions of islets, including leukocytic and eosinophilic infiltration, were demonstrated in 68% of juvenile diabetics when the pancreas was examined early after the outburst of diabetes, i.e., within a few months.[31] When the interval of time following the clinical onset of the disease is longer, the inflammatory lesions vanish, insulin-secreting cells disappear and chronic lesions of hyalinosis and fibrosis appear. This insulitis seems very similar to the adrenalitis and thyroiditis attributed to autoimmune processes. It has also been compared to the lesions of islets induced in cows by a prolonged isoimmunization against insulin.[66]

POSSIBLE ROLE OF VIRUSES IN THE INSULAR DESTRUCTION. — The clinical association between German measles and ketotic diabetes has been known for a long time.[19, 25, 60] Recent data support more specifically the concept of virus-induced diabetes: (1) the high incidence (20%) of diabetes mellitus in patients with congenital rubella and the obtention of the rubella virus from pancreatic tissue culture from these subjects;[19, 25] (2) the association of insulitis and diabetes in infants with cytomegalovirus infections;[25, 75] (3) the time-related association between juvenile diabetes and the appearance of anticoxsackie B4 antibodies;[30] (4) the association between diabetes and mononucleosis,[15] diabetes and viral hepatitis;[2] and (5) the induction of transient diabetes mellitus in mice infected with encephalomyelitis virus.[34, 69]

TABLE 1-2.—TYPES OF VIRUS SUSPECTED OF
AFFECTING THE ISLETS OF LANGERHANS

VIRUS	AFFECTED SPECIES
Mumps	Human
Infectious mononucleosis	Human
Rubella	Human
Coxsackie B4	Human
Infectious hepatitis	Human
Myxovirus	Human
Aphthous fever (foot and mouth disease)	Cow
Encephalomyocarditis	Mouse, marmoset monkey
Herpes	Mouse
Infectious necrotic pancreatitis virus	Trout
According to Ganda and Soeldner.	

Table 1-2 summarizes the virus suspected to cause diabetes. The relationship between virus and most cases of human diabetes mellitus remains, however, uncertain.

TISSUE RESISTANCE TO INSULIN

Antireceptor Antibodies

These antibodies represent a rare and exaggerated situation. A few diabetics display an extreme resistance to insulin; an immunoglobulin present in their plasma can specifically and reversibly bind the membrane adipocytes, hepatocytes and muscular cells. Acanthosis nigricans is present in most of these subjects.[41] The immunoglobulin inhibits the binding of insulin to the target cells (presumably because of a steric hindrance), but it stimulates glucose uptake by these cells: it then displays an insulin-like biologic potency of its own.[27]

Anti-insulin Antibodies

These are usually detected in insulin-treated diabetics, but their titer and avidity are generally too low to induce insulin resistance. In laboratory animals that have been immunized against heterologous insulin, circulating antibodies bind the endogenous insulin, but overt diabetes does not occur because of an oversecretion of insulin. Cows that have been immunized for a long time against isologous insulin develop discrete insulitis lesions, but no diabetes.[66] In some rare enigmatic case records, anti-insulin autoantibodies in subjects never treated with insulin coexisted with paroxysmal hypoglycemia, not with diabetes mellitus.

Obesity as a Factor of Insulin Resistance

Overweight is a far more common cause of insulin resistance.[7] The reduction of sensitivity to insulin affects the liver, muscles and adipocytes. It is related to a reduction in number (and perhaps avidity) of insulin receptors on plasma cell membranes. Glucose intolerance appears only in cases of deficient islets: most obese subjects display a normal tolerance to glucose, owing to oversecretion of insulin and a normal early insulin release. Similar schemes have been developed about uremia[9] and corticoid treatment, which induce a reduction in the number of insulin receptors.[39]

Hormonal Factors of Insulin Resistance

Acromegaly, prolactin adenomas, Cushing's syndrome or pheochromocytoma is associated with diabetes in about 30% of cases. Pregnancy and estro-progestative pills can impair glucose tolerance. Several mechanisms are involved. Corticoids, in addition to their effects on insulin receptors, increase gluconeogenesis and have a permissive effect on lipolysis. Glucagon release is increased in vivo and the glucose-induced insulin release is potentiated.[71] A vitamin B_6 deficiency is favored by corticoids and estrogens.[1] Vitamin B_6 is a cofactor for several enzymes of tryptophan metabolism: in case of deficiency, less picolinic acid (hypoglycemic) is formed from tryptophan and more xanthurenic acid appears (which may impair insulin biologic potency).

Nutritional Environment

The epidemiologic study of some population groups has demonstrated quasi-experimentally the role of the nutritional environment. Diabetes mellitus is far more common in the Pima Indians, who are often obese and overfed on carbohydrates, than in the Eskimo Indians, who are closely related by race but have a frugal diet, consisting predominantly of meat.[84] Yemenite Jews before and after their installation in Israel and Pendjabi Indians before and after transplantation to South Africa showed an increased incidence of diabetes when their feeding habits were modified, without any substantial modification of the genomes. Insulin resistance seems to play a primary role in this impairment of glucose tolerance. Important deductions for a preventive policy can be drawn from these facts.

Chronic Complications of Diabetes and the Choice of a Therapeutic Strategy

These aspects are largely debated in other chapters of this book. The problem of chronic complications will be considered from a synthetic point of view in order to facilitate the choice of a long-term therapeutic attitude.

PREVENTION OF DIABETES

To date, prevention is limited to the avoidance of diabetogenic treatments (corticoids, contraceptive pills) and overweight in subjects at high risk (subjects with both parents diabetic, monozygotic twins of diabetics, and mothers of several children with a birth weight of 4 kg or more).

NO DEFINITE CURE FOR DIABETES

Pancreas implantation has been limited to less than 100 attempts;[45] islet implantation and the mixed artificial pancreas have not been attempted in human patients.[18] The miniaturized implantable artificial pancreas is still experimental.[13]

PALLIATIVE DAILY TREATMENT OF DIABETES

The enthusiasm and perseverance necessary for a long-term palliative treatment require (for the patient and for the physician) a clear definition of goals, valid indices of the biologic state and efficient therapeutic tools.

The Goals of Treatment

Beyond the short-term aims (prevention of ketosis and hyperosmolarity, suppression of heavy glucosuria and its infectious complications), the long-range goals of treatment consist of: (1) the prevention or delay of angiopathy and neuropathy; (2) the obtention of a normal daily life (professional, personal, sexual) with the feeling of well-being; (3) obtention of a normal life expectancy; and (4) the prevention of iatrogenic complications (hypoglycemia, lactic acidosis and cardiovascular death).

Many arguments substantiate the goal of normal (or near normal) 24-hour blood glucose levels in order to prevent or delay the chronic complications of diabetes. These arguments, as briefly summarized, are drawn from the experimental induction of renal microangiopathy in diabetic animals and its reduction when the diseased kidney is reexposed to normoglycemia;[54] epidemiologic prospective studies that have demonstrated a better vascular prognosis in the better-controlled patients;[63] and the study of the biochemical mechanisms underlying neuropathy and microangiopathy. The metabolic neuropathy in diabetic patients is related to sorbitol accumulation in nerves, which itself depends directly on hyperglycemia.[28] The normalization of blood glucose and the slow retrodiffusion of sorbitol out of the nerves are accompanied by the restoration of nerve conduction. The same biochemical mechanism (sorbitol pathway) is involved in the appearance of the diabetic cataract.[28]

The diabetic microangiopathy is related to the synthesis in capillary basal membranes of glycoproteins that have an abnormal amino acid composition and an abundance of osidic side chains.[73] The glucosyltransferase that catalyzes the linkage of these side chains is enhanced by the lack of insulin in diabetic animals and partially inhibited by early insulin therapy.

Some factors distinct from hyperglycemia (and/or insulin lack) presumably contribute to the appearance of microangiopathy, such as growth hormone excess[46] and a genetic predisposition.[12]

Valid Indices of the Biochemical and Anatomical Status

Fasting and postprandial blood glucose levels do not reflect the diurnal variations of blood glucose levels, particularly in insulin-treated diabetics. An integrated index of serial blood glucose concentrations would be preferable, particularly for the long-term correlation between control and the appearance of angiopathy. The measurement of *hemoglobin A1$_6$* is promising in this regard: The $A1_6$ fraction of hemoglobin results from post-synthetic addition of glucose to the hemoglobin molecule. This glycosylation is proportionate to the blood glucose level during the life span of the red cell, i.e., 120 days.

Estimation of microangiopathy and neuropathy in diabetics relies on clinical findings, e.g., diabetic retinopathy, and estimates of proteinuria and creatinine clearance. Retinal fluorography has become essential because of its high sensitivity. Similarly, the measurement of nerve conduction velocity gives an objective and reproducible estimation of neuropathy in diabetics. The poor sensitivity of conventional measurements, e.g., proteinuria, to evaluate early glomerular microangiopathy is well known.[46] The radioimmunoassay of proteinuria may become a more sensitive and noninvasive index of glomerular status.[82]

Available Therapeutic Modalities

The apparent failure of insulin therapy to prevent complications long-term,[72] the criticism recently developed about sulfonylureas[80] and biguanides,[5, 6] and the expectation of new treatments may disturb some patients and practitioners.

The classification of therapeutic modalities, even if temporary, must take into account better use of conventional treatments and the rapid evolution of more recent treatments.

BETTER USE OF CONVENTIONAL TOOLS.—*Insulin therapy.*—Intermittent, subcutaneous insulin injections can reproduce neither the fine adjustments of plasma insulin induced in normal subjects by meals and acute blood glucose level variations, nor the physiologic portacaval gradient. Because of the persistence of an endogenous residual insulin secretion, acceptable results are sometimes obtained by the use of long-acting insulin, injected once a day subcutaneously.[70] Better control is often obtained by multiple daily insulin injections,[78] and prevention of microangiopathy by this schedule of treatment seems possible.[38]

The choice between multiple or single daily injection schedules depends largely on the patient's compliance, his physical and intellectual capacities and the importance of rigid control. Multiple injections are indicated in young subjects who are intelligent and socially well settled, and in those who develop progressive complication of diabetes. A single daily injection schedule is more adaptable to extremely old subjects, or when the performance of injections is impeded by blindness, neurologic disease, lack of cooperation or lack of comprehension. Education of the patient and his family and the prescription of glucagon (to be reserved for severe hypoglycemic episodes) must be associated with the starting of insulin therapy.

Sulfonylureas and biguanides. — Sulfonylureas augment and accelerate the release of insulin when B cells are still present in the islets; they are inefficient on the biosynthesis of insulin and the replication of insulin-secreting cells. Biguanides reduce glucose output from the liver and increase ketogenesis in the liver. It appeared logical to prescribe sulfonylureas to non-fat, non-insulin-deficient adult diabetics, and biguanides to obese diabetics. In these circumstances, short-term efficiency and an increase in comfort are often observed. However, the long-term benefits are not so obvious and the legitimacy of their use has been recently reconsidered. The UGDP report (albeit controversial) has illustrated the dangers of prescribing tolbutamide in the absence of appropriate weight reduction and of aiming at normal blood glucose values in subjects at increased cardiovascular risk. Awareness of biguanide-induced lactic acidosis has similarly led to a severe restriction of these drugs, if not their suppression, in many countries.[5, 6]

The overall treatment of the diabetic patient. — Insulin and hypoglycemic tablets are but a part of the treatments: attaining normal to low body weight, proper dietary regulation of carbohydrates, physical exercise and the education of the patients and family are other important elements, together with consideration of the patient's psychological and socioeconomic problems.

NEW THERAPEUTIC TOOLS. — The artificial pancreas is emerging from the experimental stage as a temporary external prosthesis.[3] Setting up a miniaturized implantable prosthesis seems to belong to a more remote future.[13]

Some pancreas transplantations have been performed; the implantation of islets of Langerhans is still at the experimental stage. In addition to the immunologic problems, this technique will be limited because of scarcity of potential donors and the low yield of islet collection from one single pancreas. The mixed pancreas (islet culture developed around a network of artificial capillaries) is also still experimental.

Somatostatin is another potential therapeutic approach. This tetradecapeptide, present in the hypothalamus, the digestive tract and pancreas, inhibits the release of growth hormone and glucagon. Furthermore, it reduces postprandial hyperglycemia by reducing the splanchnic blood flow and slowing down the digestive absorption of carbohydrates. Its short half-life in plasma and its many side effects are serious limitations at the present time. The synthesis of long-acting and selective analogues may facilitate its use in diabetics.

The addition to the foodstuff of pectins, cellulose fibers or amylase inhibitors may be another therapeutic approach. Will bran ingestion prevent the postprandial glucose peaks better than somatostatin? This question, far from being facetious, illustrates a pragmatic preoccupation shared by most diabetologists: the obstinate search for normoglycemia, whichever the means.

Conclusion

In the current absence of a way to completely normalize blood glucose levels in all diabetic patients, some pragmatic proposals can be stated. Meticulous regulation of blood glucose levels seems advisable. Many diabetics can and must be treated by low-calorie diet alone. The prescription of hypoglycemic tablets in such cases encourages a lax attitude regarding the diet, is distracting and may serve as an excuse for deficient dietary regulation. Insulin therapy is compulsory in cases of ketotic diabetes. Its transient use is legitimate in maturity-onset diabetics when severe neuropathy or retinopathy is present. The prescription of hypoglycemic tablets for nonketotic diabetics must be avoided in cases of renal failure.

References

1. Adams, P. W., Wynn, V., Folkard, J., and Seed, M.: Influence of oral contraceptives, pyridoxine (vitamin B6) and tryptophan on carbohydrate metabolism, Lancet 1:759, 1976.
2. Adi, F. C.: Diabetes mellitus associated with epidemic of infectious hepatitis in Nigeria, Br. Med. J. 1:183, 1974.
3. Albisser, A. M.: An artificial endocrine pancreas, Diabetes 23:389, 1975.
4. Antoniades, H. N., Beigelman, P. M., Tranquada, R. B., and Gundersen, K.: Studies on the state of insulin in blood: free insulin and insulin complexes in serum and their in vitro biological properties, Endocrinology 69:46, 1961.
5. Assan, R., Heuclin, C., Girard, J. R., Lemaire, F., and Attali, J. R.: Phenformin-induced lactic acidosis in diabetic patients, Diabetes 24:791, 1975.

6. Assan, R., Heuclin, C., Ganeval, D., Daniel, F., Bismuth, C., George, J., and Girard, J. R.: Metformin-induced lactic acidosis in the presence of acute renal failure, Diabetologia 13:211, 1977.
7. Assimacopoulos-Jeannet, F., and Jeanrenaud, B.: The hormonal and metabolic basis of experimental obesity, Clin. Endocrinol. Metabol. 5:337, 1976.
8. Aydin, I., Raskin, P., and Unger, R. H.: The effect of short-term intravenous insulin administration on the glucagon response to a carbohydrate meal in adult onset and juvenile type diabetes, Diabetologia 13:629, 1977.
9. Bagdade, J. D.: Disorders of carbohydrate and lipid metabolism in uremia, Nephron 14:153, 1975.
10. Banting, F. G., and Best, C. H.: The internal secretion of the pancreas, J. Lab. Clin. Med. 7:251, 1975.
11. Barnes, A. J., and Bloom, S. R.: Pancreatectomized man: a model for diabetes without glucagon, Lancet 1:219, 1976.
12. Becker, B., Shin, D. H., Burgess, D., Kilo, Ch., and Miller, W. V.: Histocompatibility antigens and diabetic retinopathy, Diabetes 26:997, 1977.
13. Bessman, S. P., and Schultz, R. D.: Sugar electrode sensor for the artificial pancreas, Horm. Metab. Res. 4:413, 1972.
14. Bottazzo, G. F., Florin-Christensen, A., and Doniach, D.: Islet-cell antibodies in diabetes mellitus with autoimmune polyendocrine deficiencies, Lancet 2:1279, 1974.
15. Burgess, J. A., Kirkpatrick, K. L., and Menser, M. A.: Fulminant onset of diabetes mellitus during an attack of infectious mononucleosis, Med. J. Aust. 2:706, 1974.
16. Cahill, J. F., Etzwiler, D. D., and Freinkel, N.: "Control" and diabetes, N. Engl. J. Med. 294:1004, 1976.
17. Cerasi, E., and Luft, R.: Follow-up of nondiabetic subjects with normal and decreased insulin response to glucose infusion, Horm. Metab. Res. 5(Suppl.): 113, 1974.
18. Chick, W. L., Like, A. A., Lauris, V., Galletti, P. M., Richardson, P. R., Panol, G., Mixt, W., and Colton, C. K.: A hybrid artificial pancreas, Trans. Am. Soc. Artif. Intern. Organs 21:8, 1975.
19. Craighead, J. E.: The role of viruses in the pathogenesis of pancreatic disease and diabetes mellitus, Prog. Med. Virol. 19:161, 1975.
20. Cudworth, A. G., and Woodrow, J. C.: HL-A system and diabetes mellitus, Diabetes 24:345, 1975.
21. Day, J. L., and Tattersall, R. B.: Glucagon secretion in unaffected monozygotic twins of juvenile diabetics, Metabolism 24:145, 1975.
22. Eschwege, E., Valleron, A. J., Rosselin, G. E., Claude, J. R., Warnet, J. M., and Richard, J. L.: Diabetes and Coronary Heart Disease Epidemiological Study, in Gutsche, H., and Holler, H. D. (eds.): *Diabetes Epidemiology in Europe* (Stuttgart: Georg Thieme, 1975), pp. 124–27.
23. Feingold, J.: Genetics of diabetes mellitus, Diabete Métab. 1:123, 1975.
24. Felig, P., Wahren, J., Sherwin, R., and Hendler, R.: Insulin, glucagon and somatostatin in normal physiology and diabetes mellitus, Diabetes 25:1091, 1976.
25. Forrest, M., Menser, M. A., and Burgess, J. A.: High frequency of diabetes mellitus in young adults with congenital rubella, Lancet 2:332, 1971.
26. Freychet, P., and Tchobroutsky, G.: L'hyperglycémie provoquée par voie digestive, *J. Ann. Diabetol. Hôtel-Dieu* (Paris: Flammarion, 1968), p. 249.
27. Freychet, P., Le Marchand, Y., Gorden, P., and Kahn, R.: Antibodies against the insulin receptor inhibit insulin binding and stimulate glucose metabolism in skeletal muscle, Diabetologia 13:393, 1977.
28. Gabbay, K.: Hyperglycemia, polyol metabolism, and complications of diabetes mellitus, Annu. Rev. Med. 26:521, 1975.
29. Gabbay, K., De Luca, K., Fisher, J., Mako, M. E., and Rubenstein, A. H.: Familial hyperproinsulinemia: an autosomal dominant effect, N. Engl. J. Med. 294:911, 1976.
30. Gamble, D. R., Taylor, K. W., and Cumming, H.: Coxsackie viruses and diabetes mellitus, Br. Med. J. 4:260, 1973.

31. Gepts, W.: Pathologic anatomy of the pancreas in juvenile diabetes mellitus, Diabetes 14:619, 1965.
32. Gerich, J. E., Langlois, M., Noacco, C., Karam, J. H., and Forsham, P. H.: Lack of glucagon response to hypoglycemia in diabetes: evidence for an intrinsic pancreatic alpha cell defect, Science 182:171, 1973.
33. Harris, H. F.: A case of diabetes mellitus quickly following mumps, Boston Med. Surg. J. 140:465, 1899.
34. Hayashi, K., Boucher, W., and Notkins, A. L.: Virus-induced diabetes mellitus. II. Relationship between beta cell damage and hyperglycemia in mice infected with encephalomyocarditis virus, Am. J. Pathol. 75:91, 1973.
35. Huang, S. W., and Mac Laren, N. K.: Insulin-dependent diabetes: a disease of auto-aggression, Science 192:64, 1976.
36. Ingelfinger, F. J.: Debates on diabetes, N. Engl. J. Med. 296:1228, 1977.
37. Irvine, W. J., Mac Callum, C. B., Gray, R. S., Campbell, C. J., Duncan, L. J. P., Farquhar, J. W., Vaughan, H., and Morris, P. J.: Pancreatic islet cell antibodies in diabetes mellitus correlated with the duration and type of diabetes, coexistent autoimmune disease, and HLA type, Diabetes 26:138, 1977.
38. Job, D., Eschwege, E., Guyot-Argenton, C., Aubry, J. P., and Tchobroutsky, G.: Effect of multiple daily insulin injections on the course of diabetic retinopathy, Diabetes 25:463, 1976.
39. Johansen, K., and Hansen, A. P.: Diurnal serum growth hormone levels in poorly and well controlled juvenile diabetics, Diabetes 20:239, 1971.
40. Johansen, K., et al.: Serum insulin and growth hormone response patterns in monozygotic twin siblings of juvenile diabetics, N. Engl. J. Med. 293:57, 1975.
41. Kahn, C. R., Flyer, J. S., Bar, R. S., Archer, J. A., Gorden, P., Martin, M. M., and Roth, J.: The syndromes of insulin resistance and acanthosis nigricans, N. Engl. J. Med. 294:739, 1976.
42. Koenig, R. J., Peterson, C. M., Jones, R. L., Saudek, C., Lehrman, M., and Cerami, A.: Correlation of glucose regulation and hemoglobin A_{Ic} in diabetes mellitus, N. Engl. J. Med. 295:417, 1976.
43. Kohner, E. M., Joplin, G. F., Blach, R. K., Cheng, H., and Fraser, T. R.: Pituitary ablation in the treatment of diabetic retinopathy, Trans. Ophthalmol. Soc. U.K. 92:79, 1972.
44. Krall, L.: Clinical Evaluation of Prognosis, in Marble, A., White, P., Bradley, R. F., and Krall, L. P. (eds.): *Joslin's Diabetes Mellitus* (Philadelphia: Lea & Febiger, 1971).
45. Lillehei, R. C., Simmons, R. L., Najarian, J. S., Weil, R., Uchida, H., Ruiz, J. O., Kjellstrand, C. M., and Goetz, F. C.: Pancreatico-duodenal allotransplantation. Experimental and clinical experience, Ann. Surg. 172:405, 1970.
46. Lundbaek, K.: Recent contributions to the study of diabetic angiopathy and neuropathy, Advan. Metab. Disord. 6:99, 1972.
47. Lyra de Lacerda, S. N., Feingold, J., Bernades, P., Lenriot, J. P., Mathieu, M., Cohen-Solal, C., and Tchobroutsky, G.: Diabetogenic factors in 262 patients with chronic pancreatitis, Diabetes 26:406, 1977.
48. Mac Cuish, A. C., et al.: Cell-mediated immunity to human pancreas in diabetes mellitus, Diabetes 23:693, 1974.
49. Mac Devitt, H. O., and Bodmer, W. F.: HL-A immune-response genes and disease, Lancet 1:1269, 1974.
50. Mac Donald, M. J.: Equal incidence of adult-onset diabetes among ancestors of juvenile diabetics and non-diabetics, Diabetologia 10:767, 1974.
51. Mac Intyre, N., Holdsworth, C. D., and Turner, D.: New interpretation of oral glucose tolerance test, Lancet 2:20, 1964.
52. Marble, A.: Late complications of diabetes. A continuing challenge, Diabetologia 12:193, 1976.
53. Matas, A. J., Sutherland, D. E. R., and Najarian, J. S.: Current states of islet and pancreas transplantation in diabetes, Diabetes 25:785, 1976.

54. Mauer, S. M., Steffes, M. W., Sutherland, D. E. R., Najarian, J. S., Michael, A. F., and Brown, D. M.: Studies on the rate of regression of the glomerular lesions in diabetic rats treated with pancreatic islet transplantation, Diabetes 24:280, 1975.

55. Maugh, T. H.: Diabetes: epidemiology suggests a viral connection, Science 188:347, 1975.

56. Neel, J. V.: The genetics of diabetes mellitus, Advan. Metab. Disord. 1(Suppl. 1):3, 1970.

57. Nerup, J., *et al.*: Antipancreatic cellular hypersensitivity in diabetes mellitus, Diabetes 20:424, 1971.

58. Nerup, J., *et al.*: HL-A antigens and diabetes mellitus, Lancet 2:864, 1974.

59. Olefsky, J. M., Johnson, J., Lin, F., Yen, P., and Reaven, G. M.: The effects of acute and chronic dexamethasone administration on insulin binding to isolated rat hepatocytes and adipocytes, Metabolism 24:517, 1975.

60. Om, P., Ganda, O. P., and Soeldner, S. S.: Genetic, acquired and related factors in the etiology of diabetes mellitus, Arch. Intern. Med. 137:461, 1977.

61. Palmberg, P. F.: Diabetes retinopathy, Diabetes 26:703, 1977.

62. Palumbo, P. J., Elveback, L. R., Chu-Pin Chu, Connolly, D. C., and Kurland, L. T.: Diabetes mellitus: incidence, prevalence, survivorship and causes of death in Rochester, Minnesota, 1945–1970, Diabetes 25:566, 1977.

63. Pirart, J.: Diabéte et complications dégénératives. Présentation d'une étude prospective portant sur 4.400 cas observés entre 1947 et 1973, Diabete Métab. 3:245, 1977.

64. Rabinovitch, A., Gutzeit, A., Grill, V., Kikuchi, M., Renold, A. E., and Cerasi, E.: Defective insulin secretions in the spiny mouse *(Acomys cahirinus)*. Possible value in the study of the pathophysiology of diabetes, Isr. J. Med. Sci. 11:730, 1975.

65. Rabinovitch, A., Gutzeit, A., Kikuchi, M., Cerasi, E., and Renold, A. E.: Defective early phase insulin release in perifused isolated pancreatic islets of spiny mice *(Acomys cahirinus)*, Diabetologia 11:457, 1975.

66. Renold, A. E., Soeldner, J. S., and Steinke, J.: Immunological studies with homologous and heterologous pancreatic insulin in the cow, Ciba Found. Symp. 15:122, 1964.

67. Report of the National Commission on Diabetes to the Congress of the United States. Vol. 1: The long-range plan to combat diabetes. DHEW Publication No. 76-1018.

68. Rimoin, D. L., and Schimke, R. N.: *Genetic Disorders of the Endocrine Glands* (St. Louis: C. V. Mosby Co., 1971).

69. Ross, M. E., *et al.*: Virus-induced diabetes mellitus. IV. Genetic and environmental factors influencing the development of diabetes after infection with the M variant of encephalomyocarditis virus, Diabetes 25:190, 1976.

70. Rubenstein, A. H., Block, M. B., Starr, J., Melani, F., and Steiner, D. F.: Proinsulin and C-peptide in blood, Diabetes 21(Suppl. 2):661, 1972.

71. Shafrir, E., Krausz, Y., Bar-On, H., Gordin, M., Lilling, S., Khassis, S., and Benchimol, A.: Les influences des glucorticoïdes sur la cétogénèse, la lipogénèse et l'hyperlipidémie: rôle de l'insulinémie et de la glucagonémie secondaire, in *J. Ann. Diabetol. Hôtel-Dieu* (Paris: Flammarion, 1977), p. 272.

72. Siperstein, M. D., Foster, D. W., and Knowles, H. C., Jr.: Control of blood glucose and vascular disease, N. Engl. J. Med. 296:1060, 1977.

73. Spiro, R. G.: Search for a biochemical basis of diabetic microangiopathy, Diabetologia 12:1, 1976.

74. Spiro, R. G., and Spiro, M. J.: Effects of diabetes on the biosynthesis of the renal glomerular basement membrane. Studies on the glucosyltransferase, Diabetes 20:641, 1971.

75. Steinke, J., and Taylor, K. W.: Viruses and the etiology of diabetes, Diabetes 23:631, 1974.

76. Tattersall, R. B., and Fajans, S. S.: Prevalance of diabetes and glucose intolerance in 199 offspring of 37 conjugal diabetic parents, Diabetes 24:452, 1975.

77. Tattersall, R. B., and Pyke, D. A.: Diabetes in identical twins, Lancet 2:1120, 1972.
78. Tchobroutsky, G.: How to achieve better diabetes control? Studies with insulin three-times a day, in Malaisse, W. J., Pirart, J., and Vallance-Owen, J. (eds.): *Diabetes* (Amsterdam: Excerpta Med., 1974), p. 667.
79. Unger, R. H.: Diabetes and the alpha-cell, Diabetes 25:136, 1976.
80. University Group Diabetes Program. A study of the effects of hypoglycemic agents on vascular complications in patients with adult-onset diabetes. I–II, Diabetes 19(Suppl. 2): F 47, 1970; III, J. Am. Diab. Assoc. 217:1400, 1971; IV, J. Am. Diab. Assoc. 218:777, 1971; V, Diabetes 24(Suppl. 1):65, 1971.
81. Vallance-Owen, J.: The inheritance of essential diabetes mellitus from studies of the synalbumin insulin antagonist, Diabetologia 2:248, 1966.
82. Vittinghus, E., Mogensen, C. E., and Søling, K.: Abnormal albumin excretion during exercise in diabetes. A provocation test for early abnormalities. Development and mechanism, Diabetologia 13:438, 1977.
83. Wahren, J., Felig, P., Cerasi, E., and Luft, R.: Splanchnic and peripheral glucose and aminoacid metabolism in diabetes mellitus, J. Clin. Invest. 51:1870, 1972.
84. West, K. M.: Diabetes in American Indians and other native populations of the new world, Diabetes 23:841, 1974.
85. Zonana, J., and Rimoin, D. L.: Current concepts: inheritance of diabetes mellitus, N. Engl. J. Med. 295:603, 1976.

2

Animal Models of Diabetic Nephropathy

S. MICHAEL MAUER, M.D., MICHAEL W. STEFFES, M.D., AND DAVID M. BROWN, M.D.

University of Minnesota School of Medicine, Minneapolis, Minnesota

Thirty to 50% of patients with juvenile- or maturity-onset diabetes mellitus develop clinically evident diabetic nephropathy within 10–20 years of the onset of this metabolic disease.[24, 38, 63] Among patients whose age of onset is less than 15 years, almost 60% will develop renal failure, despite insulin therapy.[45]

The pathology of human diabetic nephropathy includes glomerular capillary basement membrane (GBM) thickening,[60] accompanied late in the disease by thickening of tubular basement membranes (TBM) and Bowman's capsule.[79] There is increased localization of plasma proteins, especially IgG and albumin, in all renal extracellular membranes.[57] At the time of GBM thickening, accumulation of mesangial matrix material begins[60] and ultimately results in diffuse and nodular (Kimmelstiel-Wilson) forms of glomerulosclerosis.[34, 37] Mesangial thickening is accompanied by increased quantities of mesangial smooth muscle proteins.[66] Glomerular hyaline nodular (exudative) deposits[34, 37] and hyaline arteriolar degeneration, especially of

---

Supported by NIH grants HL0613 and AM17697-03.

23

afferent and efferent glomerular arterioles,[7, 34] are frequently present in cases of well-established diabetic nephropathy.

The mechanisms responsible for the development of these lesions are poorly understood.[54] Although there is an extensive literature exploring factors that could contribute to the microvascular complications of diabetes,[56] many questions remain unanswered. In this chapter we attempt to examine the relevance of animal models of diabetic nephropathy to the understanding of human diabetic renal disease. As we hope will become clear, animal studies have value in suggesting or supporting avenues of research in humans.

Diabetic Glomerulopathy in the Dog

More than 30 years ago Lukens and Dohan reported that a dog made diabetic by the administration of bovine pituitary growth hormone and maintained on insulin for five years developed nodular glomerulosclerosis similar to the classical Kimmelstiel-Wilson lesion.[44] Bloodworth extended these studies in dogs given either alloxan or bovine pituitary growth hormone, and he demonstrated that long-term survivors with diabetes developed renal lesions typical of human diabetic glomerulopathy.[10] Within one to six years, irrespective of the mode of induction of diabetes, all animals developed diffuse glomerulosclerosis and thickening of TBM and Bowman's capsules. Seven of ten dogs had nodular (Kimmelstiel-Wilson) glomerulosclerosis (Fig. 2–1,B) and six exhibited glomerular exudative lesions. Both alloxan and growth hormone diabetic animals had significantly increased GBM thickness compared with normal animals (Fig. 2–2).[12] Dogs whose diabetes was carefully controlled with insulin developed little glomerular pathology (Fig. 2–1,A,C).[11] Patz *et al.* described dogs with spontaneous diabetes of shorter duration than those in Bloodworth's studies. These animals had diffuse glomerulosclerosis, GBM, TBM and Bowman's capsular thickening but did not develop Kimmelstiel-Wilson nodules.[62]

Diabetic Glomerulopathy in the Monkey

Bloodworth *et al.* studied rhesus monkeys with alloxan diabetes.[12] All animals developed diffuse glomerulosclerosis, while a few developed nodular disease. Although precise measurements

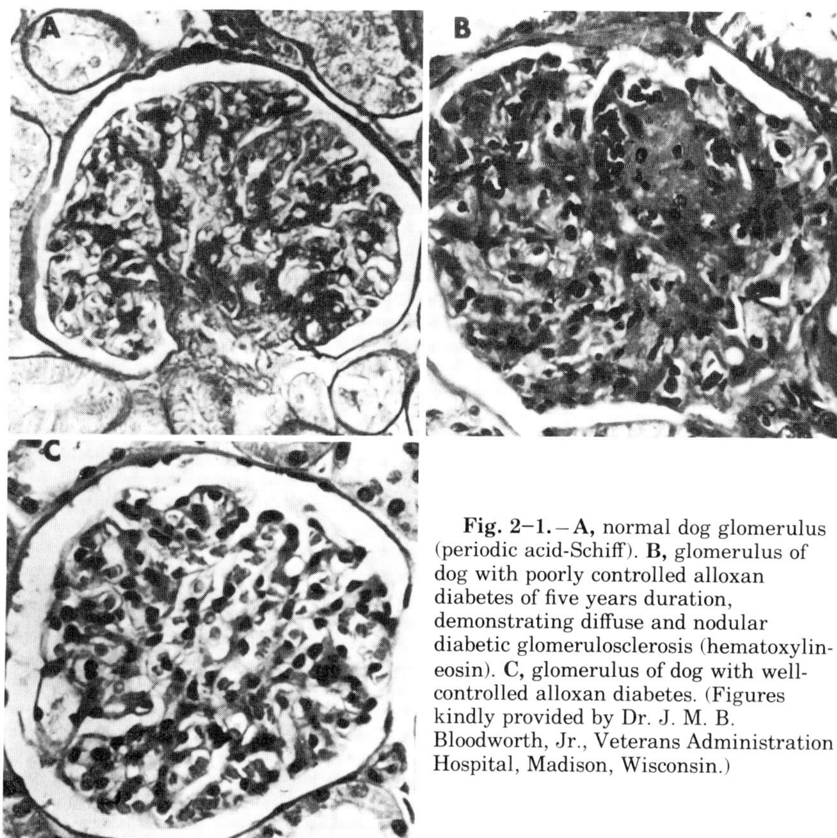

Fig. 2–1. — A, normal dog glomerulus (periodic acid-Schiff). B, glomerulus of dog with poorly controlled alloxan diabetes of five years duration, demonstrating diffuse and nodular diabetic glomerulosclerosis (hematoxylin-eosin). C, glomerulus of dog with well-controlled alloxan diabetes. (Figures kindly provided by Dr. J. M. B. Bloodworth, Jr., Veterans Administration Hospital, Madison, Wisconsin.)

were not performed, electron microscopic studies showed "unquestionably thickened" GBM. From these monkey and dog experiments, the authors concluded that diabetic nephropathy essentially identical with that seen in humans resulted from the diabetic state no matter what its cause. They rejected the concept that the secondary complications of diabetes resulted from a separately inherited disorder that was genetically linked but independent of the metabolic abnormalities of this disease.

Diabetic Glomerulopathy in the Rat

Experimental diabetes has been produced in rats by the administration of B-cell toxins, alloxan[9] or streptozotocin,[48] by

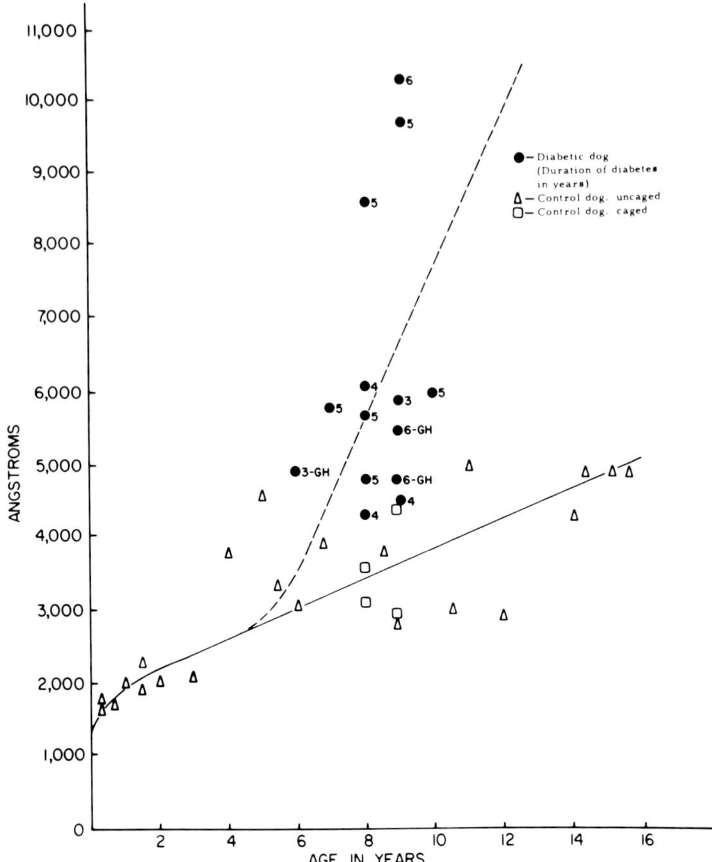

Fig. 2–2.—Dog glomerular capillary width. All tissues embedded in Epon. (From Bloodworth, J. M. B., Jr., and Engerman, R. L.: Spontaneous and induced diabetic microangiopathy, Acta Diabetol. Lat. 8(Suppl. 1):263, 1971. Courtesy of Dr. J. M. B. Bloodworth, Jr.)

pancreatectomy[26] or by the feeding of high-sucrose diets to genetically selected animals.[18, 65] Light microscopic glomerular changes in rats with these various models of diabetes are remarkably similar.[26, 48, 59, 65] There is progressive periodic acid-Schiff (PAS)-positive thickening of the glomerular mesangium, which becomes apparent after four to six months of diabetes (Fig. 2–3, A). This thickening extends down to and surrounds the intraglomerular portions of the afferent and efferent arterioles at the glomerular hilus. These mesangial changes, at first focal in distribution, become generalized and associated with glomerulosclerosis after 12 months of diabetes. In addition, crescent-shaped or nodular hyaline deposits may be seen peripherally and centrally within glomeruli after four to six months. With time (12-16 months) these "exudative" lesions may become very extensive, virtually obliterating the glomerulus.

Immunopathologic studies of rats made diabetic by alloxan or streptozotocin have demonstrated progressive localization of IgG (Fig. 2-3, C), IgM and C3 within the mesangium.[33, 39, 48, 82]

Fig. 2-3. – **A,** glomerulus from a rat diabetic for six months before transplantation into a normal recipient, demonstrating increased mesangial matrix material (periodic acid-Schiff). **B,** glomerulus from kidney of the rat in A, two months after transplantation into a normal rat, demonstrating a decrease in mesangial matrix material (periodic acid-Schiff). **C,** glomerulus from a rat diabetic for six months before transplantation into a normal recipient, demonstrating intense mesangial staining for rat IgG. **D,** glomerulus from kidney of rat in C, two months following transplantation into a normal rat, demonstrating complete disappearance of rat IgG from the mesangium. (From Lee, C. S., Mauer, S. M., Brown, D. M., Sutherland, D. E. R., Michael, A. F., and Najarian, J. S.: Renal transplantation in diabetes mellitus in rats, J. Exp. Med. 139:793, 1974.)

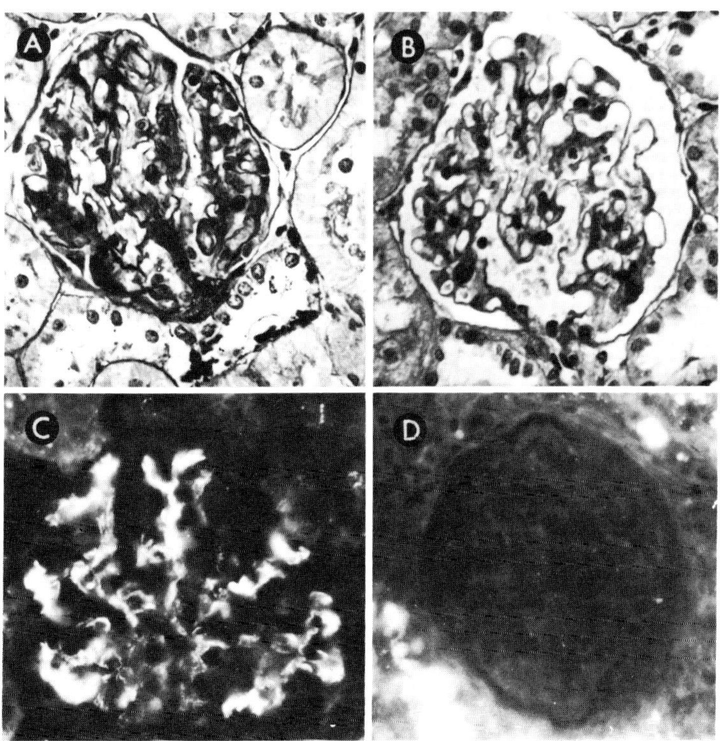

Unlike the light microscopic changes, these immunopathologic changes are generalized. There is no evidence that they represent specific immunologic injury, as the mesangium in these diabetic rats does not fix heterologous complement and significant mesangial cell proliferation is not present.[48] Further, treatment with cyclophosphamide or neonatal thymectomy has little influence on the development of these immunohistochemical lesions.[32] The hyalin nodules described above also stain for immunoglobulins and complement; however, as in human diabetes,[14] these nodules do fix heterologous complement. The significance of this finding is unclear. Increased width of mesangial staining for smooth muscle proteins occurs in diabetic rats[67] as it does in diabetic humans.[66]

The electron microscopic appearance of mesangial matrix ("basement membrane like") thickening, mesangial intracellular inclusions and hyaline nodular lesions in rats with long-standing diabetes is similar to that seen in humans.[1, 61, 82] In addition we have confirmed that progressive statistically significant GBM thickening indistinguishable from that seen in humans occurs in diabetic rats.[15, 30]

Thus, although the glomerular pathology of diabetes in the rat does not mimic human changes as closely as do diabetic glomerular changes in the dog or monkey, the similarities between rat and human diabetic glomerulopathy are striking.[9, 48, 59, 74] This is true no matter what the cause of diabetes in these various species.[5, 9, 18, 22, 26, 48, 62, 65, 83] It is therefore reasonable to postulate that diabetic glomerular disease is a manifestation of the fundamental disturbances of metabolism in cases of diabetes, and that the differences in the morphologic expression of glomerular disease in various diabetic animals and humans represent species differences in the tissue responses to these metabolic disturbances and, perhaps, differences in the duration of disease.

We have derived further evidence to support these hypotheses from manipulating the metabolic environment of the kidneys of highly inbred Lewis rats. Two to four months following transplantation of normal kidneys into streptozotocin diabetic rats, we saw PAS-positive mesangial matrix thickening, hyaline nodular glomerular deposits and mesangial and hyaline nodular immunoglobulin and complement deposition.[39] These studies are analogous to observations made in normal kidneys transplanted into diabetic humans. Within two to four years following transplantation, we noted a high incidence of glomerular arteriolar hyaline degenerative changes.[46] Further, increased GBM, TBM and Bowman's capsule immunohistochemical staining for IgG and albumin developed in these kidneys.[49]

The corollary of the above observations has been tested only in animals. We transplanted kidneys from Lewis rats diabetic for six months into their metabolically normal littermates. Within two months following transplantation, there was a marked decrease in mesangial matrix thickening and mesangial IgG, IgM and C3 localization compared with biopsy specimens of these same kidneys obtained at the time of transplantation (Fig. 2–3, A–D). These studies provide strong support for the argument that the glomerulopathy of diabetes in rats is secondary to the abnormal metabolic environment in which the kidney resides.

Further evidence to support this conclusion comes from our studies of pancreatic islet transplantation in diabetic rats. Lewis rats diabetic for six months had their diabetes cured by successful transplantation of neonatal pancreatic tissue using the method of Leonard et al.[41] Within a few weeks there was marked improvement in the glomerular alterations of diabetes as seen by light and immunofluorescent microscopy compared with biopsies performed in these same animals at the time of islet transplantation.[52, 53] By nine weeks after islet transplantation, mesangial immunofluorescent findings were indistinguishable from those from nondiabetic age-matched littermate controls. However, compared with these controls, minimal mesangial matrix thickening persisted in the transplanted animals (Table 2–1). Nontransplanted diabetic animals observed over this same time period demonstrated progressive diabetic glomerular changes. It is interesting that the glomerular hyaline nodules and their immunopathologic staining characteristics did not change following the transplantation of a kidney from a diabetic to a normal host or following reversal of the diabetic state by islet transplantation. Our findings of regression of diabetic glomerular lesions following islet transplantation have been confirmed by Federlin et al. using intraportal transplantation of isogenic islets.[25] Furthermore, Weil et al.[81] and Gray and Watkins[29] have shown that islet transplantation performed two to six weeks after streptozotocin administration prevented the

TABLE 2-1.—RESULTS OF LIGHT MICROSCOPIC STUDIES
OF MESANGIAL THICKENING

	INDEX OF MESANGIAL THICKENING*	p VALUE COMPARING PRE- AND POST-TRANSPLANT RESULTS	
		UNPAIRED t TEST	PAIRED t TEST
Pre-transplant (No.=10)	1.8 ± 0.3†		
1-2 wk post-transplant‡ (No.=10)	1.1 ± 0.3	<0.0005	<0.005, >0.0005
3-4 wk post-transplant (No.=9)	0.9 ± 0.5	<0.0005	<0.01, >0.005
6-9 wk post-transplant (No.=7)	1.1 ± 0.5	<0.005, >0.0005	<0.005, >0.0005

*Index for each biopsy represents the mean of scores provided by three observers as compared with normal age-matched littermates. (From reference 52.)
†Mean of indices ± SD.
‡Where two biopsies were available, the index was taken to be the mean of all the scores for both biopsies.

development of diabetic glomerulopathy in rats. Although insulin therapy has been shown to decrease the rate of development of mesangial thickening, mesangial IgG and C3 localization and GBM thickening, this treatment was unable to prevent the development of these lesions in rats with chronic alloxan diabetes.[31] Preliminary evidence from our laboratory suggests that GBM thickening in rats with long-standing diabetes may not be rapidly reversible by islet transplantation.[76] Whether islet transplantation performed early after the induction of diabetes in rats would prevent GBM thickening is presently unknown.

It is clear from the studies in rats that the development of several components of diabetic glomerulopathy is intimately tied to the presence of the diabetic state. Evidence in humans, including studies of kidneys transplanted into diabetic patients[46, 49] and studies of muscle capillary[86] and GBM thickness,[60] points in the same direction, but rigorous scientific proof of this thesis remains elusive. Nonetheless, even if we were to accept this thesis, the question of how the metabolic perturbations of diabetes cause the microangiopathy, including the nephropathy of diabetes, remains to be answered. An excellent review of this subject has recently been presented by McMillan, in which he explores several categories of changes in diabetic humans and speculates on their role in contributing to the secondary complications of diabetes.[54] Some of these categories have been explored in experiments with rats.

GLOMERULAR BASEMENT MEMBRANE BIOCHEMISTRY IN DIABETIC RATS

Important questions regarding the pathogenesis of increased GBM thickness and permeability in subjects with diabetes remain unanswered. A variety of investigative approaches have been undertaken to determine whether changes in thickness and permeability are related to each other, whether GBM chemistry is normal or abnormal and whether there are disturbances in GBM synthesis or degradation or both. It is clear that in juvenile-onset diabetes in humans[60] and experimental diabetes in rats, GBM thickness is normal at the onset of diabetes but increases to the abnormal range with time.[15, 30]

Spiro suggested that GBM composition in patients with long-term diabetes is abnormal based on findings of an increase in hydroxylysine content and in glucose and galactose components known to be associated with the disaccharide linked to hydroxylysine.[72] He further found a reciprocal decrease in lysine residues, smaller but significant increases in the amounts of GBM hydroxyproline and glycine and decreases in valine and tyrosine levels. However, Westberg and Michael found a decreased cystine and sialic acid content of diabetic GBM,[85] and Kefalides found a decreased half-cystine content,[35] but neither of these laboratories could confirm the increased hydroxylation of lysine noted by Spiro. Obviously, methodologic problems may be contributing to these different results[72, 84] and further studies in human diabetic GBM chemistry are required.

Unfortunately, animal studies have not provided clear-cut answers to this important controversy. Studies in rats have suggested increased rates of basement membrane synthesis. Spiro and Spiro, studying whole rat kidney cortex, found increased levels of glucosyltransferase activity in alloxan diabetic rats.[73] Since this enzyme appears to represent an index of the rate of basement membrane synthesis,[71] the authors concluded that the activity of basement membrane production was increased in these animals. Further, these authors found that this increase in enzyme activity could be reversed to normal by careful insulin treatment.[71] In addition Risteli *et al.* found significant increases in the activities of propylhydroxylase, lysylhydroxylase, collagen galactosyltransferase and collagen glucosyltransferase in the supernatant of kidney homogenates of rats diabetic for 12 weeks.[64] However, extrapolation from studies of whole renal cortex to GBM synthesis may be unwarranted. Cohen and Voght found that diabetic (pancreatectomized) rats have increased incorporation of radiolabeled lysine in subcellular fractions of isolated glomeruli.[19] Further, Khalifa and Cohen reported increased lysylhydroxylase activity in the supernatant fractions of isolated glomeruli from streptozotocin diabetic rats.[36] However, Wahl *et al.* could find no increased radiolabeled glucose incorporation into the GBM of isolated diabetic rat glomeruli.[77] Furthermore, Beisswenger found that the GBM chemical composition of rats with long-term streptozotocin diabetes did not differ significantly from normal.[6] In preparing isolated glomeruli, he was unable to confirm increased hydroxylation of lysine in diabetic rats. Thus this area of research remains confused, with contradictory data that may not be clarified until in vivo GBM amino acid and carbohydrate incorporation studies are performed. Further, the specificity of changes in basement membrane chemistry in cases of diabetes must be proved by more carefully controlled studies. It is known that streptozotocin diabetic rats undergo renal hypertrophy at rates correlatable with blood glucose concentrations.[69] Other causes of renal hypertrophy, such as unilateral nephrectomy, and other methods for producing long-term osmotic diuresis should be studied simultaneously to determine the specificity of any alterations in enzyme activity that may be found in diabetes.

Role of Hemodynamics in the Development of Diabetic Glomerulopathy in Rats

Among the categories listed by McMillan as possibly contributing to diabetic microangiopathy is that of alterations in microcirculatory hemodynamics.[54] Ditzel has pointed out that patients with diabetes have impaired tissue oxygenation based upon increased hemoglobin A_1C concentrations, significantly reduced P_{50} values and incomplete compensation by increased red blood cell 2,3-diphosphoglycerate levels because of relative hypophosphatemia.[20, 21] He argues that this results in an auto-regulatory alteration in microcirculatory flow-pressure relation-ships, resulting in increased tissue perfusion which over long periods of time could damage small vessels. McMillan[55] and Schmid-Schönbein and Vogler[68] have emphasized the potential importance of increased plasma viscosity, increased red blood cell aggregation and decreased red blood cell deformability in the development of diabetic microangiopathy. There is evidence that nephron hemodynamics are abnormal in human diabetics. Mogensen has reported increased renal size, glomerular filtra-tion rate (GFR) and filtration fraction early in cases of juvenile diabetes.[58] This increased filtration fraction probably represents increased filtration pressure. The exercise-induced albuminuria noted in recent-onset juvenile diabetes may also be secondary to increased glomerular filtration pressures.[58] Although direct measurements of glomerular capillary pressures cannot be per-formed in humans, preliminary micropuncture studies in Mu-nich-Wistar rats made diabetic by subtotal pancreatectomy dis-closed increased glomerular capillary pressures obtained direct-ly using a servo-nulling transducer.[2] Further, Lucas and Foy reported that the proportion of cardiac output received by the kidneys of diabetic rats was increased as measured by the ra-diolabeled microsphere technique.[43]

In order to further test the hypothesis that alterations in nephron hemodynamics can influence the development of dia-betic glomerulopathy, we studied the effects of unilateral ne-phrectomy on the renal pathology of diabetic rats. Unilateral ne-phrectomy, known to lead to increased glomerular blood flow and capillary pressure,[3] resulted in the accelerated development of diabetic glomerular lesions in these animals.[75] In fact, a marked increase in mesangial matrix thickening and mesangial IgG and C3 deposition occurred within three months in unine-phrectomized diabetic as compared with intact diabetic rats (Figs. 2–4 and 2–5). Further, the increased width of mesangial actomyosin staining that develops in intact diabetic rats is even more pronounced in uninephrectomized diabetic animals.[67]

Christlieb has focused on the increased incidence of hyperten-sion in human diabetics.[16] Accelerated deterioration in renal function occurs in diabetic patients with hypertension as com-pared with diabetics successfully treated with antihypertensive agents.[58] An interesting experiment of nature was reported by

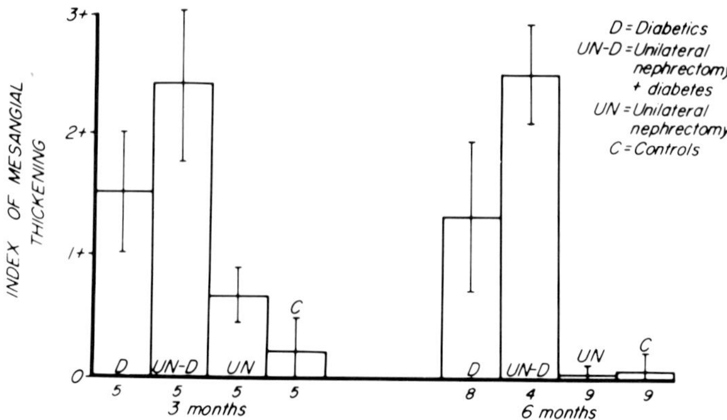

Fig. 2–4.—Mesangial thickness in control and experimental rats at three and six months following unilateral nephrectomy (mean ± 1 SD). (From Steffes, M. W., Brown, D. M., and Mauer, S. M.: Diabetic glomerulopathy following unilateral nephrectomy in the rat, Diabetes, in press.)

Berkman and Rifkin.[8] A patient with unilateral renal artery stenosis and diabetes had only ischemic changes in the stenotic kidney, whereas the kidney exposed to hypertension showed advanced nodular diabetic glomerulosclerosis. We examined the development of diabetic nephropathy in rats made hypertensive by the placement of a constrictive silver slip around one renal artery.[51] After four months of diabetes, the glomeruli of the un-clipped kidneys of hypertensive diabetic rats had greatly increased diabetic changes, including thickening of the mesangial matrix and mesangial localization of immunoglobulins (IgG and IgM) and complement (C3), when compared with glomeruli of the contralateral clipped kidneys of hypertensive diabetic rats and the kidneys of normotensive diabetic animals. Further, the clipped kidneys of diabetic hypertensive animals had less mesangial thickening and, especially, less IgG, IgM and C3 staining compared with kidneys of normotensive diabetic rats. Azar *et al.* found that one-kidney "post salt" hypertensive rats had large increases in glomerular blood flow, glomerular capillary pressure and single-nephron GFR compared with normal and non-hypertensive unilaterally nephrectomized rats.[3] It is reasonable to assume that these alterations in nephron hemodynamics contributed to the accelerated development of diabetic changes in the unclipped kidneys and to protection from these changes in the clipped kidneys in our experiments. Nondiabetic animals

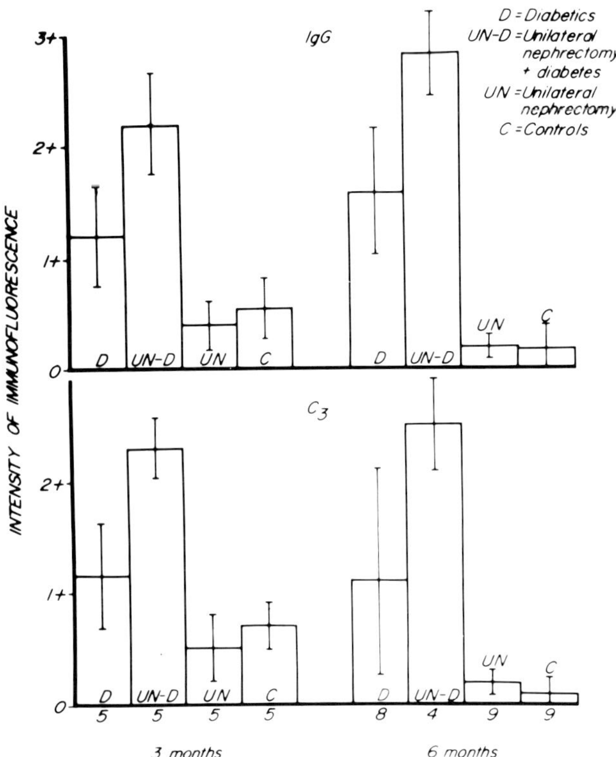

Fig. 2–5.— Intensity of mesangial IgG and C3 staining in control and experimental rats at three and six months following unilateral nephrectomy (mean ± 1 SD). (From Steffes, M. W., Brown, D. M., and Mauer, S. M.: Diabetic glomerulopathy following unilateral nephrectomy in the rat, Diabetes, in press.)

with clip hypertension did not develop similar glomerular lesions in their unprotected kidneys. Thus, the diabetic state represents a necessary cofactor for the glomerulopathy seen in hypertensive diabetic rats. How alterations in nephron hemodynamics combine with the diabetic state to influence the rate of development of diabetic glomerular lesions in these animals is unknown. It is interesting that the incidence of hyaline nodular glomerular lesions and tubular glycogen vacuolar changes was similar in unclipped kidneys of diabetic rats as compared with clipped kidneys in these animals and with kidneys of normotensive diabetic rats. Thus, these lesions of diabetic nephropathy are not influenced by hemodynamics.

MESANGIAL FUNCTION IN DIABETIC RATS

The function of the glomerular mesangium is incompletely understood. However, one relatively well-defined role of the mesangium is in the uptake and disposal of a variety of macromolecular materials.[47] In this regard, the mesangial system may be responsible for the disposal of products of GBM turnover,[78] and interference with the function of this system could have a role in GBM thickening. As the mesangial structure is prominently changed as a result of diabetes in animals and humans, it appears reasonable to study the function of the mesangium in diabetic rats. In normal rats, intravenously injected colloidal carbon is taken up at the periphery of the mesangium and migrates slowly to the glomerular hilus.[23] After four to six weeks much of the colloidal carbon has been cleared from the peripheral mesangium and significant quantities of this material are seen in the extraglomerular portion of the mesangium, in the lacis area of the juxtaglomerular apparatus. Rats diabetic for six months were given colloidal carbon and the glomerular distribution was compared to that seen in age-matched normal rats. As mentioned above, mesangial thickening after six months of diabetes is frequently focal and segmental in distribution. In those areas of the mesangium thickened by the diabetic process, large quantities of colloidal carbon accumulated in aggregated lumps and remained for several weeks.[50] However, in these diabetic rats the uptake, distribution pattern and clearance of colloidal carbon in areas of the mesangium that appeared normal by light microscopy were no different from those seen in controls. These semiquantitative studies of mesangial function in diabetic rats suggest that dysfunction of the mesangium in the uptake and processing of macromolecules is secondary to structural pathology within this system. It is unlikely that disturbed mesangial function leads to mesangial thickening in the early stages of diabetic glomerulopathy. However, it is possible that as mesangial function becomes impaired, this leads to further mesangial pathology and, possibly, to increasing rates of GBM thickening.

Diabetic Nephropathy in Other Animals

Although kidney changes have been described in several animal species in addition to those described above, the most extensive literature focuses on spontaneous diabetes in the mouse and Chinese hamster. Like *et al.* described mesangial and GBM thickening in C57 BL/KS mice that had diabetes for 6–15 months.[42] In addition to these changes, Wehner *et al.* described intense mesangial staining for IgG in the mesangium and in glomerular hyalin nodules.[80] We have also noted markedly increased mesangial IgG and C3 staining in C57/BLKsJ-db/db congenitally diabetic mice.[50] In these animals the immunofluorescent staining also involved the extraglomerular portion of the mesangium and extended into distal tubular cells at the level of the macula densa. There is evidence in the mouse that macromolecules taken up by the mesangium leave the glomerulus via the distal tubule in the area where this latter structure comes into intimate contact with mesangial cells of the lacis zone.[4, 40] We have noted glycogen vacuolation of the distal tubule at the macula densa level in cases of uncontrolled diabetes in rats, mice and humans (Fig. 2–2, A), and similar changes have been found in spontaneously diabetic Chinese hamsters.[70] The importance of these findings in the genesis of mesangial disease or the disordered function of the juxtaglomerular apparatus in subjects with diabetes remains to be determined.[17] Although it is possible to reverse the diabetic state in genetically diabetic mice with islet transplantation,[27, 28] the effects of this treatment on nephropathy in these animals has not yet been assessed.

Conclusions

The secondary complications of diabetes have not been prevented by currently available techniques. It is therefore imperative to obtain a clearer understanding of the pathophysiology of these complications and to develop treatment programs that can delay or prevent these destructive processes. Studies in humans are limited by considerations of research ethics and by the long periods of observation required to determine the efficacy of various therapeutic modalities on the development of diabetic microangiopathy. In this chapter we have presented evidence that animals with diabetes from various causes develop renal lesions identical or very similar to those seen in humans. Differences in species response may be more important than the nature of the pathophysiologic processes in determining the morphologic expressions of nephropathy in cases of long-term diabetes.

Evidence derived from animal studies and from observations in humans strongly supports the argument that diabetic nephropathy is a consequence of the diabetic state rather than a separately inherited but closely linked genetic disorder. Animal studies indicate that insulin therapy retards but does not prevent diabetic nephropathy. Successful reversal of the diabetic state in rats leads to improvement in mesangial thickening and immunopathology. Careful morphometric studies of GBM thickness in animals cured of diabetes have not been completed. Thus, the question of whether GBM thickening can be prevented or reversed cannot be answered at this time.

Studies in animals have permitted the development of pathophysiologic hypotheses that can be further tested in studies of animals and humans. Clearly, in the diabetic rat, alterations in glomerular hemodynamics can influence the rate of development of diabetic glomerulopathy. The role of other variables, such as alterations in basement membrane chemistry, blood rheology, coagulation parameters, tissue oxygen delivery and hormonal balance, can also be explored in animal model systems and can provide directions for future research in human diabetes mellitus.

Acknowledgments

We wish to thank our many colleagues who have been involved in our work, including Drs. Alfred Michael, Alfred Fish, John Najarian, Robert Vernier, Richard Simmons, Frederick Goetz, Jose Barbosa, David Sutherland and Chue Shue Lee. We also wish to acknowledge the excellent technical assistance of Susan Kupcho-Sandberg, John Basgen, Mary Stahlman and Merlene Knotts.

References

1. Anjo, A., and Couturier, E.: Mesangial changes in the renal glomerulus in long-term diabetic rats, Pathol. Eur. 10:21, 1975.
2. Azar, S.: Personal communication.
3. Azar, S., Johnson, M. A., Hertel, B., and Tobian, L.: Single-nephron pressures, flows and resistances in hypertensive kidneys with nephrosclerosis, Kidney Int. 12:28, 1977.
4. Barajas, L.: The ultrastructure of the juxtaglomerular apparatus as disclosed by three-dimensional reconstructions from serial sections. The anatomical relationship between the tubular and vascular components, J. Ultrastruct. Res. 33:116, 1970.

5. Becker, D., and Miller, M.: Presence of diabetic glomerulosclerosis in patients with hemochromatosis, N. Engl. J. Med. 263:367, 1960.

6. Beisswenger, P. J.: Glomerular basement membrane. Biosynthesis and chemical composition in the streptozotocin diabetic rat, J. Clin. Invest. 58:844, 1976.

7. Bell, E. T.: A postmortem study of vascular disease in diabetes, Arch. Pathol. 53:444, 1952.

8. Berkman, J., and Rifkin, H.: Unilateral nodular diabetic glomerulosclerosis (Kimmelstiel-Wilson): Report of a case, Metabolism 22:715, 1973.

9. Beveridge, J. M. R., and Johnson, S. E.: Studies of diabetic rats: The production of cardiovascular and renal lesions in diabetic rats, Br. J. Exp. Pathol. 31:285, 1950.

10. Bloodworth, J. M. B., Jr.: Experimental diabetic glomerulosclerosis. II. The dog, Arch. Pathol. 79:113, 1965.

11. Bloodworth, J. M. B., Jr.: Personal communication.

12. Bloodworth, J. M. B., Jr., Engerman, R. L., and Anderson, P. J.: Microangiopathy in the experimentally diabetic animal, in Camerini-Dávalos, R. A., and Cole, H. S. (eds.): *Vascular and Neurological Changes in Early Diabetes* (New York: Academic Press, 1973), pp. 245–50.

13. Bloodworth, J. M. B., Jr., Engerman, R. L., and Powers, K. L.: Experimental diabetic microangiopathy. 1. Basement membrane statistics in the dog, Diabetes 18:455, 1969.

14. Burkholder, P. M.: Immunohistopathologic study of localized plasma proteins and fixation of guinea pig complement in renal lesions of diabetic glomerulosclerosis, Diabetes 14:755, 1965.

15. Cameron, D. P., Amherdt, M., Leuenberger, P., Orci, L., and Stauffacher, W.: Microvascular alterations in chronically streptozotocin-diabetic rats, in Camerini-Dávalos, R. A., and Cole, H. S. (eds.): *Vascular and Neurological Changes in Early Diabetes* (New York: Academic Press, 1973), pp. 257–69.

16. Christlieb, A. R.: Diabetes and hypertensive vascular disease, Am. J. Cardiol. 32:592, 1973.

17. Christlieb, A. R.: Renin-angiotensin-aldosterone system in diabetes mellitus, Diabetes 25(Suppl. 2):820, 1976.

18. Cohen, A. M., Teitelbaum, A., and Saliternik, R.: Genetics and diet as factors in development of diabetes mellitus, Metabolism 21:235, 1972.

19. Cohen, M. P., and Voght, C.: Evidence for enhanced basement membrane synthesis and lysine hydroxylation in renal glomerulus in experimental diabetes, Biochem. Biophys. Res. Commun. 49:1542, 1971.

20. Ditzel, J.: Oxygen transport impairment in diabetes, Diabetes 25(Suppl. 2):832, 1976.

21. Ditzel, J., and Standl, E.: The problem of tissue oxygenation in diabetes mellitus. 1. Its relation to the early functional changes in the microcirculation of diabetic subjects, Acta Med. Scand. 578(Suppl.):49, 1975.

22. Doyle, A. P., Balcerzak, S. P., and Jeffrey, W. L.: Fatal diabetic glomerulosclerosis after total pancreatectomy, N. Engl. J. Med. 270:623, 1964.

23. Elema, J. D., Hoyer, J. R., and Vernier, R. L.: The glomerular mesangium: uptake of intravenously injected colloidal carbon, Kidney Int. 9:395, 1976.

24. Fanconi, G., Botstejn, A., and Kousmine, C.: Nephropathie beim kindlichen diabetes mellitus, Helv. Paediatr. Acta 3:341, 1948.

25. Federlin, K., Bretzel, R. G., and Schmidtchen, U.: Islet transplantation in experimental diabetes of the rat. V. Regression of glomerular lesions in diabetic rats after intraportal transplantation of isogenic islets, Horm. Metab. Res. 8:404, 1976.

26. Folgia, V. G., Mancini, R. E., and Cardeza, A. F.: Glomerular lesions in the diabetic rat, Arch. Pathol. 50:75, 1950.

27. Gates, R. J., Hunt, M. I., Smith, R., and Lazarus, N. R.: Further studies on the amelioration of the characteristics of New Zealand obese (NZO) mice following implantation of islets of Langerhans, Diabetologia 10:401, 1974.

28. Gates, R. J., Hunt, M. I., Smith, R., and Lazarus, N. R.: Return to normal of blood-glucose, plasma-insulin, and weight gain in New Zealand obese mice after implantation of islets of Langerhans, Lancet 2:567, 1972.

29. Gray, B. N., and Watkins, E., Jr.: Prevention of vascular complications of diabetes by pancreatic islet transplantation, Arch. Surg. 111:254, 1976.

30. Hägg, E.: Glomerular basement membrane thickening in rats with long-term alloxan diabetes. A quantitative electron microscopic study, Acta Pathol. Microbiol. Scand. 82:211, 1974.

31. Hägg, E.: Influence of insulin treatment on glomerular changes in rats with long-term alloxan diabetes, Acta Pathol. Microbiol. Scand. 82:228, 1974.

32. Hägg, E.: Influence of cyclophosphamide treatment and neonatal thymectomy on glomerular changes in rats with long-term alloxan diabetes, Acta Pathol. Microbiol. Scand. 82:349, 1974.

33. Hägg, E.: Occurrence of immunoglobulin and complement in the glomeruli of rats with long-term alloxan diabetes, Acta Pathol. Microbiol. Scand. 82:220, 1974.

34. Heptinstall, R. H.: *Pathology of the Kidney* (Boston: Little, Brown, 1974), pp. 939, 949.

35. Kefalides, N. A.: Biochemical properties of human glomerular basement membrane in normal and diabetic kidneys, J. Clin. Invest. 53:403, 1974.

36. Khalifa, A., and Cohen, M. P.: Glomerular protocollagen lysyl-hydroxylase activity in streptozotocin diabetes, Biochem. Biophys. Acta 386:332, 1975.

37. Kimmelstiel, P.: Diabetic nephropathy, in Becker, E. L. (ed.): *Structural Basis of Renal Disease* (New York: Harper & Row, 1968), p. 468.

38. Knowles, H. C., Guest, G. M., Lampe, J., Kessler, M., and Skillman, T. G.: The course of juvenile diabetes treated with immeasured diet, Diabetes 14:239, 1965.

39. Lee, C. S., Mauer, S. M., Brown, D. M., Sutherland, D. E. R., Michael, A. F., and Najarian, J. S.: Renal transplantation in diabetes mellitus in rats, J. Exp. Med. 139:793, 1974.

40. Leiper, J. M., Thomson, D., and MacDonald, M. K.: Uptake and transport of imposil by the glomerular mesangium of the mouse, Lab. Invest., in press.

41. Leonard, R. J., Lazarow, A., and Hegre, O. D.: Pancreatic islet transplantation in the rat, Diabetes 22:413, 1973.

42. Like, A. A., Lavine, R. L., Poffenbarger, P. L., and Chick, W. L.: Studies in the diabetic mutant mouse. VI. Evolution of glomerular lesions and associated proteinuria, Am. J. Pathol. 66:193, 1972.

43. Lucas, P. D., and Foy, J. M.: Effects of experimental diabetes and genetic obesity on regional blood flow in the rat, Diabetes 26:786, 1977.

44. Lukens, F. D. W., and Dohan, F. C.: Experimental pituitary diabetes of five years duration with glomerulosclerosis, Arch. Pathol. 41:19, 1946.

45. Marble, A.: The future of the child with diabetes, J. Am. Diet. Assoc. 33:569, 1957.

46. Mauer, S. M., Barbosa, J., Vernier, R. L., Kjellstrand, C. M., Buselmeier, T. J., Simmons, R. L., Najarian, J. S., and Goetz, F. C.: Development of diabetic vascular lesions in normal kidneys transplanted into patients with diabetes mellitus, N. Engl. J. Med. 295:916, 1976.

47. Mauer, S. M., Fish, A. J., Blau, E. B., and Michael, A. F.: The glomerular mesangium. 1. Kinetic studies of macromolecular uptake in normal and nephrotic rats, J. Clin. Invest. 51:1092, 1972.

48. Mauer, S. M., Michael, A. F., Fish, A. J., and Brown, D. M.: Spontaneous immunoglobulin and complement deposition in glomeruli of diabetic rats, Lab. Invest. 25:488, 1972.

49. Mauer, S. M., Miller, K., Goetz, F. C., Barbosa, J., Simmons, R. L., Najarian, J. S., and Michael, A. F.: Immunopathology of renal extracellular membranes in kidneys transplanted into patients with diabetes mellitus, Diabetes 25:709, 1976.

50. Mauer, S. M., Steffes, M. W., and Brown, D. M.: Manuscript in preparation.

51. Mauer, S. M., Steffes, M. W., Azar, S., Kupcho-Sandberg, S., and Brown, D. M.: The

effects of Goldblatt hypertension on the development of glomerular lesions of diabetes mellitus in the rat, submitted for publication.

52. Mauer, S. M., Steffes, M. W., Sutherland, D. E. R., Najarian, J. S., Michael, A. F., and Brown, D. M.: Studies of the rate of regression of the glomerular lesions in diabetic rats treated with pancreatic islet transplantation, Diabetes 24:280, 1975.

53. Mauer, S. M., Sutherland, D. E. R., Steffes, M. W., Leonard, R. J., Najarian, J. S., Michael, A. F., and Brown, D. M.: Pancreatic islet transplantation. Effects on the glomerular lesions of experimental diabetes in the rat, Diabetes 23:748, 1974.

54. McMillan, D. E.: Deterioration of the microcirculation in diabetes, Diabetes 24:944, 1975.

55. McMillan, D. E.: Plasma protein changes, blood viscosity and diabetic microangiopathy, Diabetes 25(Suppl. 2):858, 1976.

56. McMillan, D. E., and Ditzel, J. (eds.): Proceedings of a conference on diabetic microangiopathy, Diabetes 25(Suppl. 2):805, 1976.

57. Miller, K., and Michael, A. F.: Immunopathology of renal extracellular membranes in diabetes mellitus. Specificity of tubular basement membrane immunofluorescence, Diabetes 25:701, 1976.

58. Mogensen, C. E.: Renal function changes in diabetes, Diabetes 25(Suppl. 2):872, 1976.

59. Ørskov, H., Steen Olsen, T., Nielsen, K., Rafaelsen, O. J., and Lundbaek, K.: Kidney lesions in rats with severe long-term alloxan diabetes, Diabetologia 1:172, 1965.

60. Østerby, R.: Morphometric studies of the peripheral glomerular basement membrane in early juvenile onset diabetes. 1. Development of initial basement membrane thickening, Diabetologia 8:84, 1972.

61. Østerby Hansen, R., Lundbaek, K., Steen Olsen, T., and Ørskov, H.: Kidney lesions in rats with severe long-term alloxan diabetes, Lab. Invest. 17:675, 1967.

62. Patz, A., Berkow, J. W., Maumenee, A. E., and Cox, J.: Studies on diabetic retinopathy. II. Retinopathy and nephropathy in spontaneous canine diabetes, Diabetes 14:700, 1965.

63. Ramel, C.: The kidney in diabetes, Schweiz. Med. Wochenschr. 95:416, 1965.

64. Risteli, J., Koivisto, V. A., Åkerblom, H. K., and Kivirikko, K. I.: Intracellular enzymes of collagen biosynthesis in rat kidney in streptozotocin diabetes, Diabetes 25:1066, 1976.

65. Rosenmann, E., Teitelbaum, A., and Cohen, A. M.: Nephropathy in sucrose-fed rats. Electron and light microscopic studies, Diabetes 20:803, 1971.

66. Scheinman, J. I., Fish, A. J., and Michael, A. F.: The immunohistopathology of glomerular antigens: The glomerular basement membrane, collagen and actomyosin antigens in normal and diseased kidneys, J. Clin. Invest. 54:1144, 1974.

67. Scheinman, J. I., Steffes, M. W., Brown, D. M., and Mauer, S. M.: The immunohistopathology of glomerular antigens. III. Increased mesangial actomyosin in experimental diabetes in the rat, Diabetes, in press.

68. Schmid-Schönbein, H., and Vogler, E.: Red-cell aggregation and deformability in diabetes, Diabetes 25(Suppl. 2):897, 1976.

69. Seyer-Hansen, K.: Renal hypertrophy in experimental diabetes: relation to severity of diabetes, Diabetologia 13:141, 1977.

70. Soret, M. G., Dulin, W. E., and Gerritson, G. C.: Microangiopathy in animals with spontaneous hypertension, in Camerini-Dávalos, R. A., and Cole, H. S. (eds.): *Vascular and Neurological Changes in Early Diabetes* (New York: Academic Press, 1973), pp. 291–98.

71. Spiro, M. J., and Spiro, R. G.: Studies on the biosynthesis of the hydroxylysine-linked disaccharide unit of basement membrane and collagens. 1. Kidney glucosyltransferase, J. Biol. Chem. 246:4899, 1971.

72. Spiro, R. G.: Search for a biochemical basis of diabetic microangiopathy. Claude Bernard lecture, Diabetologia 12:1, 1976.

73. Spiro, R. G., and Spiro, M. J.: Effect of diabetes on the biosynthesis of the renal

glomerular basement membrane. Studies on the glucosyltransferase, Diabetes 20: 641, 1971.

74. Steen Olsen, T., Ørskov, H., and Lundbaek, K.: Kidney lesions in rats with severe long-term alloxan diabetes. II. Histochemical studies. Comparison with human glomerular lesions, Acta Pathol. Microbiol. Scand. 66:1, 1966.

75. Steffes, M. W., Brown, D. M., and Mauer, S. M.: Diabetic glomerulopathy following unilateral nephrectomy in the rat, Diabetes, in press.

76. Steffes, M. W., Brown, D. M., and Mauer, S. M.: Unpublished observations.

77. Wahl, R., Deppermann, D., Descher, W., Fuchs, E., and Rexroth, W.: The metabolism of the isolated renal glomerulus and its basement membranes, in Camerini-Dávalos, R. A., and Cole, H. S. (eds.): *Vascular and Neurological Changes in Early Diabetes* (New York: Academic Press, 1973), pp. 147–153.

78. Walker, F.: The origin, turnover and removal of glomerular basement-membrane, J. Pathol. 110:233, 1973.

79. Warren, S., Le Compte, P. M., and Legg, M. A.: *The Pathology of Diabetes* (Philadelphia: Lea & Febiger, 1966), pp. 231–46.

80. Wehner, H., Höhn, O., Faix-Schade, U., Huber, H., and Walzer, P.: Glomerular changes in mice with spontaneous hereditary diabetes, Lab. Invest. 27:331, 1972.

81. Weil, R., III, Nozawa, M., Koss, M., Weber, C., Reemtsma, K., and McIntosh, R. M.: Pancreatic transplantation in diabetic rats: Renal function, morphology, ultrastructure, and immunohistology, Surgery 78:142, 1975.

82. Weil, R., III, Nozawa, M., Koss, M., Weber, C., Reemtsma, K., and McIntosh, R. M.: The kidney in streptozotocin diabetic rats. Morphologic, ultrastructure, and function studies, Arch. Pathol. Lab. Med. 100:37, 1976.

83. Wellmann, K. F., and Volk, B. W.: Nodular intercapillary glomerulosclerosis in diabetes secondary to chronic calcific pancreatitis, Diabetes 25:714, 1976.

84. Westberg, N. G.: Biochemical alterations of the human glomerular basement membrane in diabetes, Diabetes 25(Suppl. 2):920, 1976.

85. Westberg, N. G., and Michael, A. F.: Human glomerular basement membrane: Chemical composition in diabetes mellitus, Acta Med. Scand. 194:39, 1973.

86. Williamson, J. R., and Kilo, C.: Current status of capillary-basement membrane disease in diabetes mellitus, Diabetes 26:65, 1977.

3

Early and Late Changes in the Diabetic Kidney

H. J. G. GUNDERSEN, M.D., C. E. MOGENSEN, M.D., K. SEYER-HANSEN, M.D., R. ØSTERBY, M.D., AND K. LUNDBÆK, M.D.

The Second Department of Internal Medicine, the Laboratory of Endocrine Research, the Electronmicroscopic Laboratory of Diabetes Research and the Institute of Experimental Clinical Research, Kommunehospitalet, Aarhus, Denmark

The renal abnormalities occurring in diabetic patients can be divided into four kinds: glomerulopathy, pyelonephritis, papillary necrosis and glycogen nephrosis. This chapter deals exclusively with glomerulopathy. We will present and discuss some recent results from studies of the morphology of the glomerulus, the glomerular filtration rate (GFR) and renal plasma flow (RPF), and urinary protein excretion in patients with diabetes mellitus.

Historically the study of diabetic glomerular disease was inaugurated by Kimmelstiel's and Wilson's demonstrations of the specific nodular changes in the glomeruli of diabetic patients.[21] This phenomenon occurs in some patients after many years of diabetes. When it is present, renal insufficiency either is manifest or can be predicted to set in shortly.

During recent years there has been much interest in the *early* changes occurring many years before the appearance of clinically significant renal damage. In this survey the emphasis is on those early changes.

43

Onset of Diabetes and the First Years

Shortly after the acute clinical onset of juvenile diabetes a characteristic renal abnormality can be observed. Examining patients before or a few weeks or months after the institution of diet plus insulin therapy, in the usual moderately controlled metabolic state, it appears that the renal glomeruli are enlarged, involving an increase in filtering area, GFR is increased to greater than normal levels and the filtration fraction (FF) is high. However, the amount of resting or basal albumin excretion is not increased.

This pattern remains constant for many years, while at the same time a gradual increase in the thickness of the glomerular basement membrane can be demonstrated.

EARLY RENAL HYPERTROPHY

The first indications of an expansion of renal tissue in patients with early diabetes came in 1973 from the radiologic demonstration of an increased kidney size by Mogensen and Andersen.[42] The weight of the kidney was estimated from measurements on pyelograms from young diabetics with a mean duration of diabetes of five years and from normal subjects of the same age. As shown in Figure 3–1, in the diabetics the kidney weight was 22% higher than that in the normal subjects.[42]

To see whether this enlargement affected glomerular structures, Østerby and Gundersen performed a morphometric study of the glomeruli in kidney biopsy specimens from recent juvenile diabetics, patients one to six years after the onset of diabetes and control subjects.[48] In newly diagnosed diabetics the mean glomerular volume and the capillary lumen per glomerulus were enlarged, with both quantities being nearly twice as great as in the nondiabetics (Fig. 3–2). The solid volume (cells and extracellular material) was also enlarged, whereas the number of cells was identical in the two groups, indicating cellular hypertrophy. In patients with a duration of diabetes of one to six years, no significant regression of these changes occurred.

The increase in the area of the capillary lumen was further elucidated by a recent stereologic study by Kroustrup, Gundersen and Østerby, demonstrating an 80% increase in the capillary wall area in subjects with early diabetes (Fig. 3–3).[22]

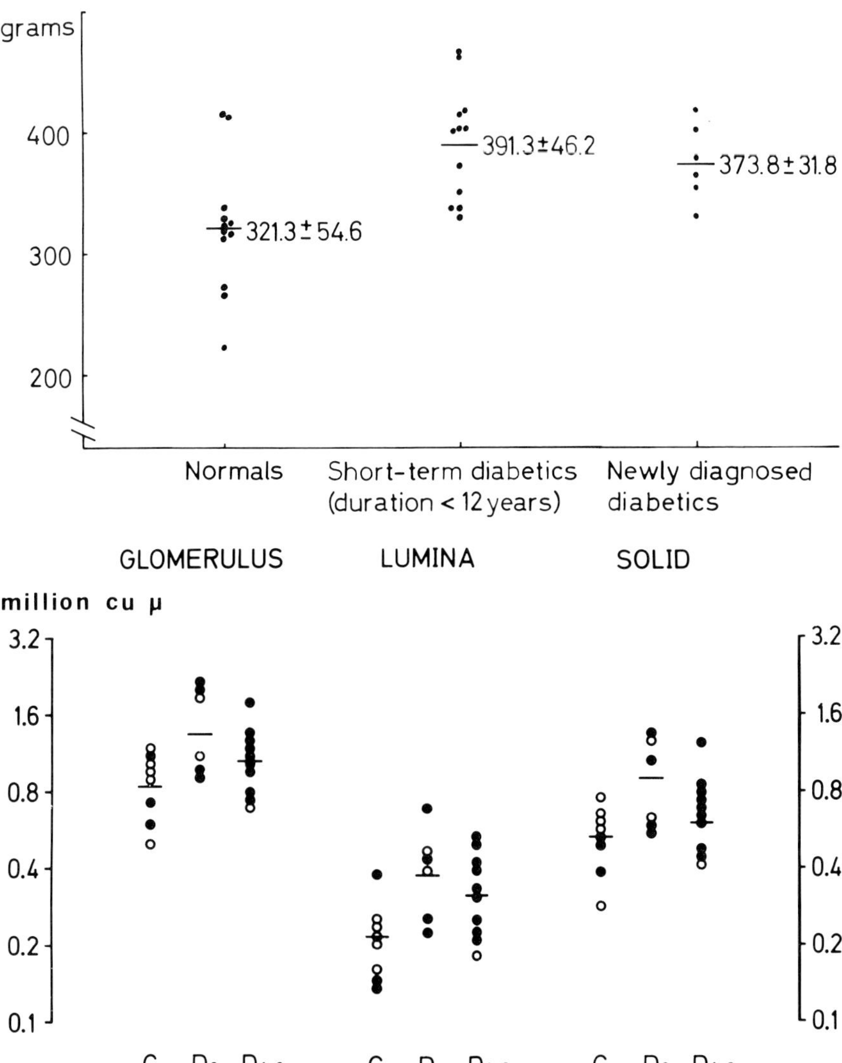

Fig. 3–1 (top). – Calculated kidney weight (corrected to 1.73 sq m) in 12 normal and 18 diabetic subjects. (From Mogensen, C. E., and Andersen, M. J. F.: Increased kidney size and glomerular filtration rate in early juvenile diabetics, Diabetes 22:706, 1973.)

Fig. 3–2 (bottom). – Volumes of the total glomerular tuft, of the capillary lumen and of the solid part of the glomerulus (millions of cubic microns per 1.73 sq m). Abbreviations: C, controls; D_0; newly diagnosed diabetics; D_{1-6}, patients with 1–6 years duration of diabetes; open circles, females; filled circles, males. The horizontal bars indicate mean values. (From Østerby, R., and Gundersen, H. H. G.: Glomerular size and structure in diabetes mellitus. I. Early abnormalities, Diabetologia 11:225, 1975.)

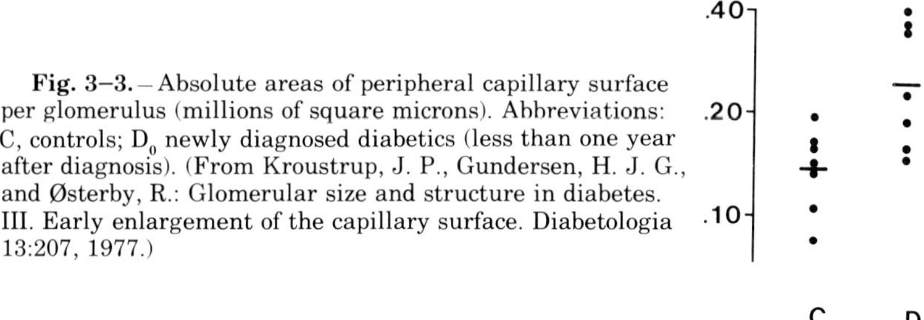

Fig. 3–3.—Absolute areas of peripheral capillary surface per glomerulus (millions of square microns). Abbreviations: C, controls; D_0 newly diagnosed diabetics (less than one year after diagnosis). (From Kroustrup, J. P., Gundersen, H. J. G., and Østerby, R.: Glomerular size and structure in diabetes. III. Early enlargement of the capillary surface. Diabetologia 13:207, 1977.)

The early morphological deviations in juvenile diabetes are determined by metabolic factors. This is demonstrated by the fact that three months of very strict control of the blood glucose level results in a significant decrease in the radiologically determined kidney size.[43]

Animal studies performed in our laboratory have shown that the kidney weight increases a few days after the induction of diabetes by streptozotocin in rats.[52, 53] The increase in kidney weight is accompanied by an increase in the protein-DNA as well as the RNA/DNA ratio, indicating an increase in protein synthesis and cellular hypertrophy.[53] The same conclusions can be drawn from earlier studies of amino acid incorporation by kidney ribosomes.[50]

In Seyer-Hansen's study the acute changes in kidney weight and the parameters of protein synthesis could be inhibited by early insulin administration.[53] This same result appears from another study of streptozotocin diabetes in the rat, where the results of badly versus strictly controlled diabetic states were observed after six months.[51] This study shows an increase in glomerular volume in the streptozotocin diabetic rats and an inhibition of this change by near normalization of the blood glucose.

BASEMENT MEMBRANE THICKNESS IN EARLY DIABETES

It appears from the above discussion that at the clinical onset of juvenile diabetes the glomeruli are enlarged, involving a commensurate increase in the *total amount* of basement membrane. On the other hand, at this same time the *thickness* of the glomerular basement membrane remains normal, as shown earlier in a series of studies by Østerby.[46, 47]

Over the years the basement membrane becomes thickened, leading eventually to the total occlusion of many glomeruli as seen in patients with long-term diabetes. We shall discuss the results of our studies on basement membrane thickness later because of their particular importance for understanding the pathogenesis of diabetic glomerulopathy.

EARLY RENAL HYPERFUNCTION

The kidney function is increased in patients with early diabetes. Stalder *et al.* showed that GFR is high in children and young patients after a few years of diabetes.[59, 60] Several later studies by Ditzel and Schwartz,[8] Hirose and Tojo[17] and Mogensen[35, 36] have confirmed and extended this observation. Using various filtration markers — inulin, cyanocobalamin, iothalamate — the authors reported values that are 20 – 30% higher than the levels found in normal subjects of the same age.

Our results of studies of RPF have varied somewhat, from normal to slightly elevated values, probably depending on the technique used, para-aminohippurate (PAH) or ^{131}I-hippuran. In all studies the FF was found to be somewhat increased.[7, 36, 39]

Tm_G is increased by about 20% and a correlation exists between the increases in GFR and in Tm_G in diabetic patients, thus indicating that the tubuloglomerular balance is intact.[37]

It is of particular interest that the elevation of GFR persists for many years in diabetic patients.[39] As shown by Mogensen, a high GFR is still present in the initial stage of proteinuria ("intermittent proteinuria").[41]

MECHANISMS INVOLVED IN RENAL HYPERTROPHY-HYPERFUNCTION

The elevated renal function in patients with diabetes mellitus was demonstrated and studied in detail several years before the structural changes came into focus.

Two possible explanations of the increase in GFR were envisaged: an increase in the filtration pressure or a change in the quality of the filtering membrane.

The first of these possibilities seemed to be supported by the common tendency for an increase in the FF. The second was tentatively rejected on the basis of clearance studies using a wide range of low- and high-molecular-weight dextrans.

The results of radiologic studies and the general experience from morphological examinations of the glomeruli suggested a hitherto neglected possibility: an increase in the filtration area. When this was shown in histologic studies, it became reasonable to accept it as the main reason for the increased GFR in diabetic patients. At the same time, the idea of an increase in filtration pressure causing the increased GFR had to be given up, as it presupposes an unchanged area of filtration.

Results of clinical and animal studies of kidney size and weight are compatible with the conclusion that the increased filtration rate is due to an increase in filtering structures. There is a positive correlation between kidney function — GFR and RPF — and the size of the kidney in diabetic patients as well as in nondiabetics.[42] Moreover, during strict diabetes control, when the radiologically determined kidney size is being reduced, a concomitant decrease in GFR is observed (Fig. 3 – 4).[43] After one

Fig. 3–4.—Glomerular filtration rate and calculated kidney weight in six newly diagnosed diabetics before and three months after the start of insulin treatment. (From Mogensen, C. E., and Andersen, M. J. F.: Increased kidney size and glomerular filtration rate in untreated juvenile diabetics. Normalization by insulin treatment, Diabetologia 11:221, 1975.

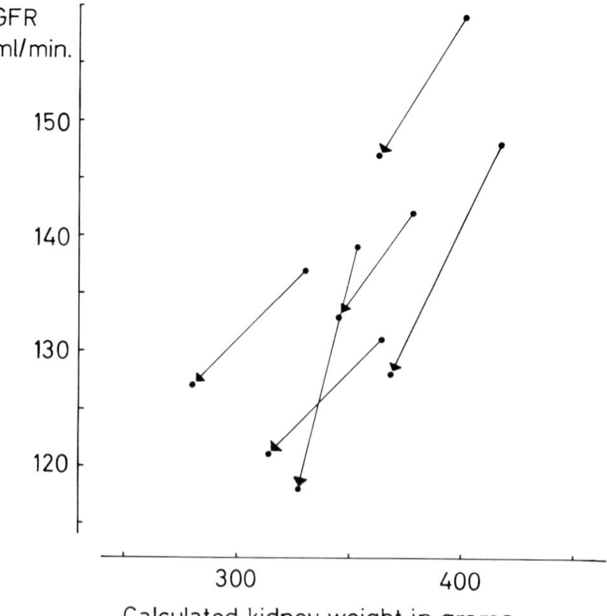

week of diabetes in rats there is a very close correlation between kidney weight and blood glucose.[54]

These findings strongly suggest that it is the acute metabolic changes that cause the enlargement of renal structures and the increase in various renal functions.*

If this is accepted, then the question arises as to which feature in the biochemical and hormonal disorders of diabetic patients is the causative agent or stimulus for growth. There is no answer to this question today, but in all probability it is a change in an energy-requiring process, either in the cells of the glomerulus or in the tubular cells. The significance of these alternatives is further discussed in the final section of this chapter.

PROTEIN EXCRETION

It is well known that diabetic patients in severe ketoacidosis or diabetic coma may have slight proteinuria. Apart from that, the urine of young patients with early diabetes does not contain protein, as determined by the usual clinical methods such as precipitation tests or Albustix.

The introduction of radioimmunologic techniques has provided new insight into the renal handling of proteins in cases of diabetes.

Albumin excretion, normally occurring to the extent of 5–20 μg/minute, is not elevated in the basal nonstimulated state in early diabetes if the patients are in the usual well-controlled state, but even moderate loss of control may be associated with albumin values of 30 μg/minute and even up to 100 μg/minute. This is about where the Albustix reaction results become positive (75–125 μg/minute).[38]

It might have been expected that the use of radioimmunologic techniques would disclose a gradual increase in the amount of albumin excretion over the years, concomitant with the gradual increase in basement membrane thickness. This is, however, not the case. Mogensen has shown that basal albumin excretion lev-

---

*Recent micropuncture studies of glomerular ultrafiltration in the Munich-Wistar rat by Brenner and co-workers have led to the conclusion that an increased filtration surface would be of relatively small importance for the GFR, because filtration equilibrium normally takes place at the efferent end of the glomerular capillary.[4] Whether this holds true also for the human kidney is not known. Measurements on Munich-Wistar rats with experimental diabetes might help to settle the question of which factors determine the increased kidney function in diabetes.

els remain normal for many years and are elevated only in patients who have already developed clinical proteinuria (Albustix). The exact timing of these events is not known, but there is no doubt that many patients have normal amounts of albumin excretion year after year, while at the same time the basement membrane grows thicker and thicker.[41]

This apparent paradoxical dissociation of form and function is resolved, at least partially, by studying the patients during exercise. Strenuous exercise results in proteinuria in normal subjects; at a moderate work load (600 kpm/minute for 20–30 minutes) no change in albumin excretion occurs in normal subjects, but a marked increase is seen in patients with diabetes of only a few years duration (Fig. 3–5). On the other hand, the amount of β_2-microglobulin, which is filtered freely, shows no increase, indicating that there is no change in tubular reabsorption. These studies by Mogensen and Vittinghus make it seem reasonable to assume that it is the higher filtration pressure obtained during exercise that discloses the functional abnormality of thickened basement membrane.[44]

Fig. 3–5. – Urinary albumin excretion during exercise in 11 normals (N), 6 diabetics (D_a = 0–1 year duration of diabetes), 18 diabetics (D_b = 2–11 years duration) and 7 diabetics (D_c = 16–20 years duration).

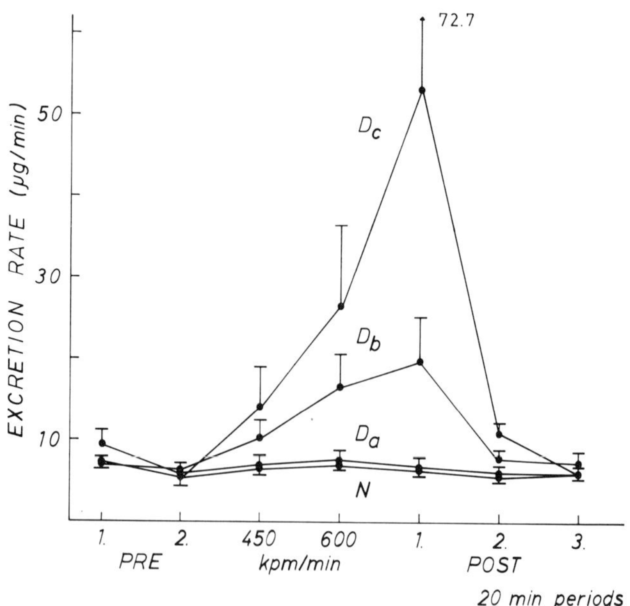

It still remains a mystery, however, what it is that happens when after many years the amount of albumin excretion seems to suddenly increase to values many times normal levels, and eventually reaches the extremely high values characterizing the Kimmelstiel-Wilson syndrome.

A new facet has recently been added to the problem of urinary protein excretion in cases of diabetes mellitus. It has been shown in studies on diabetic patients that intravenous insulin administration, causing a moderate decrease in the level of blood glucose without hypoglycemia, results in a decrease of GFR and RPF with a concomitant increase in the amount of albumin excretion. The mechanism involved is probably increased sympathetic activity due to hypovolemia occurring after insulin administration, as recently described by Gundersen and Christensen.[11]

The Kidney in Long-Term Diabetes

We are not going to dwell on the form and function of the renal structures in patients with long-term diabetes. Nearly all our information about these problems comes from classic studies dating back 20 or 30 years.

We shall mention only three recent aspects: the problem of the heterogeneity of glomerular size in long-term diabetes, intermittent proteinuria and the problem of elevated arterial blood pressure.

Size of Individual Glomeruli

At light microscopy *severe* diabetic glomerulosclerosis presents a very *heteromorphic picture*, a mixture of open and occluded glomeruli, with many of the open ones being much larger than normal. The mechanism behind the occurrence of the large glomeruli in patients with long-term diabetes was elucidated in a recent morphometric study, which concluded that the glomeruli are a result of a compensatory hypertrophy, rather than of an excessive deposition of basement membrane material.[12]

Complete closure of glomeruli, due either to accumulation of basement membrane or to arteriolar lesion, is seen only after one or two decades, but thereafter the proportion of destroyed glomeruli appears to increase rapidly. This process may well play a role in the suddenness of the appearance of clinical nephropathy and the swiftness of its progression, once established.[12]

INTERMITTENT PROTEINURIA

The classical concept of "intermittent proteinuria" as a forerunner of persistent proteinuria in patients with diabetes mellitus has been mentioned above. It appears on the laboratory sheet of the case records of patients in diabetes clinics, e.g., as urines reported to contain 0.2 gm/L at one visit, no protein one month later, and 0.4 gm/L the following month. It probably just means very mild proteinuria as defined by some simple and rough clinical test. Zero values may mean a particularly large diuresis that day, and high values may be caused by extra muscular exercise.

Intermittent proteinuria is, however, a very real phenomenon, and it must be distinguished from constant proteinuria because of the difference in the relationship of these two kinds of proteinuria to renal function and also to prognosis.

In cases of permanent proteinuria the amount of protein excretion may remain moderate for many years. On the average it increases year by year.[34, 49] In some patients eventually very high values are seen – 10 – 15 gm/L.

BLOOD PRESSURE

Blood pressure is on the whole normal in diabetic patients.[10, 19] However, in long-term diabetic patients with proteinuria, both systolic and diastolic pressures are slightly elevated, in accordance with the degree of proteinuria.[19] In this period the rate of decrease in the GFR is positively correlated to diastolic blood pressure levels, and the progression rate can be predicted from repeated measurements of GFR.[40, 41] An increase in blood pressure during exercise in diabetic patients with normal resting values has been reported by Karlefors.[18]

In the last month of life *severe* arterial hypertension is often seen in patients with multiple signs and symptoms of diabetic angiopathy.[64]

Pathogenesis of Diabetic Glomerulopathy

The pathogenesis of diabetic glomerulosclerosis cannot be separated from that of vascular lesions in other organs of the body. Glomerulosclerosis is the renal expression of generalized diabetic angiopathy. This was shown many years ago by a study of a large unselected series of long-term diabetic patients in which the statistical links between the occurrence of various organ lesions were demonstrated.[25] This conclusion has been confirmed and extended in several later studies of patients with renal, retinal and cardiac abnormalities.[23, 24, 61]

Long-term diabetic angiopathy in the kidney as well as in other organs of the body is secondary to the metabolic, i.e., biochemical and hormonal, abnormalities characterizing the diabetic state. The arguments supporting the "metabolic theory" of diabetic angiopathy in general are as follows:

1. Clinical studies (e.g., ophthalmoscopic investigations) as well as quantitative electron microscopic studies show normal vascular structures at the moment of acute onset of diabetes.

2. Many large studies of the effect of "good control" versus "bad control" on the development of diabetic angiopathy have indicated a beneficial effect of "good control," although not a large effect.

3. Diabetic angiopathy occurs in patients after many years in secondary diabetes (in chronic pancreatitis, for example).

4. Lesions very similar to those of diabetic angiopathy develop after many months or years in animals with severe alloxan or streptozotocin diabetes. The development of diabetic retinopathy can be suppressed in the alloxan diabetic dog by careful insulin treatment, as seen with the ophthalmoscope.[9] The same conclusion can be drawn from recent studies of the basement membrane *thickness*, which is the fundamental microscopic abnormality in subjects with diabetic microvascular disease. Studies by Rasch in our laboratory showed that treatment of diabetic rats, leading to near normalization of blood glucose levels, prevents the development of basement membrane thickening seen in the poorly controlled diabetic rats.[51] The well-controlled rats also failed to develop an abnormal increase in the amount of protein excretion. The enzyme abnormalities of renal tissue supposedly leading to accumulation of basement membrane can be prevented by insulin administration.[56]

The concept of diabetic angiopathy as a secondary phenomenon implies that if patients could be studied at the time of onset of diabetes there should be no demonstrable signs of glomerulosclerosis, not even mild ones. This possibility exists in cases of juvenile diabetes, because it appears acutely in the space of weeks or a few months. Some years ago Østerby made an extensive study of the renal glomeruli obtained by kidney biopsy from such patients.[46, 47] Her studies were prompted by casual reports in the literature claiming that the glomerular basement membrane was thickened in early diabetes and even in the prediabetic state.

The thickness of the peripheral glomerular basement membrane was estimated from measurements obtained from total glomerular cross-sections, produced as photomontages of electron micrographs. The measuring points (on the average 1,000 per cross-section) were randomly selected, but only at places of perpendicular sectioning so that the recorded values represent true basement membrane thickness. Measurements from each cross-section showed right-skewed distributions. A transformation leading to normal distributions was determined,[47] and mean values from these normal distributions were used for the statistical analyses.

Applying these procedures to a group of young diabetics with newly diagnosed disease and to a comparable group of nondiabetics, it was found that the basement membrane thickness is completely normal in subjects at the acute onset of juvenile diabetes mellitus, and therefore also, by implication, in prediabetics.[46, 47] It was further shown that a thickening of the peripheral basement membrane was demonstrable in patients after 1½ to 2½ years of diabetes (Fig. 3 – 6).[47]

The mesangial regions were also measured. The relative amount of mesangial tissue in a glomerulus was determined by measuring the mesangial area as a fraction of the area of the whole tuft. Planimetric measurements of the individual compartments of the tuft performed on the electron microscopic photomontages mentioned above showed that the mesangial regions are normal in patients at the onset of diabetes, both in relative size and in relative content of basement-membrane-like material.[47]

These results strongly support the idea that the thickening of the glomerular capillary wall is secondary to the metabolic

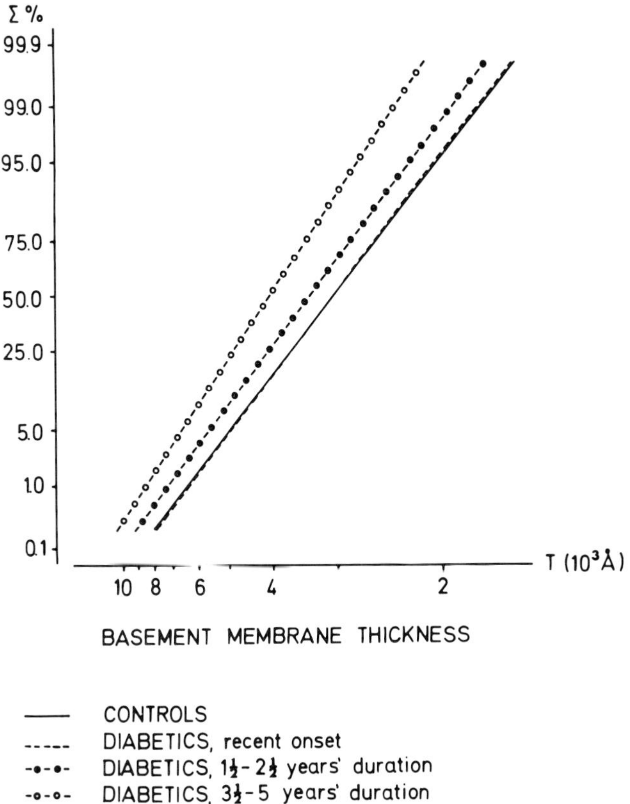

Fig. 3–6. — Basement membrane thickness; transformed values (1/√thickness); cumulative frequency scale. (From Østerby, R.: Early phases in the development of diabetic glomerulopathy. A quantitative electron microscopic study, Acta. Med. Scand. [Suppl.] 574:1, 1975.

changes characterizing diabetes mellitus. Thickening is absent in patients at the clinical onset of diabetes and develops slowly over the years. There is no reason to doubt that the same pattern applies for less easily measurable capillaries of other regions of the body. Competent studies of the muscle capillaries have shown results similar to those obtained in studies of renal glomeruli.[65]

Recent studies of the biochemistry of the glomerular basement membrane have given a new dimension to diabetic kidney research and to the study of diabetic vascular disease in general.

They have also provided biochemical evidence supporting the concept of diabetic angiopathy being a secondary phenomenon.

We are not going to discuss in detail the pioneer studies of Spiro on the chemistry and biochemistry of renal basement membrane,[56-58] or the subsequent developments in this field. There are a number of controversial points today, but it can hardly be doubted that the synthesis of the glycoprotein making up the basement membrane is abnormal in patients with diabetes, and also that this abnormality may be prevented or at least inhibited by proper insulin treatment.

We do not know which particular element or elements of the complicated metabolic and hormonal disturbances are actually responsible for the abnormality of glycoprotein synthesis and the consequent thickening of the basement membrane. This is a large problem in diabetes research in general. Here we shall limit ourselves to a few words about growth hormone and glucose as possible causal factors.

Growth hormone may be involved.[26, 27] The level of plasma growth hormone is high in patients with diabetes mellitus,[13-15] and pituitary ablation, followed by substitution with steroid, thyroid and gonadal hormones, inhibits the development of diabetic retinopathy and normalizes skin capillary resistance.[5, 28] Growth-hormone-deficient dwarfs with diabetes mellitus show very little sign of diabetic vascular disease.[32, 33]

Glucose itself may also be involved. The vascular wall is metabolically non-insulin-dependent, and hyperglycemia may enhance the synthesis of the disaccharide unit of the basement membrane polysaccharide. It has been shown that the incorporation of glucose into the capillary basement membrane in isolated glomeruli is linearly related to the glucose concentration in the incubation medium.[63] The enhancing effect of glucose on the synthesis of basement membrane is independent of insulin, a relationship that has recently been demonstrated also for collagen production by human fibroblasts.[62]

The effects of increased growth hormone and hyperglycemia are combined in the glucose-growth hormone hypothesis, according to which "growth hormone increases the synthesis of the peptide chain and perhaps enhances hydroxylase activity, while glucose increases the activity of the specific glycosyltransferases."[2, 57]

EARLY AND LATE RENAL CHANGES: TWO PHASES OR TWO ENTITIES?

After the discovery and elaboration of the early hypertrophy-hyperfunction stage, one wonders if this pattern should be regarded as a forerunner of long-term diabetic glomerulosclerosis or if the two should be thought of as independent entities.

The early expansion of renal tissue is very similar in magnitude and time course to that seen after unilateral nephrectomy.[55] The mechanisms behind the two conditions may, however, be different. While compensatory hypertrophy probably is caused by some renotropic humoral factors, the diabetic hypertrophy may be triggered by the increased osmolar work load imposed on the tubular cells by hyperglycemia.

In this perspective the glomerular changes, including the increase in *total* basement membrane material, would in some way be secondary to tubular changes. We know that the growth of the renal structures ceases at a certain time, after a few weeks of hyperglycemia, probably when a new balance is reached between opposing factors governing renal form and function. Basement membrane thickening, proceeding to severe and life-threatening glomerulosclerosis, could then be regarded as an entirely different process, progressing more slowly and demonstrable only after some years of diabetes.

However, an alternative, unitary hypothesis is also imaginable. According to this, the primary event would be an increase in the total area of the capillary basement membrane, i.e., a lengthening without thickening. The trigger mechanism might be a change in glomerular cell function, leading to an increase in basement membrane synthesis. Thus changes in tubular and other renal structures would be secondary or unrelated phenomena.

After cessation of the acute increase in area of the glomerular basement membrane, the growth stimulus still persisting may lead to a slow and gradual increase in basement membrane *thickness*, which is distinguishable only after some years of diabetes. Finally, the elevated plasma growth hormone characterizing diabetic patients may be a causal factor in the early as well as the late developments.

There is today no evidence for choosing between these two alternative hypotheses. They may have different consequences, but it seems to be too early to discuss them in detail. A few points should, however, be mentioned.

First, the results obtained from enzymatic studies of kidney tissue from animals with experimental diabetes of rather short duration are not necessarily related to the development of life-threatening diabetic glomerulosclerosis.[6, 20, 58] They may just as well be related to the acute early expansion of all the components of the kidney described above. An exception to this statement may be the increase in the level of glycosyltransferases observed by Spiro four to five months after the induction of diabetes.[58]

Second, in discussing the relevance of the biochemical studies for the understanding of diabetic vascular disease in human subjects, considerable emphasis has been placed on the notion of a very slow turnover time of basement membrane glycoprotein. Once a certain degree of thickening of the basement membrane had occurred, it was difficult to achieve a regression, indicating the extreme importance of attempts to normalize the diabetic state from the time of the onset of diabetes. Admittedly, however, the available literature on this point does not permit any definite conclusion about the turnover time of basement membrane glycoproteins.[31, 57]

Prophylaxis and Therapy

The problems of the prophylaxis and treatment of diabetic renal disease are parts of the problems of diabetic angiopathy in general. It is not possible in this chapter to discuss them in detail. Suffice it to say that our presentation leads logically to the conclusion that stricter control should be attempted and that alternative ways of treatment should be sought.

In the present situation stricter attention to diet, several injections of insulin and shorter intervals between control visits constitute a practical possibility.

Further developments are expected and hoped for along three lines: (1) transplantation of the pancreas or of islets;[30] (2) complete regulation of blood glucose by an automatic device implanted under the skin;[3] and (3) growth hormone and glucagon suppression by long-acting and specific analogues to be developed from somatostatin.[16, 29]

The therapeutic measures aiming directly at the kidney include antihypertensive treatment and renal transplantation.

When the nephropathy is already established clinically by the finding of proteinuria, the renal and cardiovascular situation of the patients should be followed carefully. Development of high blood pressure, which is seen in some patients, is associated with the rapid progression of nephropathy. Antihypertensive treatment, given over two years in a small series of patients, reduced the rate of decrease in the GFR, thus probably postponing the onset of uremia.[40] The insulin requirement decreases in many cases with advanced uremia. Biguanides should be strictly avoided, since they accumulate in patients with renal failure and lactic acidosis may develop. Other oral agents may also be hazardous due to the accumulation and development of severe hypoglycemia.

In patients in the final state of renal insufficiency, hemodialysis or kidney transplantation may be contemplated. In many cases, however, diabetic cardiopathy and neuropathy, including encephalopathy, preclude any major action taken against uremia. In 1976 the Renal Transplant Registry reported three-year survival rates of 57% (cadaver graft) and 74% (living related donor graft) in a total of 193 presumably selected cases.[1] The results of Najarian and co-workers on patients without "overwhelming complications" are even better.[45] All in all, these results seem to us to be similar to those obtained from nondiabetic uremic recipients. But a definite conclusion cannot be made because of the various programs of selection for operation used in various centers.

References

1. ACS-NIH Organ Transplant Registry, April 1976.
2. Alberti, K. G. M. M., and Hockaday, T. D. T.: The biochemistry of the complications of diabetes mellitus, in Keen, H., and Jarrett, J.: *Complications of Diabetes* (London: Eduard Arnold, 1975), p. 221.
3. Albisser, A. M., Leibel, B. S., Ewart, T. G., Davidovac, Z., Botz, C. K., and Zingg, W.: An artificial endocrine pancreas, Diabetes 23:389, 1974.
4. Brenner, B. M., Baylis, D., and Deen, W. M.: Transport of molecules across renal glomerular capillaries, Physiol. Rev. 56:502, 1976.
5. Christensen, N. J., and Terkildsen, A. B.: Quantitative measurements of skin capillary resistance in hypophysectomized long-term diabetics, Diabetes 20:297, 1971.
6. Cohen, M. P., and Vogt, C.: Evidence for enhanced basement membrane synthesis and lysine hydroxylation in renal glomerulus in experimental diabetes, Biochem. Biophys. Res. Commun. 49:1542, 1972.

7. Ditzel, J., and Junker, K.: Abnormal glomerular filtration rate, renal plasma flow, and renal protein excretion in recent and short-term diabetics, Br. Med. J. 2:13, 1972.

8. Ditzel, J., and Schwartz, M.: Abnormally increased glomerular filtration rate in short-term insulin-treated diabetic subjects, Diabetes 16:264, 1967.

9. Engerman, R. L., and Bloodworth, J. M. B.: Role of diabetes control in microvascular disease, in Abstracts, 8th Congress of the International Diabetes Federation, Series no. 280 (Amsterdam: Excerpta Medica, 1973), p. 188.

10. Freedman, P., Moulton, R., and Spencer, A. G.: Hypertension and diabetes mellitus, Q. J. Med. 27:293, 1958.

11. Gundersen, H. J. G., and Christensen, N. J.: Intravenous insulin causing loss of intravascular water and albumin and increased adrenergic nervous activity in diabetics, Diabetes 26:551, 1977.

12. Gundersen, H. J. G., and Østerby, R.: Glomerular size and structure in diabetes mellitus. II. Late abnormalities, Diabetologia 13:43, 1977.

13. Hansen, Aa. P.: Serum growth hormone patterns in juvenile diabetes, Dan. Med. Bull. 19 (Suppl. 1):3, 1972.

14. Hansen, Aa. P.: Serum growth hormone patterns in female juvenile diabetics, J. Clin. Endocrinol. Metab. 36:638, 1973.

15. Hansen, Aa. P.: Abnormal serum growth hormone response to exercise in maturity onset diabetes, Diabetes 22:619, 1973.

16. Hansen, Aa. P., and Lundbæk, K.: Somatostatin. A review of its effects, especially in human beings, Diabete Metab. 2:203, 1976.

17. Hirose, K., and Tojo, S.: Abnormally increased glomerular filtration rate in diabetic patients, in Abstracts, 8th Congress of the International Diabetes Federation, Series no. 280 (Amsterdam: Excerpta Medica, 1973), p. 189.

18. Karlefors, T.: Exercise test in male diabetics. II. Heart rate and systolic blood pressure, Acta Med. Scand. 180 (Suppl. 449):19, 1966.

19. Keen, H., Track, N. D., and Sowry, G. S. C.: Arterial pressure in clinically apparent diabetics, Diabete Metab. 1:159, 1975.

20. Khalifa A., and Cohen, M. P.: Glomerular protocollagen lysyl-hydroxylase activity in streptozotocin diabetes, Biochim. Biophys. Acta 386:332, 1975.

21. Kimmelstiel, P., and Wilson, C.: Intercapillary lesions in glomeruli of kidney, Am. J. Pathol. 12:83, 1936.

22. Kroustrup, J. P., Gundersen, H. J. G., and Østerby, R.: Glomerular size and structure in diabetes. III. Early enlargement of the capillary surface, Diabetologia 13:207, 1977.

23. Kuhlmann, H., Mehnert, H., and Langer, E.: Retinopathie und Glomerulosklerose bei Diabetikern, Med. Klin. 64:747, 1969.

24. Ledet, T.: Histological and histochemical changes in the coronary arteries of old diabetic patients, Diabetologia 4:268, 1968.

25. Lundbæk, K.: *Long-Term Diabetes — The Clinical Picture in Diabetes Mellitus of 15 to 25 Years Duration with a Follow-up of a Regional Series of Cases* (the ophthalmological section in collaboration with V. A. Jensen) (Copenhagen: Munksgaard, 1953).

26. Lundbæk, K., Christensen, N. J., Jensen, V. A., Johansen, K., Olsen, T. S., Hansen, Aa. P., Ørskov, H., and Østerby, R.: Diabetes, diabetic angiopathy and growth hormone, Lancet 2:131, 1970.

27. Lundbæk, K., Christensen, N. J., Jensen, V. A., Johansen, K., Olsen, T. S., Hansen, Aa. P., Ørskov, H., and Østerby, R.: The pathogenesis of diabetic angiopathy and growth hormone, Dan. Med. Bull. 18:1, 1971.

28. Lundbæk, K., Malmros, R., Andersen, H. C., Rasmussen, J. H., Bruntse, E., Madsen, P. H., and Jensen, V. A.: Hypophysectomy for diabetic angiopathy: A controlled clinical trial, in Goldberg, M. F., and Fine, S. L.: Symposium on the treatment of diabet-

ic retinopathy. U.S. Public Health Service Publ. No. 1890 (Washington, D. C.: Government Printing Office, 1969), p. 291.

29. Lundbæk, K., and Hansen, Aa. P.: Diabetes mellitus and somatostatin, Dan. Med. Bull. 24:1, 1977.

30. Matas, A. J., Sutherland, D. E. R., and Najarian, J. S.: Current status of islet and pancreas transplantation in diabetes, Diabetes 25:785, 1976.

31. Mauer, S. M., Sutherland, D. E. R., Steffes, M. W., Leonard, R. J., Najarian, J. S., Michael, A. F., and Brown, D. M.: Pancreatic islet transplantation: Effects of the glomerular lesions of experimental diabetes in the rat, Diabetes 23:748, 1974.

32. Merimee, T. J., Fineberg, S. E., McKusick, V. A., and Hall, J.: Diabetes mellitus and sexual ateliotic dwarfism: a comparative study, J. Clin. Invest. 49:1096, 1970.

33. Merimee, T. J., Fineberg, S. E., and Hollander, W.: Vascular disease in the chronic HGH-deficient state, Diabetes 22:813, 1973.

34. Miki, E., Kuzuya, T., Idé, T., and Nakao, K.: Frequency, degree and progression with time of proteinuria in diabetic patients, Lancet 1:922, 1972.

35. Mogensen, C. E.: Kidney function and glomerular permeability to macromolecules in early juvenile diabetes, Scand. J. Clin. Lab. Invest. 28:79, 1971.

36. Mogensen, C. E.: Glomerular filtration rate and renal plasma flow in short-term and long-term juvenile diabetes mellitus, Scand. J. Clin. Lab. Invest. 28:91, 1971.

37. Mogensen, C. E.: Maximum tubular reabsorption capacity for glucose and renal hemodynamics during rapid hypertonic glucose infusion in normal diabetic subjects, Scand. J. Clin. Lab. Invest. 28:101, 1971.

38. Mogensen, C. E.: Urinary albumin excretion in early and long-term juvenile diabetes, Scand. J. Clin. Lab. Invest. 28:183, 1971.

39. Mogensen, C. E.: Kidney function and glomerular permeability to macromolecules in juvenile diabetes with special reference to early changes, Dan. Med. Bull. 19(Suppl. 3):1, 1972.

40. Mogensen, C. E.: Progression of nephropathy in long-term diabetics with proteinuria and effect of initial antihypertensive treatment, Scand. J. Clin. Lab. Invest. 36:383, 1976.

41. Mogensen, C. E.: Renal function changes in diabetes, Diabetes 25(Suppl. 2):872, 1976.

42. Mogensen, C. E., and Andersen, M. J. F.: Increased kidney size and glomerular filtration rate in early juvenile diabetics, Diabetes 22:706, 1973.

43. Mogensen, C. E., and Andersen, M. J. F.: Increased kidney size and glomerular filtration rate in untreated juvenile diabetics. Normalization by insulin treatment, Diabetologia 11:221, 1975.

44. Mogensen, C. E., and Vittinghus, E.: Urinary albumin excretion during exercise in juvenile diabetes. A provocation test for early abnormalities, Scand. J. Clin. Lab. Invest. 35:295, 1975.

45. Najarian, J. S., Kjellstrand, C. M., Simmons, R. L., Buselmeier, T. J., Hartitzsch, B. V., and Goetz, F. C.: Renal transplantation for diabetic glomerulosclerosis, Ann. Surg. 178:477, 1973.

46. Østerby Hansen, R.: A quantitative estimate of the peripheral glomerular basement membrane in recent juvenile diabetes, Diabetologia 1:97, 1965.

47. Østerby, R.: Early phases in the development of diabetic glomerulopathy. A quantitative electron microscopic study, Acta Med. Scand. [Suppl.]574:1, 1975.

48. Østerby, R., and Gundersen, H. J. G.: Glomerular size and structure in diabetes mellitus. I. Early abnormalities, Diabetologia 11:225, 1975.

49. Panzram, G., Anger, G., and Wölner, H.: Untersuchungen über die physiologische Proteinurie beim Diabetes mellitus, Dtsch. Med. Wochenschr. 92:1013, 1967.

50. Peterson, D. T., Greene, W. C., and Reaven, G. M.: Effect of experimental diabetes on kidney ribosomal protein synthesis, Diabetes 20:649, 1971.

51. Rasch, R.: The effect of diabetic control on kidney weight, glomerular volume and glomerular basement membrane thickness, Diabetologia 13:426, 1977 (Abstract).
52. Ross, J., and Goldman, J. K.: Effect of streptozotocin-induced diabetes on kidney weight and compensatory hypertrophy in the rat, Endocrinology 88:1079, 1971.
53. Seyer-Hansen, K.: Renal hypertrophy in streptozotocin diabetic rats, Clin. Sci. Mol. Med. 51:551, 1976.
54. Seyer-Hansen, K.: Renal hypertrophy in experimental diabetes: Relation to severity of diabetes, Diabetologia 13:141, 1977.
55. Seyer-Hansen, K.: Renal hypertrophy in experimental diabetes: a comparison to compensatory hypertrophy, in press.
56. Spiro, R. G.: Chemistry and metabolism of the basement membrane, in Ellenberg, M., and Rifkin, H.: *Diabetes Mellitus: Theory and Practice* (New York: McGraw-Hill, 1970), p. 210.
57. Spiro, R. G.: Search for a biochemical basis of diabetic microangiopathy. Claude Bernard lecture, Diabetologia 12:1, 1976.
58. Spiro, R. G., and Spiro, M. J.: Effect of diabetes on the biosynthesis of the renal glomerular basement membrane. Studies on the glycosyltransferase, Diabetes 20: 641, 1971.
59. Stalder, G., and Schmid, R.: Severe functional disorders of glomerular capillaries and renal hemodynamics in treated diabetes mellitus during childhood, Ann. Paediatr. 193:129, 1959.
60. Stalder, G., Schmid, R., and Wolff, M. V.: Funktionelle Mikroangiopathie der Nieren beim behandelten Diabetes mellitus im Kindesalter, Dtsch. Med. Wochenschr. 85: 346, 1960.
61. Thomsen, Aa. Chr.: *The Kidney in Diabetes Mellitus.* (Copenhagen: Munksgaard, 1965).
62. Villee, D. B., and Powers, M. L.: Effect of glucose and insulin on collagen secretion by human skin fibroblasts in vitro, Nature 268:156, 1977.
63. Wahl, P., Deppermann, D., Deschner, W., Fuchs, E., and Rexroth, W.: The metabolism of the isolated renal glomerulus and its basement membranes, in Camerini-Dávalos, R. A., and Cole, H. S.: *Vascular and Neurological Changes in Early Diabetes* (New York: Academic Press, 1973).
64. Watkins, P. J., Blainey, J. D., Brewer, D. B., Fitzgerald, M. G., Malins, J. M., O'-Sullivan, D. J., and Pinto, J. A.: The natural history of diabetic renal disease. A follow-up study of a series of renal biopsies, Q. J. Med. 41:437, 1972.
65. Williamson, J. R., Vogler, N. J., and Kilo, C.: Basement membrane thickening in muscle capillaries. Observations on diabetics and non-diabetics with both parents diabetic, in Srow R. O., Ebling, F. J. G., and Henderson, I. W. (eds.): Proceedings of the Fourth International Congress on Endocrinology, Washington, D.C., 1972, Series no. 273 (Amsterdam: Excerpta Medica, 1973), p. 1122.

4

Prevention and Treatment of Diabetic Nephropathy

GEORGES TCHOBROUTSKY, M.D.

Université Pierre et Marie Curie and Hôpital Hôtel-Dieu, Paris, France

The acute metabolic complications of diabetes mellitus cause only about 1% of the deaths from this disease.[70] In addition, most metabolic complications are avoidable by proper training of diabetic patients and the rational organization of diabetic departments.[77] The major cause of death from diabetes mellitus is coronary artery disease.[11] In the study by the Joslin Clinic, the overall mortality due to renal insufficiency was 5.7% of 6,800 deaths,[4] but the mortality was 53% in patients whose diabetes was diagnosed before they were 20 years old.[69]

Diabetic glomerulopathy is related to the duration of the diabetes and is inevitably present after 20 years or more of the disease.[114] Nevertheless, the question is still unanswered whether a causal relationship exists between chronic hyperglycemia and the late glomerular and retinal complications of this disorder. In other words, is it possible to prevent or limit the evolution of these vascular lesions by keeping the blood sugar levels relatively normal over a period of years? If the capillary lesions responsible for late diabetic microangiopathy are inevitable consequences of diabetes mellitus itself and unrelated to the level of blood sugar, then it is obviously useless to try to keep the blood

63

0084-5957/79/080063-24$3.75

sugar level within normal limits. If, on the other hand, the capillary lesions are secondary to chronic hyperglycemia and/or to its consequences and/or to the insulin deficiency, it is reasonable to attempt to normalize blood sugar levels as much as possible. Meticulous attention to blood sugar regulation, however, creates additional problems for the diabetic patient, in particular psychological problems[58] and the risks of episodic hypoglycemia. Furthermore, in the best of situations, regulation of blood sugar levels is imperfect, and in adult-onset diabetes it is often started late in the natural history of the disease. Even in prospective studies, criteria differ with regard to the diagnosis of diabetes mellitus, the quantification of complications and the assessment of control.

These facts explain, in part, why it has been impossible until now, despite 50 years of insulin therapy, to affirm or deny that in the diabetic careful control of blood glucose levels may forestall the development of diabetic microangiopathy. A large-scale, prospective randomized study is not feasible because of ethical considerations. In experimental diabetes in animals, the specificity of the lesions is disputed.[105]

Despite the lack of unequivocal scientific proof, I am convinced that: (1) the lesions of diabetic microangiopathy are secondary to the diabetes mellitus itself and are statistically correlated to the cumulative degree of chronic hyperglycemia, and (2) meticulous long-term control of blood glucose levels decreases the frequency, delays the appearance, decreases the severity and stops the evolution of the lesions of diabetic microangiopathy in humans.

This chapter will examine the arguments both for and against the cause and effect relationship between the degree of blood glucose control and microangiopathy. It will include clinical studies in humans, epidemiologic data, biochemical data, functional studies and experimental diabetes mellitus.

Diabetic Glomerulopathy: Consequence or Symptom of Diabetes Mellitus?

A number of current hypotheses will be examined to see whether the available evidence does or does not support these hypotheses.

Hyperglycemia is not the only cause of microangiopathic complications.

Heredity plays an important role independent of hyperglycemia.[105] Pyke and Tattersall studied 23 sets of identical twins; in 13 of them both siblings had diabetes.[94] They showed that the twins of whom both had diabetes had more severe forms of retinopathy than did the diabetic twins of the mixed sets. They note that "because of the small number of subjects studied, the differences do not reach conventional levels of statistical significance but they suggest that genetic factors may also be important in the etiology and time of appearance of diabetic retinopathy." They do not think that diabetic retinopathy could be related to factors other than diabetes itself, and they reason: "If there are any patients who might be expected, because of their heredity, to show diabetic retinopathy without diabetes it is the unaffected identical twins of diabetics. We have not found any sign of retinopathy in the nine unaffected identical twins of diabetics reported here." These authors are persuaded that the diabetes is responsible for the retinal lesions because "if a wholly environmentally determined form of diabetes does exist, one would expect to find it in the diabetic twins of discordant pairs. The fact that five or ten of our discordant twins showed retinopathy suggests that it is the condition of diabetes itself rather than genetic factors which leads to the retinopathy."

Two other studies of twins[53] and of triplets[37] have shown the absence of microangiopathy in nondiabetic propositi.

Glomerular (and/or retinal) lesions exist in the absence of hyperglycemia in nondiabetic humans.

The supporters of the hypothesis, according to which the complications of microangiopathy are not directly linked to hyperglycemia, report glomerular and/or retinal lesions in nondiabetic subjects.[9, 19, 25, 42, 43, 50, 67, 83, 111] A careful review of published articles shows, with only two exceptions,[42, 111] that either the lesions are not characteristic of diabetes or that the subjects are, or were, with certainty or with a very strong probability, previously diabetic. An excellent analysis of these cases was done by Lauvaux and Pirart.[63, 90]

One of the two observations showing the existence of diabetic glomerulosclerosis in the nondiabetic is that of Strauss, Argy and Schreiner.[111] In a 29-year-old man whose maternal grandmother was diabetic, examination did not show any anomaly in his glucose tolerance except for slightly abnormal cortisone-glucose test results. However, under the electron microscope, there were renal lesions quite "characteristic" of diabetes, including mesangial deposits and diabetic nodules. Retinal angiography with fluorescence dye showed normal results, as well as normal motor conduction velocity. Hyalin deposits in the basement membranes were thickened. The subject presented with a nephrotic syndrome. The other very precise observation is that of Harrington and colleagues.[42] This is a case of a 59-year-old man with normal glucose regulation whose father had died of diabetes. The man's previous weight is unknown, but a loss of 4.5 kg in one year is mentioned. The fundi were normal. A nephrotic syndrome with renal insufficiency was responsible for his death during an intercurrent infection. The kidneys, which weighed 140 gm and 120 gm, showed diffuse glomerulosclerosis and nodular lesions characteristic of diabetes. The slides were reviewed by Paul Kimmelstiel.

Besides the fact that it is difficult to believe that diabetics can develop nephrotic syndrome and advanced glomerular lesions without retinopathy or neuropathy, these observations* posed the question of whether these so-called diabetic glomerular lesions are specific or only highly suggestive.

As stated by Cameron and colleagues, "It is now agreed that the nodule is confined to, and pathognomonic of, diabetes mellitus and that early reports to the contrary were a consequence either of mistaking lobular nephritis or exudative glomerular lesions with the nodule, or to a failure to detect clinically mild disturbances of carbohydrate metabolism in so-called nondiabetics."[16] In fact, it is highly probable that the Kimmelstiel-Wilson nodule is not limited to diabetes, since similar lesions have been reported by several authors in patients with multiple myeloma and the benign monoclonal gammapathies.[80]

On the other hand, many observations have reported retinopathy or glomerulopathy in patients with recently discovered diabetes mellitus, as was studied for the retina by Pyke and

---

*Other unpublished cases of diabetic renal lesions without diabetes certainly exist, and the author has knowledge of two such observations.[81]

Roberts,[93] as well as cases of retinopathy or nephropathy in very moderate diabetics.[23, 40] These cases are not very troublesome because diabetic remissions are not uncommon,[91] and because of the asymptomatic character of moderate chemical diabetes and the variability of glucose tolerance tests in moderate diabetics. Fajans and colleagues have shown in young patients presenting moderate and inapparent clinical forms of diabetes, that glucose tolerance test results could be periodically normal or abnormal, and that an unquestionable thickening of the basement membranes took place in some diabetic subjects.[30]

Thus, the observations reporting glomerular and/or retinal lesions in the absence of diabetes mellitus are: (1) very rare, (2) very debatable insofar as diabetes cannot really be excluded, and (3) nonspecific, except in two well-analyzed observations, but the specificity of the so-called diabetic glomerular lesions is not absolutely certain.

Studies done on the Pima Indians, where more than 40% of the subjects 35 years or older are affected by diabetes, also present solid arguments against the existence of diabetic nephropathy without diabetes. Kamenetzky and colleagues studied 1848 Pima Indians.[51] At the autopsy of 105 subjects, 43 diabetics and 62 nondiabetics, no nodular glomerulosclerosis or exudative glomerular lesions were found in the nondiabetics, whereas the frequency in the diabetics was 55.8% and 44.1%, respectively. Diffuse lesions of moderate or severe glomerulosclerosis were observed in 65.1% of the diabetics and 3% of the nondiabetics. Clinically, the nondiabetic Pima Indians showed a frequency of proteinuria of the same order reported for control populations, whereas among the diabetics proteinuria was 3.3 times more frequent and the increase of serum creatinine clearance was 9 times more frequent than in the nondiabetics.

In humans, thickening of the capillary basement membranes is observed before or at the time of diagnosis of diabetes, does not increase with the duration of the disease and is not seen in cases of secondary diabetes.

Siperstein and colleagues have described a quantitative method of measuring the mean thickness of the quadriceps muscle capillary basement membrane in humans; it consists of placing a clear piece of plastic over the electron microscope photograph and measuring the thickness of the basement membrane in about a dozen places, using different angles and avoiding a slanted pinpoint measurement.[103] These authors observed that the basement membranes of adult diabetics were thickened from the moment the diagnosis of diabetes was made, were normal in patients with diabetes secondary to acquired pancreatic disease and, finally, that 74% of the prediabetic subjects (genetically susceptible to diabetes) had thickened basement membranes without overt diabetes. Let us emphasize the fact that 98% of the diabetics had a thickened basement membrane, of which 92% were above the 95th percentile of the normal distribution. Utilizing other fixation methods, Williamson and colleagues measured the thickening of the muscular capillary basement membrane at its thinnest point and showed that the basement membrane was of normal thickness at the beginning of the diabetes and increased in width with the progression of the disease.[121] They also showed a thickening of the basement membrane with respect to age in both diabetic and nondiabetic subjects. Since 1971, the disagreement continues between these two groups. The reader may consult the review by Williamson and Kilo, which appeared in 1977 and updates this controversy.[124] According to Williamson and colleagues,[122] Siperstein's facts are linked to tangential measurements. Siperstein published a refined study in 1973 complete with a solid mathematical appendix in order to show his disagreement (a maximum of 10% erroneous). The fixation technique was itself the object of heated controversy.

Troublesome is the fact that diabetics younger than 20 years old, as studied by the Siperstein group,[97] do not have the same frequency of basement membrane thickening as do those over 20 years of age—an average of 40% as compared with 98%. The younger the child, the less frequent the thickening: no thickening is seen in diabetics from 4 to 5 years old. Other studies of the capillary basement membrane in children also disagree. Jackson and colleagues, using Williamson's method, showed that the basement membrane thickness was normal when the diagnosis of diabetes was made and thickened with its progression, and that there was a significant relationship between the quality of diabetic control and the integrity of the basement membrane.[47] Sheikholislam and colleagues[100, 101] used the two methods of Siperstein and Williamson. They showed that: (1) their handling of the two methods correlated well, (2) basement membrane lesions were not correlated with age or with the duration of diabetes, (3) the diabetics had definite, but insignificantly thicker basement membranes than the nondiabetics, and (4) an important inverse relationship existed between the basement membrane thickness and the glucose tolerance. A study done with the Pima Indians did not show basement membrane thickening in prediabetics (Williamson's method).[3]

Thus, it appears difficult to believe that there is thickening of the basement membrane in prediabetic adults (not hyperglycemic) but not in diabetic children if this disease is genetically transmitted. The observation in a pair of discordant twins that only the diabetic twin has thickening of the muscular basement membrane[53] is hard to explain; could it be a nongenetic diabetes affecting only one twin? In that case, why would the diabetic have thickening of the basement membrane if this is a characteristic of genetic diabetes? Finally, clinicians are familiar with the lesions of diabetic nephropathy and/or retinopathy in cases of diabetes secondary to chronic pancreatitis and hemochromatosis. Ireland and colleagues have shown glomerular capillary basement membrane thickening in patients with secondary diabetes.[45]

Above all, it appears that the decisive fact is that the studies of muscular basement membranes contradict those done on glomerular capillary basement membranes. The muscular capillary is probably a poor quantitative element to study. Pardo and colleagues have described the focal and segmental fluctuations in the thickness of the muscular basement membrane, which make this capillary, according to them, unsuitable for the early, sensitive or consistent identification of diabetic individuals.[88] Cameron and colleagues insist on the difficulty in identifying the indistinct external limit of the muscular capillary basement membrane.[16] On the other hand, "if the glomerular basement membrane thickening may be variable, it is neither focal nor segmental. Moreover, by analysis of variance it can be shown that results from individual glomeruli are reproducible and therefore representative of the patient's glomerular population."

The study of glomerular capillaries showed that the glomerular capillary basement membrane was of normal thickness at the time of diagnosis of diabetes, thickened with progression of the disease and was seen in patients with secondary diabetes of moderate or long duration.[45, 46, 64, 85] These facts strongly suggest that the alterations of glomerular capillaries in diabetics are secondary to the metabolic alterations of the disease. Østerby has shown by a quantitative electron microscope study that the glomerular basement membrane thickness was normal at the beginning of acute-onset juvenile diabetes but that thickening was demonstrable about 1½ years later.[85] According to a recent review of this work, this very short interval "indicates that such thickening must have started even before this time."[105] But these were subjects who were biopsied twice, and the author affirms that the glomerular basement membranes had normal thickness at the first biopsy.[85]

Thus, it is unlikely that the capillary basement membranes were really thickened in the absence of chronic hyperglycemia. The majority of existing data in humans support a cause and effect relationship between the metabolic manifestations of diabetes (hyperglycemia and/or its consequences) and the thickening of the capillary basement membranes, which precede the late glomerular and retinal lesions.

The individual progression of microangiopathy is unpredictable in humans. Severe diabetes may be accompanied by minimal lesions, minimal diabetes by severe lesions.

It is indisputable that individual progression can be surprising with regard to retinal lesions. Spontaneous regression or stabilization of serious forms of diabetic retinopathies is known. Kohner and Dollery, in their exhaustive review,[62] recall that "Beetham (1963) found that 10% of his patients with proliferative retinopathy arrested spontaneously after many years of visual turmoil. Most of these patients maintained useful vision. Caird and Draper (personal communication) found that, even among blind patients, there was a 4.8% chance of improving vision to better than 6/60."

There have been reports of patients with known duration of diabetes of more than 40 years who are free of proteinuria and sometimes even retinopathy. Such small groups of patients (generally less than 100) have been reported in Great Britain and in the United States.[16] But the progression in a few individuals does not modify the average progression of the population. The evolution of diabetic retinopathy and nephropathy is usually marked by "an increase of the incidence, the prevalence and the severity of the complications in parallel to the duration of the diabetes."[63, 90]

Individual variations in progression of retinal and/or glomerular lesions may depend on permissive or modulating factors of which only a very small number are beginning to be known. Severe myopia, intraocular hypertension and insufficient secretion of growth hormone seem to protect diabetics from the development of microangiopathy, or at least from its most severe forms. The argument that severe diabetics (poorly equilibrated?) have few lesions while benign diabetics (without marked hyperglycemia) have serious ones is reasonable. What do "benign" and "severe" diabetes really signify? Is it more serious to be affected with insulin-dependent diabetes that is unstable and oscillating from frank hyperglycemia to hypoglycemia, or with obese diabetes that is unknown for 20 years and characterized by moderate but constant hyperglycemia? With respect to the damage created by the hyperglycemia, it is probable that it is cumulative and correlated with the periods of hyperglycemia, in particular during the first years of the disease.[13, 22] Thus, the periods of "desugaring," which may be sporadic in the history of an apparently unstable diabetes, probably do not contribute to the buildup of the long-term complications, whereas in "benign" diabetes, the permanent hyperglycemia slowly and progressively alters the capillaries (which explains the frequency with which retinal lesions exist at the time of diagnosis of previously unknown mature-onset diabetes).[93]

In addition, assessment of the quality of control is difficult; and how can the real duration of diabetes discovered in an overweight adult be known? Thus, comparisons of the degree of retinal and/or renal lesions with the severity of the diabetes in an individual patient are impossible. It is equally important, in order to compare the individual events leading to blindness (objective fact), to know of which lesions one is speaking: serious, widespread but peripheral lesions are infinitely less dangerous for the vision than is a lesion, even localized, that affects the macula, as in macula edema.

Lesions that are reversible after the cure of experimental diabetic animals are not "diabetic."

It has been written that renal lesions obtained from experimental diabetes in the dog or rat do not have "thickening of the glomerular basement membrane, lesions generally held to be the sine qua non of diabetic nephropathy."[105] (This topic is discussed in more detail below and in Chapter 2 of this volume.) But it must be emphasized that many authors have described thickening of the glomerular or retinal capillary basement membrane in experimental diabetes in the rat, dog and monkey.[7, 15, 28, 31, 33, 41, 66, 68, 95, 106, 109] It is possible that the rat is not the best model for such a study, which Klein and colleagues have recently noted.[57] In addition, alloxan and streptozotocin have induced retinopathy in animals.[66]

Clinical Studies

As emphasized above, it is impossible to compare two well-defined populations, the mild versus the severe diabetics. It is possible only to study various degrees of imperfect control (equilibrium) in a continuum of patients.

Even such a task is difficult because of our limits and inherent bias in studying groups of human beings. The reason for the controversies of the past 50 years is that most of the reports suffer from the difficulties inherent in all retrospective studies. Of several exhaustive reviews analyzing the degree of control and its relationship to microangiopathy,[14, 21, 52, 59, 62, 63, 90, 92, 110] two[52, 59] drew negative conclusions, i.e., no relation between the quality of control on the development of renal and/or retinal lesions. In 1964, Knowles, in a review of more than 300 articles, concluded that "information sufficient to arrive at any conclusion is not yet at hand."[59] Almost ten years later, Kaplan and Feinstein analyzed the methods used in 149 studies.[52] They very pessimistically concluded that "a predominantly statistical approach to therapeutic trials cannot be expected to resolve the existing scientific controversies about treatment." But the other analysts conclude that good diabetic control is "probably" beneficial.[14, 21, 62, 63, 90, 92, 110] Pirart and Lauvaux, aside from their own material (4,400 cases over almost 30 years), consider that only 44 publications are methodologically usable.[63, 90] Their opinion is essentially based on prospective studies. The recent study by Francois and colleagues of 203 children shows the existence of permanent proteinuria in 7% of the cases where diabetic control is good, as compared with 15% where it is fair and 39% where it is poor.[34] Four older, negative studies are often cited.[20, 26, 78, 82] They were well analyzed by Lauvaux and Pirart:[63, 90] "Methodology does not resist even a superficial criticism." An excellent retrospective study done by Constam[22] proposed for the first time the idea, which was later confirmed,[13] that the first years of treatment play an important role; during the first five years of their illness, well-controlled diabetics developed fewer vascular lesions than those who were poorly controlled.

Among the 20 or so prospective studies considered to be accurate and favoring a positive relationship between the quality of control and the decreased development of lesions, two do not show any relationship between the incidence of retinopathy or glomerulopathy and the quality of control of blood glucose levels.[60, 116] The first study was by Knowles and colleagues in 1965.[60] Overall, it concerns very poorly controlled children and adolescents. As emphasized by Pirart, "not having a group of patients normally well controlled, the authors were limited to comparing 22 cases without retinopathy to 25 cases with lesions."[90] It is possible that within the very poorly controlled group, certain patients were relatively protected and others aggravated by unknown permissive and/or protective factors; it is also possible, as emphasized above, that "poorly controlled" describes many different situations. A similar situation exists in the population studied by Gerritzen.[38] The other negative prospective analysis is the recent report of the UGDP,[116] which includes the following comments and conclusions: "These results suggest that attempts to normalize blood glucose levels in the adult-onset diabetic will not alter the incidence of renal impairment, retinal changes, or the other common complications of diabetes. Of course, it must be recognized that few patients were found to have renal or ocular disorders over the period covered by this report, and longer periods of follow-up may yield different results with respect to these vascular changes."

Of a group of prospective studies on the evolution of glomerular and/or retinal lesions already present at the start of the investigation,[10, 13, 24, 27, 32, 35, 49, 61, 63, 75, 76, 90, 99, 112, 116] ten showed a beneficial effect of good control on further progression and four had negative results. Davis *et al.* report instances of spontaneous improvement of proliferative retinopathy without evidence of any improvement in the quality of control of the diabetes.[24] Schlesinger and colleagues,[99] as well as Burditt and colleagues,[13] could not relate quality of control to the frequency of the aggravation of existing lesions. Kohner and Dollery noted that the progression of retinopathy in these two studies is probably due to the progression of one type of retinopathy to another type rather than to the aggravation of a particular type of lesion.[62]

All of the other studies conclude that good or very good control slows the progression and decreases the severity of the existing lesions. In particular, the following prospective studies done on the evolution of constituted glomerular lesions should be cited: references 12, 63, 76, 90. The retinal studies by Kohner and her colleagues,[61] those of our group in Paris[49] and others[35, 63, 65, 90] also suggest a beneficial effect of the best possible control of blood glucose levels.

Miki and colleagues showed that after six years of observations, 8% of well-controlled patients had increased their proteinuria versus 24% of poorly controlled diabetics.[76] Takazakura and colleagues performed serial renal biopsies in 23 diabetics at an average interval of about 52.6 months.[112] In six diabetics with good control, no vascular progression was noted. In 13 with poor or fair control, only four had no anatomical worsening. The study by Pirart and Lauvaux permitted them to affirm that "hyperglycemia together with its duration appears to be the only factor really linked to the appearance and the overall frequency, whenever the time of their appearance, of the complications of neuropathy, nephropathy and retinopathy."[63, 90]

We are in accord with this conclusion concerning the clinical studies, which despite their difficulties and limits, seem to point to the protective effect of good control.

Epidemiologic Studies

Serial, long-term epidemiologic studies on large populations show a statistically significant correlation between the degree of hyperglycemia and the frequency of lesions complicating diabetes.[48, 51, 54, 86]

We have already reviewed the results acquired from the Pima

Indians of North America.[51] The 17-year study by O'Sullivan *et al.* showed that the retinal and electrocardiographic lesions, as well as the degree of arterial hypertension and the survival rate, were all correlated to the initially elevated levels of blood sugar.[86] Another British epidemiologic study showed that diabetic retinopathy was rare in subjects who earlier presented "borderline" anomalies of glucose tolerance, as compared with those in which the blood glucose level, 2 hours after glucose ingestion, was greater than 2 gm/L.[48] Katsilambros confirmed these facts in an investigation done in Athens on 21,410 subjects.[54]

Biochemical Studies of the Glomerular Capillary Membrane

The principal protein component of the glomerular capillary basement membranes is a form of collagen, richer in hydroxyproline, hydroxylysine and glycosylhydroxylysine than the collagen of interstitial tissue.[5, 55] The disaccharide radicals are made of glucose and galactose linked to hydroxylysine.[5] As was shown by Klein and colleagues in measuring the hydroxyproline concentration, there is more collagen in human diabetic glomeruli than in those of nondiabetics.[56] Synthesis of the basement membrane from renal and glomerular collagen is increased in human diabetics and in experimentally induced diabetic animals.[64, 95, 96]

These works depend on the study of the activity of four intracellular enzymes that catalyze the hydroxylation of lysine and proline, as well as the transfer of glucose and galactose on the polypeptide chains. Differences appear, according to the study, depending on whether the study is done on the analysis of whole kidneys or the renal cortex, on animals treated with alloxan or with streptozotocin or spontaneously diabetic and, finally, on the extraction techniques used.[98, 108] Certain authors, although demonstrating an increased total enzymatic activity for the two kidneys in streptozotocin-induced diabetic rats,[98] do not find a proportionally increased enzymatic activity that permits the glycolization of the polypeptide chains. These facts agree with other publications that show neither an excess of sugar glycoproteins in diabetic glomerular capillary basement membranes with respect to those of nondiabetics, nor increased glucosyltransferase activity.[28, 55, 120]

The results of biochemical analyses of the composition are inconsistent. Spiro showed specific anomalies in diabetic humans and rats, characterized by an increase in the disaccharide radicals linked to the polypeptide chain due to the increased enzyme activity of glucosyltransferase.[108] Spiro and Spiro showed that careful treatment with insulin in these rats caused a normalization of the enzymatic activity if the insulin treatment was begun soon after the induction of diabetes.[107] Cohen and Khalifa, studying glomeruli isolated from rats, showed that diabetes increased the lysylhydroxylase activity.[17, 18] All of these studies assert that the synthesis of glomerular collagen is increased in patients with diabetes and that insulin normalizes it. If the results of Spiro's work are confirmed, it could also be suggested that diabetes increases the sugar accumulation in the capillary basement membranes, allowing in this non-insulin-dependent tissue the abnormal accumulation of gluco- and galactoglycoproteins. Let us emphasize that this concept of sugar accumulation also rests on multiple data collected from nerves, the lens, the aortic wall and the retina and on the study of plasma concentrations of glycosylated hemoglobin.[108] Insulin, in decreasing or normalizing the blood glucose level, limits the possibilities of this accumulation. As the renewal of the basement membrane is a slow metabolic process, an increased synthesis leads to the accumulation of material.

It is also possible that the degradation of the basement membrane is slowed in patients with diabetes. Brownlee[12] and others[123] suggested that the increase in the blood α_2-macroglobin levels of diabetics could be responsible for an inhibition of collagen synthesis which interferes with the degradation of the basement membrane. But McMillan criticized this hypothesis after his own investigation.[74] Fushimi and Tarui showed that in streptozotocin-induced diabetic rats, β-N-acetylglucose-aminidase activity was increased in the serum and decreased in the kidney after eight weeks of diabetes.[36] Insulin administration significantly reverses these anomalies. The authors recall that β-N-acetylglucose-aminidase is implicated in glycoprotein catabolism, principally in the lysosomes, and they suggest that the diabetic-induced anomalies contribute to glycoprotein accumulation in the diabetic kidney. Thus, many authors showed a beneficial effect of insulin on the diabetes-induced renal enzymatic anomalies. However, Archer and Kaye showed collagen hypersecretion by the fibroblasts originating from cultured skin of diabetic humans, and they suggest that a genetic defect could be responsible.[2]

Thus glycoprotein synthesis is increased in the diabetic renal glomerulus, leading to an excess of a collagen-like substance of abnormal chemical structure containing too many disaccharide radicals. Some enzymatic anomalies induced by experimental diabetes are slowed or normalized by insulin treatment.

Vascular Wall Permeability Studies

The capillary walls (or more precisely the microvessel walls) of diabetics allow an abnormal passage of certain tracers,[115] including fluorescence and albumin,[79] and in general allow the passage of plasma proteins,[89] particularly glycoproteins, whose concentrations are elevated in diabetes.[1] Spiro presumes that these functional anomalies are secondary to the anatomical and biochemical alterations of the capillary basement membranes.[108] But this has been refuted,[87, 89, 123] particularly because two studies have shown fluorescence escape after retinal angiopathy in diabetics with no ophthalmologic or angiographic signs of retinopathy.[87] This would suggest that the thickening of the capillary basement membrane could be secondary to the functional anomalies due to the diabetes, rather than being responsible for the hyperpermeability. In this sequence, the first lesions would be retinal sorbitol and fructose accumulation leading to functional damage and then to the deposition of proteins of circulatory origin on the basement membrane.

Whatever the order of events, it was established that the vascular wall permeability was normal at the time of diagnosis of juvenile diabetes and that hyperpermeability appeared and increased with the duration of the illness.[79, 115] It was also shown that the increase in vascular permeability to fluorescence in streptozotocin-induced diabetic rats was considerably reduced after normalization of blood glucose levels with insulin.[117]

Parving showed that the rate of transcapillary escape of albumin was significantly higher in recently discovered, poorly controlled young diabetics than in those with better control.[89] Mogensen showed a close correlation between the quality of control and the proteinuria induced by muscular exercise.[79] It is important to emphasize that the numerous functional anomalies observed in the kidney in patients with recently discovered and, above all, poorly controlled diabetes, as well as the increased kidney and glomerular volumes, are reversible by careful control of the diabetes.[79] The sequence of normalization is: urinary excretion of albumin and β_2-microglobulin, rate of glomerular filtration, filtration fraction, renal plasma flow and the size of the kidneys and glomeruli.

Experimental Diabetes

The bulk of animal experiments support the secondary character of the glomerular, retinal and nervous lesions. Several groups[7, 15, 28, 31, 33, 41, 66, 68, 95, 106, 109] have produced glomerular and/or retinal lesions characterized by thickening of the basement membranes, which are visible under the regular and electron microscope, thus refuting recently written reviews.[105]

The first works of the Minneapolis group[73] are detailed in Chapter 2 of this volume. They showed that transplantation of the islets of Langerhans causes normalization of blood glucose levels, followed in a few months by a decrease or disappearance of the lesions induced by the experimental diabetes. These authors have described arteriolar lesions in human kidneys of nondiabetics after transplantation into diabetics and have demonstrated that the lesions in an affected kidney from a diabetic rat disappeared after transplantation of the kidney into a healthy rat.

Many groups have obtained results showing regression of capillary basement membrane thickening secondary to experimental diabetes following insulin therapy or transplantation of the islets of Langerhans.[8, 29, 31, 33, 39, 41, 65, 68, 73, 84, 95, 106, 119] Hägg, studying alloxan-treated rats, showed that the diabetes induced thickening of the glomerular basement membranes and of the mesangial zones, as well as deposition of immunoglobulins in the mesangium.[41] Insulin treatment caused a decrease in the thickening of the basement membrane and mesangial tissue, as well as decreased deposition of IgG. Neonatal thymectomy or cyclophosphamide treatment did not protect the diabetic rats from immunoglobulin deposition. Hägg concluded that the glomerular immunoglobulin deposits are secondary to the insulin deficiency and play no pathogenic role in the development of diabetic glomerulopathy.

Sheffield's group has recently done an exhaustive study on the effect of streptozotocin and of intraperitoneal transplantation of insulin-containing tissues in the rat.[68, 106] These authors showed a thickening of the glomerular basement membranes under the electron microscope after six months of diabetes. No fusion of the epithelial pedocytes was observed. IgG deposits along all of the basement membranes were observed after one month, but without deposition of complement (agreeing with Hägg's results). Pancreatic transplantation prevented basement membrane thickening and the IgG deposits, as well as the deposition of basement-membrane-like material in the mesangial matrix. A review of this subject was published by Matas and colleagues[71] and by Slater and colleagues.[106] A Belgian group studied the capillary basement membranes of the eel swimming-bladder as related to the glucose concentration of a bathing solution. These vessels, studied in vitro, absorb glucose in proportion to its concentration. Alloxan in vivo or insulin in vitro does not change the result. In vitro glucose incorporation into the basement membrane increases greatly if the surrounding glucose concentration increases. In vivo, if the eel lives three or four months in water greatly enriched with glucose, the capillary basement membranes of its swimming-bladder significantly thicken. As Lauvaux emphasized, this experimental model could be the first example of a chronic, nondiabetic, hyperglycemic state.[63] In the retina, Engerman's work on dogs showed that well-controlled diabetes with careful insulin therapy significantly slowed the development of retinal lesions as compared with the effects of continuous insulin therapy.[29]

Mauer *et al.* concluded that "diabetic glomerular changes in the rat are secondary to the diabetic state and are reversible upon normalization of the metabolic environments of the kidney."[72]

Conclusions

The opinion of a great number of researchers and clinicians is that the microangiopathic and neuropathic complications of diabetes mellitus are secondary to insulin deficiency, hyperglycemia or their consequences. This concept mandates continuing research aimed at improving the control of blood glucose levels. This effort is justified even if lesions already exist, since they are often still responsive to good diabetic control. It is important to evaluate the risks of a rigid therapy as compared with more permissive regimens. As emphasized, little is known of the risks, especially hypoglycemic, of patients whose diabetes is meticulously controlled by insulin.[44] The psychologic restrictions can sometimes be difficult,[58] but it has been shown that children and adolescents can be taught and educated to rigidly control their insulin-dependent diabetes without major alternations in life-style. Dividing insulin therapy into several daily injections has been advised for a long time and the arguments in favor of this method are developed elsewhere.[113]

This review suggests that diabetic nephropathy can be prevented or slowed by careful diabetic therapy. As noted in this volume by Jacobs *et al.* (Chapter 6) and by others,[16, 118] it is essential to treat associated arterial hypertension, which plays an aggravating role in the evolution of nephropathy[62] and atheromas in diabetics.

The best treatment of diabetic nephropathy is careful control of blood glucose levels during the lifetime of the diabetic patient.

References

1. Alberti, K. G. M. M., and Hockaday, T. D. R.: The biochemistry of the complications of diabetes mellitus, in Keen, H. and Jarrett, H. (eds.): *Complications of Diabetes* London: E. Arnold, 1975), pp. 221–64.
2. Archer, J., and Kaye, R.: Cultured skin fibroblasts and juvenile diabetes: senescene and collagen synthesis, Diabetes 26 (Suppl. 1):361, 1977 (Abstract).
3. Aronoff, S. L., Bennett, P. H., Williamson, J. R., Siperstein, M. D., Plumer, M. E., and Miller, M.: Muscle capillary basement membrane (MCBM) measurements in prediabetic, diabetic, and normal Pima Indians and normal caucasians, Clin. Res. 24:455A, 1976.
4. Balodimos, M. C.: Diabetic nephropathy, in Marble, A., White, P., Bradley, R. F., and Krall, L. P. (eds.): *Joslin's Diabetes Mellitus* (Philadelphia: Lea & Febiger, 1971), p. 526.
5. Beisswenger, P. J., and Spiro, R. G.: Studies on the human glomerular basement membrane. Composition, nature of the carbohydrate units and chemical changes in diabetes mellitus, Diabetes 22:180, 1973.
6. Bendayan, M., Sandborne, E., and Rasio, E.: Concurrent studies on the morphology, the permeability and the metabolism of a blood capillary preparation, Diabetologia 10:358, 1974.
7. Bloodworth, J. M. B., Jr., Engerman, R. L., Camerini-Davalos, R. A., and Powers, K. L.: Variations in capillary basement membrane width produced by aging and diabetes mellitus, in Camerini-Davalos, R., and Cole, H. S. (eds.): *Early Diabetes* (New York/London: Academic Press, 1970), pp. 279–95.
8. Bloodworth, J. M. B., Jr., and Engerman, R. L.: Diabetic microangiopathy in the experimentally-diabetic dog and its prevention by careful control with insulin, Diabetes 22 (Suppl. 1):290, 1973 (Abstract).
9. Börner, E., Meissner, H. P., Städtler, F., Weinges, K., and Krück, F.: "Diabetische glomerulosklerose" ohne diabetes mellitus, Klin. Wochenschr. 49:1267, 1971.
10. Boyd, J. D., Jackson, R. L., and Allen, J. H.: Avoidance of degenerative lesions in diabetes mellitus, J.A.M.A. 118:694, 1942.

11. Bradley, R. F.: Cardiovascular disease, in Marble, A., White, P., Bradley, R. F., and Krall, L. P. (eds.): *Joslin's Diabetes Mellitus* (Philadelphia: Lea & Febiger, 1971), pp. 417–77.

12. Brownlee, M.: α 2-Macroglobulin and reduced basement-membrane degradation in diabetes, Lancet 1:779, 1976.

13. Burditt, A. F., Caird, F. I., and Draper, G. J.: The natural history of diabetic retinopathy, Q. J. Med. 37:303, 1968.

14. Caird, F. I., Pirie A., and Ramsell, T. G.: *Diabetes and the Eye* (Oxford: Blackwell Scientific, 1969).

15. Cameron, D. P., Amherdt, M., Leucnberger, P., Orci, L., and Stauffacher, W.: Microvascular alterations in chronically streptozotocin-diabetic rats, in Camerini-Davalos, R. A., and Cole, H. S. (eds.): *Early Diabetes* (New York: Academic Press, 1973).

16. Cameron, J. S., Ireland, J. T., and Watkins, P. J.: The kidney and renal tract, in Keen, H., and Jarrett, H. (eds.): *Complications of Diabetes* (London: E. Arnold, 1975), pp. 99–150.

17. Cohen, M. P., and Khalifa, A.: Effect of diabetes and insulin on rat renal glomerular protocollagen hydroxylase activities, Biochim. Biophys. Acta 496:88, 1977.

18. Cohen, M. P., and Khalifa, A.: Renal glomerular collagen synthesis in streptozotocin diabetes. Reversal of increased basement membrane synthesis with insulin therapy, Biochim. Biophys. Acta, in press.

19. Collens, W. S., Silverstein, J. M., and Dobkin, J. B.: Case of a diabetic with a Kimmelstiel-Wilson syndrome and a normal glucose tolerance, Ann. Intern. Med. 50:1282, 1959.

20. Colwell, A. R.: Observed course of diabetes mellitus and inferences concerning its origin and progress, Arch. Intern. Med. 70:523, 1942.

21. Colwell, J. A.: Effect of diabetic control on retinopathy, Diabetes 15:497, 1966.

22. Constam, G. R.: Contrôle du diabète et prévention des complications, in *Ann. Diabetol. l'Hôtel-Dieu* (Paris: Flammarion, 1972), pp. 313–20.

23. Darnaud, Ch., Denard, Y., Moreau, G., Voisin, R., and Combes, P.: Rétinopathies diabétiques, Diabète 7:142, 1959.

24. Davis, M. D., Norton, E. W. D., and Myers, F. L.: The airlie house classification of diabetic retinopathy, in Goldberg, M. F., and Fine, S. L. (eds.): *Treatment of Diabetic Retinopathy* (Washington, D.C.: U. S. Public Health Service Publ. No. 1890, 1969), p. 7.

25. Daysog, A., Dobson, H. L., and Brennan, J. C.: Renal, glomerular and vascular lesions in prediabetes and in diabetes mellitus, Ann. Intern. Med. 54:672, 1961.

26. Dolger, H.: Clinical evaluation of vascular damage in diabetes mellitus, J. A. M. A., 134:1289, 1947.

27. Dollery, C. T., and Oakley, N. W.: Reversal of retinal vascular changes in diabetes, Diabetes 14:121, 1965.

28. Duhault, J., Boulanger, M., Lebon, F., and Beert, L.: La microangiopathie diabétique expérimentale. Nouv. Presse Med. 45:3013, 1973.

29. Engerman, R. L., Bloodworth, J. M. B., Jr., and Nelson, S.: Relationship of microvascular disease in diabetes to metabolic control, Diabetes 26:760, 1977.

30. Fajans, S. S., Taylor, C. I., Floyd, J. C., Jr., and Conn, J. W.: Some aspects of the natural history of diabetes mellitus, in Malaisse, W. J., Pirart, J., and Vallance-Owan, J. (eds.): *Diabetes*, Eighth Congress of the International Diabetes Federation, Brussels (Amsterdam: Excerpta Medica, 1974), pp. 329–40.

31. Federlin, K., Bretzel, R. G., and Schmidtchen, U.: Islet transplantation in experimental diabetes of rat. 5. Regression of glomerular lesions in diabetic rats after intraportal transplantation of isogeneic islets. Preliminary results, Horm. Metab. Res. 8:404, 1976.

32. Folk, M. L., and Soskin, S.: Fundus oculi in diabetes mellitus, Am. J. Ophthalmol. 18:432, 1935.
33. Fox, Ch., Darby, S. C., Ireland, J. T., and Sönksen, P. H.: Blood glucose control and glomerular capillary basement membrane thickening in experimental diabetes, Br. Med. J. 2:605, 1977.
34. Francois, R., Mamelle, H., Leonetti, P., Jarlot, B., Gillet, P., David, L., and Tardieu, M.: Complications dégénératives après 10 ans de diabète infantile, in *J. Ann. Diabetol. Hôtel-Dieu* (Paris: Flammarion, 1976), pp. 135–156.
35. Freyler, H., *et al.:* Welche faktoren beeinfluenssen die progredienz der diabetischen retinopathie? Wien. Klin. Wochenschr. 86:621, 1974.
36. Fushimi, H., and Tarui, S.: Kidney and serum beta-N-acetyglucosaminidase activities in streptozotocin diabetic rats and their responses to insulin and glucagon, J. Biochem. 76:225, 1974.
37. Ganda, O. P., Soeldner, J. S., Gleason, R. E., Smith, T. M., Kilo, C., and Williamson, T. R.: Monozygotic triplets with discordance for diabetes mellitus and diabetic microangiopathy, Diabetes 26:469, 1977.
38. Gerritzen, F. M.: The course of diabetic retinopathy, Diabetes 22:122, 1973.
39. Gray, B. N., and Watkins, E.: Prevention of vascular complications of diabetes by pancreatic islet transplantation, Arch. Surg. 111:254, 1976.
40. Guinet, P.: Les complications vasculaires du syndrome prédiabétique, in *J. Ann. Diabetol. l'Hôtel-Dieu* (Paris: Flammarion, 1961), p. 113.
41. Hägg, E.: On the pathogenesis of glomerular lesions in the alloxan diabetic rat, Acta Med. Scand. [Suppl.] 558:1, 1974.
42. Harrington, A. R., Hare, H. G., Chambers, W. M., and Valmin, H.: Nodular glomerulosclerosis suspected during life in a patient without demonstrable diabetes mellitus, N. Engl. J. Med. 275:206, 1966.
43. Harrington, J. T., Garella, S., Stilmant, M. M., and Chazan, J. A.: Renal failure as the initial manifestation of diabetes mellitus, Arch. Intern. Med. 132:249, 1973.
44. Ingelfinger, F. J.: Debates on diabetes, N. Engl. J. Med. 296:1228, 1977.
45. Ireland, J. T., Patnaik, B. K., and Duncan, L. J. P.: Glomerular ultrastructure in secondary diabetics and normal subjects, Diabetes 16:628, 1967.
46. Ireland, J. T.: Diagnostic criteria in the assessment of glomerular capillary basement membrane lesions in newly diagnosed juvenile diabetics, in Camerini-Davalos, R. A., and Cole, H. S. (eds.): *Early Diabetes* (New York: Academic Press, 1970), pp. 273–278.
47. Jackson, R., Guthrie, R., Esterly, J., Bilginturan, N., James, R., Yeast, J., Saathof, J., and Guthrie, D.: Muscle capillary basement membrane changes in normal and diabetic children, Diabetes 24(Suppl. 2):400, 1975 (Abstract).
48. Jarrett, R. J., and Keen, H.: Hyperglycaemia and diabetes mellitus, Lancet 2:1009, 1976.
49. Job, D., Eschwege, E., Guyot-Argenton, C., Aubry, J. P., and Tchobroutsky, G.: Effect of multiple daily insulin injections on the course of diabetic retinopathy, Diabetes 25:463, 1976.
50. Johansen, K.: Diabetic angiopathy in a patient with normal glucose tolerance and plasma insulin response, Am. J. Med. 47:487, 1969.
51. Kamenetzky, S. A., Bennett, P. H., Dippe, S. E., Miller, M., and LeCompte, P. M.: A clinical and histologic study of diabetic nephropathy in the Pima Indians, Diabetes 23:61, 1974.
52. Kaplan, M. H., and Feinstein, A. R.: A critique of methods in reported studies of long-term vascular complications in patients with diabetes mellitus, Diabetes 22:160, 1973.
53. Karam, J. H., Rosenthal, M., O'Donnel, J. J., Tsalikian, E., Lorenzi, M., Gerich, J. E., Siperstein, M. D., and Forsham, P. H.: Discordance of diabetic microangiopathy in identical twins, Diabetes 25:24, 1976.

54. Katsilambros, N.: Diabetic retinopathy and blood-sugar, Lancet 2:1253, 1976.
55. Kefalides, N. A.: Biochemical properties of human glomerular basement membrane in normal and diabetic kidneys, J. Clin. Invest. 53:403, 1974.
56. Klein, L., Butcher, D. L., Sudilovsky, O., Kikkawa, R., and Miller, M.: Quantification of collagen in renal glomeruli isolated from human nondiabetic and diabetic kidneys, Diabetes 24:1057, 1975.
57. Klein, L., Yoshida, M., and Miller, M.: Does experimental diabetes in the rat produce basement membrane (BM) thickening in renal glomeruli? Diabetes 26(Suppl. 1):361, 1977 (Abstract).
58. Knibbs, S., and Jackson, J. G. L.: Social and emotional complications of diabetes, in Keen, H., and Jarrett, H. (eds.): *Complications of Diabetes* (London: E. Arnold, 1975), pp. 265–277.
59. Knowles, H. C., Jr.: The problem of the relation of the control of diabetes to the development of vascular disease, Trans. Am. Clin. Climatol. Assoc. 76:142, 1964.
60. Knowles, H. C., Guest, G. M., Lampe, J., Kessler, M., and Skillman, Th. G.: The course of juvenile diabetes treated with unmeasured diet, Diabetes 14:239, 1965.
61. Kohner, E. M., Fraser, T. R., Joplin, G. F., and Oakley, N. W.: The effect of control on diabetic retinopathy, in Goldberg, M. F., and Fine, S. L. (eds.): *Treatment of Diabetic Retinopathy* (Washington, D.C.: U. S. Public Health Service Publ. No. 1890, 1969), p. 119.
62. Kohner, E. M., and Dollery, C. T.: Diabetic retinopathy, in Keen, H., and Jarrett, H. (eds.): *Complications of Diabetes* (London: E. Arnold, 1975), pp. 7–98.
63. Lauvaux, J. P.: Le rôle de l'hyperglycémie chronique dans l'apparition et le développement de la triopathie diabétique: neuropathie, néphropathie, rétinopathie (Etude clinique). Thesis, Université Libre de Bruxelles, 1976.
64. Lazarow, A.: Glomerular basement membrane thickening in diabetes, in Ostman, J., and Milner, R. D. G. (eds.): *Diabetes*, Sixth Congress of the International Diabetes Federation (Amsterdam: Excerpta Medica, 1969), p. 301.
65. Lee, C. S., Mauer, S. M., Brown, C. M., Sutherland, D. E. R., Michael, A. F., and Najarian, J. S.: Renal transplantation in diabetes mellitus in rat, J. Exp. Med. 139:793, 1974.
66. Leuenberger, P. M., Cameron, D., and Stauffacher, W.: Ocular lesions in rats rendered chronically diabetic with streptozotocin, Ophthal. Res. 1:189, 1970.
67. Linner, E., Svanborg, A., and Zelander, T.: Retinal and renal lesions of diabetic type, without obvious disturbances of glucose metabolism in a patient with family history of diabetes, Am. J. Med. 39:298, 1965.
68. Mangnall, Y., Smythe, A., Slater, D., Milner, R. D. G., Milner, G. R., Strachan, I., McLaren, E. H., and Fox, M.: Pancreatic islet transplantation effects on the metabolic changes and secondary complications of experimental diabetes in the rat. British Diabetes Assoc., Autumn 1976 (Abstract).
69. Marks, H. H.: Longevity and mortality of diabetics, Am. J. Public Health 55:416, 1965.
70. Marks, H. H., and Krall, L. P.: Onset, course, prognosis and mortality in diabetes mellitus, in Marble, A., White, P., Bradley, R. F., and Krall, L. P. (eds.): *Joslin's Diabetes Mellitus* (Philadelphia: Lea & Febiger, 1971), pp. 209–254.
71. Matas, A. J., Sutherland, D. E. R., and Najarian, J. S.: Current status of islet and pancreas transplantation in diabetes, Diabetes 25:785, 1976.
72. Mauer, S. M., Michael, A. F., Fish, A. J., and Brown, D. M.: Spontaneous immunoglobin and complement deposition in glomeruli of diabetic rats, Lab. Invest. 27:488, 1972.
73. Mauer, S. M., Sutherland, D. E. R., Steffes, M. W., Leonard, R. J., Najarian, J. S., Michael, A. F., and Brown, D. M.: Pancreatic islet transplantation. Effects on the glomerular lesions of experimental diabetes in the rat, Diabetes 23:748, 1974.
74. McMillan, D. E.: Alpha-macroglobulin in diabetes, Lancet 2:1020, 1976.

75. Miki, E., Fukuda, M., Kuzuya, T., Kosaka, K., and Nakao, K.: Relation of the course of retinopathy to control of diabetes, age and therapeutic agents in diabetic Japanese patients, Diabetes 18:773, 1969.
76. Miki, E., Kuzuya, T., Ide, T., and Nakao, K.: Frequency, degree and progression with time of proteinuria in diabetic patients, Lancet 1:922, 1972.
77. Miller, L. V., and Goldstein, J.: More efficient care of diabetic patients in a county-hospital setting, N. Engl. J. Med. 286:1388, 1972.
78 . Mirsky, I. A.: Our challenge for the future (editorial), Diabetes Abstracts 5:71, 1946.
79. Mogensen, C. E.: Renal function changes in diabetes, Diabetes 25 (Suppl. 2):872, 1976.
80. Morel-Maroger, L.: Le rein dans les dysproteinuries, in Hamburger, J., Crosnier, J., and Grunfeld, J. P. (eds.): *Néphrologie* (Paris: Flammarion), in press.
81. Morel-Maroger, L.: Personal communication.
82. Muri, J.: Diabetic nephropathy and retinopathy, Acta Med. Scand. 149:211, 1954.
83. Nash, D. A., Rogers, P. W., Langlinais, P. C., and Bunn, S. M., Jr.: Diabetic glomerulosclerosis without glucose tolerance, Am. J. Med. 59:191, 1975.
84. Orloff, M. J., Lee, S., Charters, A. C. III, Grambort, D. E., Storck, L. G., and Knox, D.: Long term studies of pancreas transplantation in experimental diabetes mellitus, Ann. Surg. 182:198, 1975.
85. Østerby, R.: Course of diabetic glomerulopathy, Acta Diabetol. Lat. 8 (Suppl. 1):179, 1971.
86. O'Sullivan, J. B., Cosgrove, J., and McCaughan, D.: Blood sugars, vascular abnormalities and survival. The Oxford study after 17 years, Postgrad. Med. J. 44(Suppl.): 955, 1961.
87. Palmberg, P. F.: Diabetic retinopathy, Diabetes 26:703, 1977.
88. Pardo, V., Perez-Stable, E., Alzamora, D. B., and Cleveland, W. W.: Incidence and significance of muscle capillary basal lamina thickness in juvenile diabetes, Am. J. Pathol. 68:67, 1972.
89. Parving, H. H.: Increased microvascular permeability to plasma proteins in short- and long-term juvenile diabetics, Diabetes 25(Suppl. 2):884, 1976.
90. Pirart, J.: Rigueur du traitement du diabéte et complications rétiniennes, in *J. Ann. Diabetol. Hôtel-Dieu* (Paris: Flammarion, 1977), pp. 282–296.
91. Pirart, J., and Lauvaux, J. P.: Remission in diabetes, in Pfeiffer, E. (ed.): *Handbook of Diabetes Mellitus*, Vol. 2 (München: J. F. Lehmanns, 1971), p. 443.
92. Pometta, D.: La microangiopathie diabétique, Acta Endocrinol. (Kbh.) 67(Suppl. 156), 1971.
93. Pyke, D. A., and Roberts, D. S. C.: Retinopathy in early cases of diabetes mellitus, Acta Med. Scand. 163:489, 1959.
94. Pyke, D. A., and Tattersall, R. B.: Diabetic retinopathy in identical twins, Diabetes 22:613, 1973.
95. Rasch, R.: The effect of diabetic control on kidney weight, glomerular volume and glomerular basement membrane thickness (abstract), Diabetologia 13:426, 1977.
96. Rasio, E., Bendayan, M., and Sandborn, E. B.: Ultrastructure and glucose metabolism of an isolated blood capillary preparation, in Malaisse, W., and Pirart, J. (eds.): *Diabetes* (Amsterdam: Excerpta Medica, 1974), p. 396.
97. Raskin, P., Marks, J. F., Burns, H., Plumer, M. E., and Siperstein, M. D.: Capillary basement membrane width in diabetic children, Am. J. Med. 58:365, 1975.
98. Ristelli, J., Koivisto, V. A., Akerblom, H. K., and Kivirikko, K. I.: Intracellular enzymes of collagen biosynthesis in rat kidney in streptozotocin diabetes, Diabetes 25:1066, 1976.
99. Schlesinger, F. G., Franken, S., Van Lange, L. T. P., and Schwartz, F.: Incidence and progression of retinal and vascular lesions in long-term diabetes, Acta Med. Scand. 168:483, 1960.

100. Sheikholislam, B. M., Irias, J. J., Lin, H. J., Lowrey, G. H., Stephenson, S. R., Peterson, G. E., Devereux, D. F., and Volk, T. L.: Carbohydrate metabolism and capillary basement-membrane thickness in children. I. Cross-sectional studies, Diabetes 25:650, 1976.
101. Sheikholislam, B. M., Irias, J. J., Lowrey, G. H., and Lin, H. J.: Carbohydrate metabolism and capillary basement-membrane thickness in children. 2. Longitudinal studies, Diabetes 25:661, 1976.
102. Shepherd, G. R.: Diabetes mellitus of juvenile onset with 40 years' survival and no gross damage, Arch. Intern. Med. 128:284, 1971.
103. Siperstein, M. D., Unger, R. H., and Madison, L. L.: Studies of muscle capillary basement membranes in normal subjects, diabetic, and prediabetic patients, J. Clin. Invest. 47:1973, 1968.
104. Siperstein, M. D., Raskin, P., and Burns, H.: Electron microscopic quantification of diabetic microangiopathy, Diabetes 22:514, 1973.
105. Siperstein, M. D., Foster, D. W., Knowles, H. C., Jr., Levine, R., Madison, L. L., and Roth, J.: Control of blood glucose and diabetic vascular disease, N. Engl. J. Med. 1: 1060, 1977.
106. Slater, D. N., Mangnall, Y., Smythe, A., Ward, A. M., and Fox, M.: Neonatal islet cell transplantation in the diabetic rat: effect on the renal complications, Br. J. Pathol., in press.
107. Spiro, R. G., and Spiro, M. J.: Effect of diabetes on the biosynthesis of the renal glomerular basement membrane, Diabetes 20:641, 1971.
108. Spiro, R. G.: Search for a biochemical basis of diabetic microangiopathy, Diabetologia 12:1, 1976.
109. Stout, C., Kennedy, A., Solse, D., Beathard, G., Granholm, N., Padula, R., Williams, G. R., Whorton, E., Davis, E., and Kimmelstiel, P.: Glomerulosclerosis in "secondary" diabetes in baboons, Diabetes 25 (Suppl. 1):349, 1976 (Abstract).
110. Stowers, J. M.: Special features of diabetic pregnancies and their progeny, in Keen, H., and Jarrett, J. (eds.): Complications of Diabetes (London: E. Arnold, 1975), pp. 205–219.
111. Strauss, R. G., Argy, W. P., Jr., and Schreiner, G. E.: Diabetic glomerulosclerosis in the absence of glucose intolerance, Ann. Intern. Med. 75:239, 1971.
112. Takazakura, E., Nakamoto, Y., Hayakawa, H., Kawai, K., Muramoto, S., Yoshida, K., Shimizu, M., Shinoda, A., and Takeuchi, J.: Onset and progression of diabetic glomerulosclerosis, Diabetes, 24:1, 1975.
113. Tchobroutsky, G.: How to achieve better diabetic control. Studies with insulin three times a day, in Malaisse, W. J., and Pirart, J. (eds.): Diabetes, Eighth Congress of the International Diabetes Federation, Brussels (Amsterdam: Excerpta Medica, 1973), pp. 667–679.
114. Thomsen, A. C.: The Kidney in Diabetes Mellitus (Copenhagen; Munksgaard, 1965).
115. Trap-Jensen, J.: Permeability of small vessels in diabetes, Acta Diabetol. Lat. 8 (Suppl. 1):192, 1971.
116. U.G.D.P.: A study of the effects of hypoglycemia agents on vascular complications in patients with adult-onset diabetes. VI. Supplementary report on nonfatal events in patients treated with tolbutamide, Diabetes 25:1129, 1976.
117. Waltman, S. R., et al.: Blood-retinal barrier in experimental diabetes. Presented at the Spring Meeting of the Association for Research in Vision and Ophthalmology, Sarasota, Florida, April 26, 1977.
118. Watkins, P. J., Parsons, V., and Bewick, M.: The prognosis and management of diabetic nephropathy, Clin. Nephrol. 7:243, 1977.
119. Weil, R., Nozawa, M., Koss, M., Weber, C., Reemtsma, K. B., and McIntosh, R.: Pancreatic transplantation in diabetic rats: renal function, morphology, ultrastructure and immunohistology, Surgery 78:142, 1975.
120. Westberg, N. G., and Michael A. F.: Human glomerular basement membrane: chemical composition in diabetes mellitus, Acta Med. Scand. 194:39, 1973.

121. Williamson, J. R., Vogler, N. J., and Kilo, C.: Estimation of vascular basement membrane thickness, Diabetes 18:567, 1969.
122. Williamson, J. R., Rowold, E., Hoffman, P., and Kilo, C.: Influence of fixation and morphometric technics on capillary basement-membrane thickening prevalence data in diabetes, Diabetes 25:604, 1976.
123. Williamson, J. R., and Kilo, C.: Basement-membrane thickening and diabetic microangiopathy, Diabetes 25(Suppl. 2):925, 1976.
124. Williamson, J. R., and Kilo, C.: Current status of capillary basement-membrane disease in diabetes mellitus, Diabetes 26:65, 1977.

5

Disorders of Glucose Metabolism in Uremia

JOHN D. BAGDADE, M.D.

Department of Medicine, School of Medicine, University of Washington and the Providence Medical Center, Seattle, Washington

Glucose intolerance, with changes in blood glucose concentrations following the oral ingestion of glucose comparable to those found in patients with diabetes mellitus, was one of the first metabolic disturbances observed in azotemic patients.[7] Subsequently, a variety of abnormalities in glucose homeostasis have been described in patients with chronic renal failure. These range from spontaneous hypoglycemia to overt fasting hyperglycemia, even in the absence of a positive family history and lack of prior clinical or chemical evidence of diabetes mellitus. Thus, it has become increasingly apparent that uremia is associated with perturbations of glucose metabolism that can be manifested by both abnormally increased and, occasionally, markedly decreased levels of circulating glucose.

It is appropriate that this subject be considered now, for recently completed studies provide important new insights into why these disturbances in glucose homeostasis occur in cases of renal failure. I wish to bring you up to date on this subject and to suggest on the basis of a review of the new and old literature how it is possible that a given patient with renal failure might

87

0084-5957/79/080087-14$3.75

© 1979, Year Book Medical Publishers, Inc.

on one day have glucose levels in the clearly diabetic range and shortly thereafter manifest symptoms of hypoglycemia.

To do this, I have chosen to take a physiologic approach and develop an understanding of how the organs, tissues and hormones whose interactions determine minute-to-minute glucose concentrations are altered in cases of chronic uremia. Since the classic studies of Claude Bernard, the unique role of the liver in maintaining glucose homeostasis has been recognized for several reasons:[12] (1) it is an organ capable of producing as well as utilizing glucose; (2) it is exposed to concentrations of insulin and other gut hormones in the portal venous blood that exceed by three- to tenfold those found in the systemic circulation; (3) it is the sole site of the glucoregulatory action of glucagon; (4) hexoses absorbed from the gastrointestinal tract reach the liver before being delivered to muscle and adipose tissue, the other major sites of glucose utilization.

Contrary to earlier belief, resistance to the entry of glucose into peripheral tissues may not be the only cellular mechanism that causes glucose intolerance. A number of mechanisms, as will be described below, can adversely affect glucose utilization at this level. Of perhaps greater interest at this time is new information indicating that in patients with uremia the formation of new glucose from amino acid precursors continues inappropriately in the postprandial state. Thus, glucose tolerance will decrease if cellular disposal mechanisms cannot keep pace with the rate at which newly formed glucose is being added to an expanded circulating pool of glucose. Glucose intolerance resulting from a combination of sustained new glucose formation and peripheral resistance to insulin action is not unique to uremia, but resembles that which occurs in Cushing's disease and in patients receiving large doses of glucocorticosteroids. In such patients, gluconeogenesis is increased because elevated circulating levels of adrenal steroids activate systems that produce glucose from protein and glycerol, and glucose assimilation is simultaneously retarded because steroids induce cellular resistance to insulin action. Thus, the alterations in glucose homeostasis in uremic patients resemble those that occur during the administration of glucocorticoids, agents shown to increase hepatic glucose production and simultaneously to impair the capacity of both hepatic and peripheral tissues to normally assimilate and utilize glucose.

Insulin Antagonism and Secretion

Historically, a number of observations have suggested that the uremic state was associated with tissue changes that antagonized the glucose-lowering actions of insulin. Westervelt's forearm perfusion studies, demonstrating that glucose and phosphorus uptake as well as lactate production in uremic patients were only 25% of those of controls,[28] did not distinguish whether these effects resulted from a circulating insulin antagonist, a defect in insulin-mediated cell membrane transport of glucose or defective glucose phosphorylation. The fact that the amount of lactate produced per mole of glucose was similar in uremic and control subjects suggested, at least, that once glucose entered the cell and became phosphorylated, the Embden-Meyerhof pathway was intact. Further evidence for insulin antagonism in cases of uremia has been the repeated observation that the fall in blood glucose levels following both exogenous insulin[27] and tolbutamide[26] administration is frequently delayed and decreased in patients with renal failure. The restoration of sensitivity to the glucose-lowering effects of insulin following dialysis treatment suggests that some circulating dialyzable substance(s) contribute to this abnormality.[16, 21]

The increase in basal insulin levels in patients with renal failure has been presumed to result from a compensatory increase in insulin secretion similar to that occurring in patients receiving corticosteroids.[2] It appears that a delay in renal catabolism, rather than increased pancreatic secretion, is responsible for the increase in the amounts of all three measurable components of insulin (C-peptide, proinsulin and insulin itself[19]) found in most patients with renal failure. Such findings are compatible with tissue insulin antagonism, but they also indicate that renal dysfunction causes marked changes in serum β-cell peptide levels, and their relative concentration in a given patient may vary depending on the quantitative role (i.e., how much residual renal function there is) that the kidneys play in their removal.

The kidney has been shown to play a key role in the metabolism of other low-molecular-weight peptides. These include glucagon, gastrin, secretin, cholecystokinin, parathyroid hormone and thyroid-stimulating hormone (TSH). It is apparent that several immunologically similar molecular species of these substances, which vary in size and biologic action, are present in uremic patients.[19] Alterations of this type appear to result from the growing recognition that the kidney plays an important role in the degradation of several hormones. Two distinct pathways are present in the kidney to perform the metabolic transformation of these peptide hormones. The first pathway is glomerular filtration, followed by uptake and degradation by the luminal border of the renal tubular cells; the second involves uptake from the peritubular blood and degradation in tubular cells, presumably by cytosolic enzyme systems.[8] In patients with renal failure these processes are grossly impaired and, due to a decreased metabolic clearance, the levels of C-peptide, proinsulin and insulin are all increased. These findings account for the well-recognized fact that with the onset of renal failure, insulin requirements typically decline in the insulin-dependent diabetic.

The effects of delayed degradation of these other peptide hormones on glucose homeostasis has only recently become apparent. Glucagon in particular,[20] but parathyroid hormone as well, has important glucoregulatory functions, particularly in new glucose formation. Gastrin, secretin and cholecystokinin, on the other hand, have important insulinotropic effects. An imbalance in these humoral substances resulting from their altered catabolism and clearance appears to be one factor that significantly influences glucose homeostasis. The regulation of other hormones, such as growth hormone, cortisol and catecholamines, which are known to have actions antagonistic to insulin, has been shown to be abnormal in patients with renal failure. Thus, these humoral factors are also capable of contributing to glucose intolerance in uremic patients by as yet unclear mechanisms.

A number of metabolic end products that accumulate because of the inability of the kidney to excrete them normally, such as urea, creatinine, indoles, guanidines, phenols, aliphatic amines, small polypeptides and guanidinosuccinic acid, as well as other unidentified substances perhaps contained in the middle-molecule fraction,[13] have been implicated in the pathogenesis of glucose intolerance.[10] Guanidines in particular appear to inhibit several enzyme systems. If these other substances, in fact, affect cellular processes that modulate glucose metabolism, their mechanism(s) of action too remains unclear. The contributions of altered potassium and magnesium levels as well as the nutritional status of patients with renal failure are not as significant in the pathophysiology of glucose intolerance in uremia as they were once thought to be.

There is mounting evidence indicating that generalized cellular derangements in non-insulin-dependent pathways of glucose metabolism also contribute substantially to the disturbances observed in glucose transport in cases of uremia. An inhibition in the skeletal muscle glycolytic enzyme, phosphofructokinase, has been found in uremic rats;[9] serum from these animals has been found by a number of workers to uncouple mitochondrial oxidative metabolism. Defects of this type suggest that uremia itself depresses glucose-derived energy production. Such abnormalities may increase the cellular requirement for glucose and thereby activate mechanisms to accelerate new glucose formation.

In any discussion of perturbed glucose homeostasis in uremic patients, it is necessary to consider the role of insulin, the hormone most closely associated with glucose transport. Conflicting reports have appeared in the literature about whether the plasma insulin response to glucose administered intravenously and orally in uremic patients is increased or reduced.[7] Interpretation of most of these studies, however, has been limited by problems in both experimental design and methodology. At the time most of these studies were performed, it was not appreciated that the "acute insulin response" (i.e., the insulin secreted in the first three to five minutes following the administration of glucose intravenously or in the initial 15 minutes after oral intake of glucose) was the critical determinant of glucose tolerance.[22] Since most insulin measurements were obtained well after the acutely releasable insulin pool had been discharged, it is not surprising that the results of these studies are confusing and contradictory.

Methodology also has confused the interpretation of post-glucose insulin data. Most insulin radioimmunoassays used in the past lacked the precision required to accurately measure insulin amounts at the low concentrations found in subjects in the basal or overnight-fasted state. Because an accurate measurement of *basal* insulin is necessary in order to correctly estimate the *response*,[1] interpretation of insulin levels in a number of these studies is difficult. To further complicate the problem of interpreting immunoreactive insulin (IRI) measurements in uremic patients, other β-peptides that are immunologically similar but not identical with insulin have been shown to be included in the routine IRI measurement.[19] Despite these limitations, however, it can be stated with some assurance that both qualitative and quantitative alterations in the levels of insulin secretion take place in patients with renal failure.

Dialysis treatment does appear to correct, at least partially, the reduction in the early insulin response to glucose intravenously[21, 17] and is followed by improved glucose tolerance. The general lack of correlation between insulin levels and glucose tolerance found in the majority of past studies is probably attributable to the interplay of varying degrees of disturbances in insulin secretion and apparent peripheral antagonism to insulin action. The role of enteric hormones, which also stimulate insulin secretion and whose action explains why circulating insulin levels are higher after oral than after glucose administration intravenously, needs to be examined further in cases of renal failure.

Role of Liver and Muscle

The discussion thus far has dealt principally with factors relating to insulin antagonism and secretion. As stated in the introduction, it is essential that the role of the liver and muscle be considered in any discussion of glucose homeostasis. In recent studies in the laboratory of Felig and co-workers, a number of basic observations have been made that make it possible to better understand some of the cellular mechanisms in the liver that appear to alter glucose transport in cases of renal failure.

In addition to confirming the earlier observation of hyperglucagonemia in uremia,[5] not only have they shown that this elevation is the result of decreased turnover rather than hypersecretion,[24] but they also have found that sensitivity to the glucose-elevating effect of glucagon is increased in uremic patients, and this is reversed by dialysis treatment. To better understand the cellular basis for these findings, the role of glucagon and insulin receptor binding was studied in the liver plasma membranes of control and chronically uremic rats.[25] Specific binding of ^{125}I-glucagon was increased by 80–120% and glucagon-stimulated adenylate cyclase activity was reduced (Fig. 5–1), while ^{125}I-insulin binding was reduced by 40–50% compared with controls (Fig. 5–2). These changes in the binding of glucagon and insulin

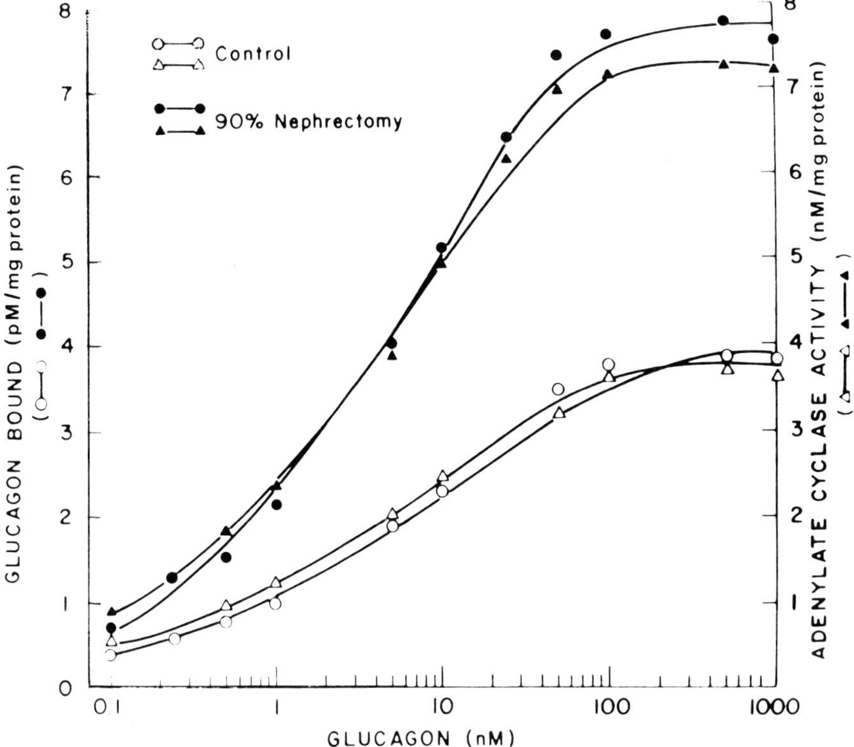

Fig. 5–1. – Correlation between glucagon binding and glucagon-stimulated adenylate cyclase activity in liver plasma membranes in both control and uremic rats (90% nephrectomy).

were found to be due to alterations in binding capacity rather than changes in affinity. These observations of oppositely directed simultaneous changes in glucagon and insulin receptor binding may account for the apparent hypersensitivity to glucagon and the resistance to insulin observed in the glucose intolerance of uremic subjects. If these observations on liver cell plasma membranes from uremic rats can be extrapolated to uremic humans, they suggest that chronic renal failure may be associated with receptor abnormalities involving both insulin and glucagon — hormones with potent influences on glucose homeostasis. If the number of insulin binding sites is also reduced in skeletal muscle and adipocyte cell membranes in uremic patients, then the long-observed resistance of peripheral tissues to

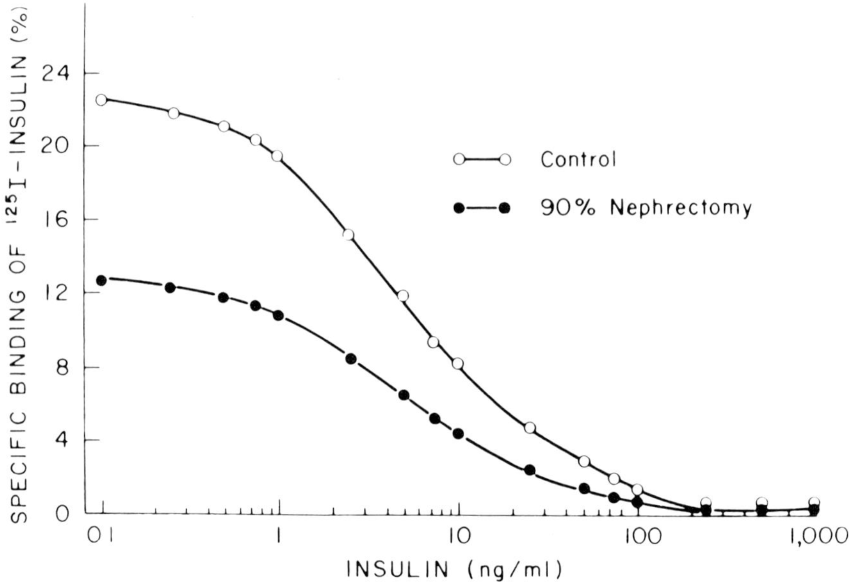

Fig. 5–2.—Binding and displacement of ^{125}I-insulin in liver plasma membranes in control and uremic rats (90% nephrectomy).

the action of insulin may be explained. If the facilitative action of insulin in promoting hepatic glucose transport is reduced markedly in cases of uremia, as this receptor data suggest, and the liver normally retains 75% of the glucose ingested during an oral glucose tolerance test, these findings partially explain why patients with renal failure demonstrate more severe disturbances in oral rather than intravenous glucose tolerance.

These alterations in hormone binding may have profound effects on fuel homeostasis in uremic patients. For example, in the liver, the major site of glucagon action, glucagon may simultaneously stimulate glycogenolysis through an adenylate-cyclase-mediated sequence of events and gluconeogenesis by facilitation of hepatic uptake of glucogenic amino acids, principally alanine.[20] Thus, receptor alterations in uremia may create a situation resembling that found in the poorly controlled diabetic patient in whom the amount of insulin is reduced and the level of glucagon increased — increased hepatic glycogenolysis, gluconeogenesis and glucose intolerance.

It is doubtful whether glucagon has any proteolytic action on skeletal muscle or lipolytic action on adipose tissue at physiologic concentrations. If, however, the number of insulin receptors in muscle is reduced, an important modulating influence on the membrane flux of amino acids will be lost, protein synthesis reduced, and proteolysis thereby indirectly enhanced. The investigations by Garber of the kinetics and production of glucose in cases of chronic renal failure have added considerably to our understanding of glucose homeostasis in uremic patients.[14] His studies indicate that despite the fact that the rate of glucose utilization is abnormally increased, it does not keep pace with the markedly enhanced rates of glucose production (Fig. 5–3).

It is interesting to speculate on whether the increased synthesis and release of alanine, the principal amino acid substrate for hepatic gluconeogenesis, from skeletal muscle found by Garber in uremic humans and animals are attributable to the combination of an increased number of membrane receptors for glucagon and a reduced number of receptors for insulin. Such a possibility is strongly suggested both by the observation from Felig's laboratory that insulin receptors may be reduced in skeletal muscle in uremic subjects, and by Garber's own finding that plasma membranes of skeletal muscle from chronically uremic rats

Fig. 5–3. – Mechanisms contributing to altered glucose kinetics in uremic patients.

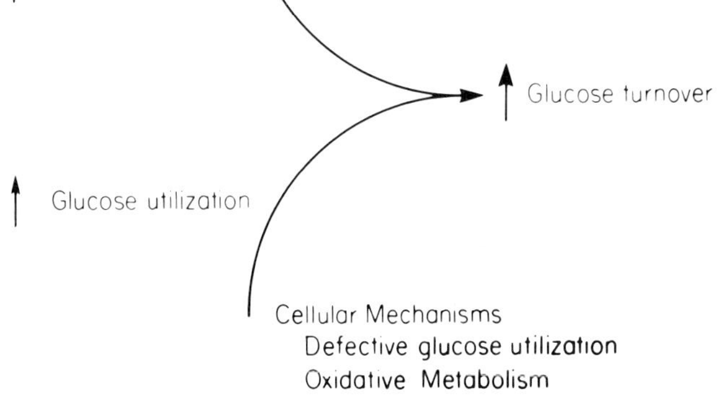

have a markedly reduced capacity (50%) to generate adenylate cyclase following stimulation with epinephrine. This latter finding suggests that intracellular levels of cyclic nucleotides may be increased as a consequence of glucagon action, and the cyclase enzyme may be secondarily reduced by feedback inhibition.

Garber's studies also suggest that elevated parathyroid hormone levels in patients with renal failure may have proteolytic effects on skeletal muscle and represent yet another humoral factor that accelerates new glucose formation. Whatever the precise mechanisms, it is clear that in chronically uremic patients there is a primary acceleration of both glucose production and utilization, and that this enhancement is derived in part from an increased rate of gluconeogenesis from alanine. Not only does an increased rate of alanine production from peripheral tissues, such as skeletal muscle, contribute to increased new glucose formation, but, in addition, there appears to be a redirection of the hepatic metabolism of alanine in uremia which preferentially increases the proportion of alanine utilized for gluconeogenesis away from other pathways of hepatic alanine disposal.

As mentioned above, Garber has shown that in patients with renal failure glucose production and utilization were both considerably increased (about 60%) prior to dialysis. Following dialysis, these parameters of glucose kinetics fell in parallel with alanine production and utilization, but between dialyses the abnormalities reappeared. Thus, hemodialysis appears to only partially correct the elevated production and utilization of glucose that characterize chronic uremia. Paradoxically, glucose intolerance in patients with renal failure seems to occur in part because the rate of glucose production exceeds the already increased rate of utilization. It is unclear why utilization is increased, but it is interesting to speculate here also that the inefficient and/or complete oxidation that might result from impaired oxidative metabolism may be contributory.[11]

Indeed, there is mounting experimental evidence suggesting that oxidative metabolism may be perturbed in cases of uremia. For example, studies with kidney slices indicate that uremic serum uncouples oxidative phosphorylation[18, 23] at the site of $NADH_2$ oxidation,[15] indicating that the generation of high-energy phosphates is inhibited during $NADH_2$ oxidation. Thus, these changes disturb the balance between adenosine triphosphate (ATP) and its metabolites (adenosine diphosphate, ADP; adenosine monophosphate, AMP; cyclic AMP; Pi), and this could serve as the stimulus for glycolysis and inhibition of gluconeogenesis. Cellular defects of this type appear to activate a number of compensatory homeostatic processes that assure a continued supply of glucose.

Why then is spontaneous hypoglycemia recognized with increasing frequency in uremic patients? It would appear that factors that upset the delicate balance between glucose production and utilization can potentially result in hypoglycemia. For example, an impairment in muscle metabolism could disturb this balance and predispose to hypoglycemia by reducing the availability of gluconeogenic amino acids for hepatic glucose production. Thus, in patients with renal failure in whom glucose turnover is increased, small changes in substrate availability may have rather profound effects on circulating glucose levels, not only during an actual fast, but even during an overnight fast when new glucose formation is generally required to maintain normal circulating glucose concentrations. Experimental evidence showing that the chronically uremic rat has reduced basal glucose and insulin levels[3] indicates that this balance is indeed upset during fasting and that glucose production cannot keep pace with the rate of utilization. In addition, after only 12 hours of fasting, the activity of phosphoenol pyruvate-carboxykinase (PEPCK), the rate-limiting enzyme in hepatic gluconeogenesis, was significantly increased, and alanine, free fatty acid and glycerol concentrations were higher than control levels in the uremic animals. These animal data are consistent with Garber's finding that glucose turnover and production are increased in both dialyzed and undialyzed patients.

The fact that pyruvate levels are elevated and pyruvate utilization is delayed in uremic patients[6] suggests that renal failure may compromise hepatic uptake and the conversion of pyruvate to phosphoenol pyruvate (PEP), a key precursor for newly formed glucose. This could also be a limiting factor in the glucose production-utilization balance. Biochemical evidence summarized by Dzurik indicates that in uremic patients a number of enzymatic abnormalities may limit the capacity of pyruvate to enter the mitochondria from its origin in the cytosol. For example, the activity of pyruvate carboxylase, an enzyme estimated to convert 90% of pyruvate to PEP, is inhibited by ADP. Thus, if a relative deficiency of high-energy phosphate is present and the ratio of ATP to ADP is altered, gluconeogenic activity may be grossly curtailed. Pyruvate carboxylase is also inactive in the absence of acetylcoenzyme A (acetyl-CoA) and the synthesis of this citric acid cycle intermediary is reduced in patients with renal failure.[11]

It is of interest that insulin inhibits the formation of both of these important gluconeogenic enzymes, pyruvate carboxylase and PEPCK. While some of the observed biochemical derangements in carbohydrate homeostasis can be explained on the basis of inadequate insulin action, it is likely that a number of other substances modulate these alterations as well. These include the guanidines,[4] but we must also consider the possibility that other heretofore poorly characterized compounds such as the polyamines (spermine, spermidine, putrescine and cadaverine), which accumulate to very high levels in patients with renal failure, may antagonize insulin action either directly or indirectly or interfere with key gluconeogenic enzyme systems.

Summary

Chronic renal failure results in a variety of metabolic derangements that perturb glucose homeostasis. These may in part result from the fact that the kidney plays a prominent role in the metabolism of insulin as well as a number of other low-molecular-weight peptide hormones that affect carbohydrate metabolism. Specific abnormalities in glucose utilization that appear to be related to alterations in membrane receptors, resulting in increased glucagon sensitivity and decreased insulin action, are a newly recognized factor in intolerance to oral glucose. Glucose production and utilization are both abnormally increased in patients with chronic uremia, and these disturbances are only partially corrected by hemodialysis treatment. The mechanism(s) contributing to these changes is unclear, but seems to involve a combination of humoral and cellular factors. These include some degree of insulin resistance, probably inadequately modulated proteolytic responses to glucagon and parathyroid hormone, and a basic defect in energy production that alters intracellular concentrations of high-energy phosphate-containing nucleotides. It is unclear whether these changes in carbohydrate tolerance pose an increased risk for the premature development of cardiovascular disease in patients with renal failure, as they appear to do in the nonuremic population. The occasional patient with renal failure may develop clinical hypoglycemia when glucose utilization continues in a setting in which the hepatic capacity to produce glucose is reduced, probably as a consequence of altered substrate delivery and/or inhibition of one or more key gluconeogenic enzymes.

References

1. Bagdade, J. D., Bierman, E. L., and Porte, D., Jr.: The significance of basal insulin levels in the elevation of the insulin response to glucose in diabetic and non-diabetic subjects, J. Clin. Invest. 46:1549, 1967.
2. Bagdade, J. D., Porte, D., Jr., and Bierman, E. L.: Hypertriglyceridemia: a metabolic consequence of chronic renal failure, N. Engl. J. Med. 269:181, 1968.
3. Bagdade, J. D., Yee, E., and Shafrir, E.: Evidence for an accelerated adaptation to starvation in chronic uremia, Metabolism 26:1107, 1977.
4. Balestri, P. L., et al.: Uremic toxins, Arch. Intern. Med. 126:843, 1970.
5. Bilbrey, G. L., Faloona, G. R., White, M. G., and Knochel, J. P.: Hyperglucagonemia of renal failure, J. Clin. Invest. 53:841, 1974.
6. Campanacci, L., et al.: Metabolic studies of acetoacetate, pyruvate, lactate and citrate in uremic acidosis, Clin. Chim. Acta 20:341, 1968.
7. De Fronzo, R. A., et al.: Carbohydrate metabolism in uremia: a review, Medicine 52: 469, 1973.
8. Duckworth, W. C., Heinemann, H., and Goessling, M.: Enzymatic mechanisms for insulin and glucagon degradation by kidney, Clin. Res. 24:359A, 1976.
9. Dzurik, R., and Valovicova, E.: Glucose utilization in muscle during uremia; in vitro study, Clin. Chim. Acta 30:137, 1970.
10. Dzurik, R., et al.: The isolation of an inhibitor of glucose utilization from the serum of uremic subjects, Clin. Chim. Acta 46:77, 1973.
11. Dzurik, R.: *Uremia: The Pathophysiology of Carbohydrate Metabolism* (Bratislava: Publishing House of the Slovak Academy of Sciences, 1973), pp. 72, 104.
12. Felig, P.: *Diabetes: Its Physiological and Biochemical Basis*, ed. J. Vallance-Owen (Baltimore: University Park Press, 1975), p. 93.
13. Furst, P., Asaba, M., and Gordon, A.: Middle molecules in uremia, Proc. Eur. Dial. Transplant Assoc. 2:417, 1974.
14. Garber, A.: Abnormalities of carbohydrate metabolism in chronic uremia, Ninth Annual Contractors' Conference: Artificial Kidney-Chronic Uremia Program, National Institute of Arthritis, Metabolism and Digestive Diseases, January 17–19, 1977, p. 3.
15. Glaze, R. P., Morgan, J. M., and Morgan, R. E.: Uncoupling of oxidative phosphorylation by ultrafiltrates of uremic serum, Proc. Soc. Exp. Biol. Med. 125:172, 1967.
16. Hampers, C. L., et al.: Effect of chronic renal failure and hemodialysis on carbohydrate metabolism, J. Clin. Invest. 45:1719, 1966.
17. Hampers, C. L., et al.: Insulin-glucose relationships in uremia, Am. J. Clin. Nutr. 21: 414, 1968.
18. Heintz, R., and Renner, D.: Über Hemmwirkugen des Serums von Kranken mit hepatorenalem Syndrom und mit chronischer Urämie auf Sauerstoffverbrauch und Kohlenhydratstoffwechsel von Nieren- und Hirngewebe der Ratte, Klin. Wochenschr. 43:1167, 1965.

19. Jaspan, J. B., Mako, M. E., Kuzuya, H., Blix, P., Horwitz, D. L., and Rubenstein, A. H.: Abnormalities in circulating beta cell peptides in chronic renal failure: comparison of C-peptide, proinsulin and insulin, J. Lab. Clin. Med. 45:441, 1977.
20. Jaspan, J. B., and Rubenstein, A. H.: Circulating glucagon: plasma profiles and metabolism in health and disease, Diabetes 26:887, 1977.
21. Kaneda, H., and Mimura, N.: Effect of dialysis treatment on glucose metabolism in uremic patients, Tohuku J. Exp. Med. 122:35, 1977.
22. Porte, D., and Bagdade, J. D.: Human insulin secretion: an integrated approach, Annu. Rev. Med. 21:219, 1970.
23. Renner, D., and Heintz, R.: Metabolic changes of kidney and brain tissue incubated in sera of chronic uremic patients, Proc. Eur. Dial. Transplant Assoc. 2:128, 1965.
24. Sherwin, R. S., *et al.*: Influence of uremia and hemodialysis on the turnover and metabolic effects of glucagon, J. Clin. Invest. 57:722, 1976.
25. Soman V., and Felig, P.: Glucagon and insulin binding to liver membranes in a partially nephrectomized uremic rat model, J. Clin. Invest. 60:224, 1977.
26. Teuscher, V. A., Frankhauser, S., and Kuffer, F. R.: Studies on carbohydrate metabolism in renal insufficiency, Klin. Wochenschr. 41:706, 1963.
27. Westervelt, F. B., and Schreiner, G. E.: The carbohydrate intolerance of uremic patients, Ann. Intern. Med. 57:266, 1962.
28. Westervelt, F. B., Jr.: Uremia and insulin response, Arch. Intern. Med. 126:865, 1968.

6

Treatment of End-Stage Renal Failure in the Insulin-Dependent Diabetic Patient

C. JACOBS, M.D., J. ROTTEMBOURG, M.D.,
P. FRANTZ, M.D., G. SLAMA, M.D., AND
M. LEGRAIN, M.D.

Service de Néphrologie, Groupe Hospitalier Pitié-Salpétrière, and Service de Diabétologie, Hôtel-Dieu, Paris, France

The population of diabetic patients with end-stage renal failure treated by regular dialysis and/or renal transplantation is rapidly increasing, notwithstanding the "sad truth" expressed some years ago about the preliminary results obtained with these methods of treatment.[9, 21] Three hundred three new diabetics were started on such treatment in Europe during 1976. They account for 3.5% of all patients with terminal renal failure who started treatment during that year.[30]

According to the policy of nonselection of patients instituted during the past five years in the Department of Nephrology of La Pitié Hospital in Paris, 32 insulin-dependent diabetic patients were treated by dialysis and/or renal transplantation between November 1972 and September 1977. They account for 10.3% of the 310 patients who were started on treatment in the center during the same period. Because of increasing pressure

Supported in part by a grant from the Association pour l'Utilisation du rein artificiel.

101

for treatment of diabetic patients, many centers may soon become involved in a similar experience. The purpose of this chapter is to outline the conditions required to optimize the results obtained from insulin-dependent diabetic patients treated by chronic dialysis and/or renal transplantation, on the basis of our personal experience and the reports available in the literature.

Patients, Methods and Results

PATIENT MATERIAL

Only four of the 36 insulin-dependent diabetics admitted to the Nephrology Department during the relevant period were excluded from treatment, either because of the severity of visceral lesions or, in two cases, because of poor psychological and environmental conditions. There were 21 men and 11 women. Mean age at commencement of treatment was 41 years (range 23 to 73). All patients had severe visceral complications associated with renal failure, as described in Table 6–1. Bilateral blindness was associated with symptoms of motor neuropathy in the lower limbs in nine patients. Before the first dialysis, the mean level of plasma creatinine was 12.6 mg/100 ml in the men and 10.3 mg/100 ml in the women.

MANAGEMENT OF DIABETES

The mode of treatment generally adopted was the following: daily caloric intake between 1,800 and 2,200 calories, with a

TABLE 6–1.—EXTRARENAL COMPLICATIONS IN 32
INSULIN-DEPENDENT DIABETIC PATIENTS WITH
END-STAGE RENAL FAILURE

COMPLICATIONS	NO. OF PATIENTS	PERCENT OF PATIENTS
Hypertension (150/95 mm Hg)	30	93.7
Previous history of myocardial infarction	5	15.6
Angina	10	31.2
Clinical symptoms of peripheral vascular disease	10	31.2
Bilateral blindness	12	37.5
Unilateral blindness	4	12.5
Clinical symptoms of motor neuropathy	12	37.5
Clinical symptoms of diabetic enteropathy	3	9.4

protein supply of at least 1 gm/kg/body weight. Daily carbohydrate intake was between 180 and 200 gm. Polyunsaturated fatty acids were given in order to increase caloric lipid intake. The effective caloric intake was actually highly variable according to overall clinical conditions. Blood glucose level was usually controlled by twice-daily injections of intermediate insulin (Rapitard). The patients or their relatives were trained to check the blood glucose concentration with an Eyetone apparatus. The usual insulin regimen was administered on the days of dialysis, with a stable glucose level maintained in the dialysis fluid. A supplement of insulin was required for patients treated with peritoneal dialysis, according to the technique described below.

TREATMENT OF RENAL FAILURE

Dialysis techniques used in the patients were hemodialysis in 28 patients and peritoneal dialysis in three. All patients except two were treated in La Pitié Hospital; 19 patients were put on the waiting list as candidates for cadaver-donor renal transplantation. Five patients received renal transplants, three from cadaver donors. This small proportion of transplanted patients was due to the scarcity of donors and also to the occurrence of frequent complications that constituted temporary contraindications to transplantation. Two patients benefited from a related living-donor kidney; and transplantation was performed without preliminary dialysis in one case.

MAINTENANCE HEMODIALYSIS. — Forty-seven vascular accesses were performed: 34 arteriovenous fistulas in the distal part of the upper limbs, five external arteriovenous shunts and eight venous homografts. Seventeen of 28 patients needed only one vascular access during their period of treatment with hemodialysis. Seventeen (50%) of the original arteriovenous fistulas have functioned during 238 patient-months. Difficulties in creating a functional vascular access and repetitive thrombosis occurred in 11 patients. Transfer to peritoneal dialysis was necessary for two of these patients.

The formula of the dialysis fluid was as follows: sodium, 138 mEq/L; potassium, 1 mEq/L; magnesium, 1.5 mEq/L; calcium, 70 mg/L. Glucose was supplied by a constant infusion pump at a rate set to keep a level of 1.20 gm/L. Various types of dialyzers were used: disposable flat plate dialyzers with cuprophane or polyacrylonitrile membranes, cuprophane coils and capillary dialyzers fitted with cellulose or cuprophane membranes. Heparin was usually supplied by continuous intravenous infusion; "minimal" heparinization (about 5,000 units per dialysis) was used for patients in whom hemorrhagic complications, especially ocular ones, were feared. The frequency of dialysis was usually thrice weekly. Duration of dialysis was between 12 and 16 hours per week, depending on the patient's weight, residual renal function and the type of dialyzer used.

PERITONEAL DIALYSIS. — This procedure was used for two different purposes. In nine patients peritoneal dialysis was carried out on a temporary basis (duration 3 – 17 days) while awaiting the proper development of a newly created vascular access for hemodialysis. In this setting, dialysis was performed with a semiautomatic apparatus, using a dialysis fluid with 15 gm glucose/L. Regular insulin diluted in human albumin was injected intravenously during dialysis with a constant infusion pump. The insulin dose was monitored according to the blood glucose level, which was checked at regular intervals with the Destrostix method.

Three patients were treated with chronic peritoneal dialysis according to the technique described by Tenckhoff, with fully automatic dialysis equipment fitted with a reverse osmosis unit.[69, 70] Glucose content of the dialysis fluid was 15 – 25 gm/L. The frequency of dialysis was twice or thrice weekly, with each dialysis session lasting 8 – 10 hours. Control of the blood glucose level during the dialysis session was achieved with a supplementary subcutaneous injection of regular insulin — approximately half of the usual morning dose.

RENAL TRANSPLANTATION. — The operative procedure and immunosuppressive therapy (azathioprine and prednisone) were identical with those used for the nondiabetic patients treated in the transplant unit. The usual doses of insulin were given in the preoperative periods. Control of blood glucose levels was achieved during and after surgery in four patients with a continuous infusion of insulin. In one patient monitoring the blood glucose level was carried out with the assistance of an artificial pancreas during transplantation and for the first 48 hours after operation. Rejection crises were treated with an intravenous bolus of methylprednisolone, 1 gm/day for three days. Continuous infusion of regular insulin was also administered with these very high doses of steroids.

RESULTS

In the 31 patients treated with dialysis, the cumulative duration of treatment was 436 patient-months. Their survival rate is shown in Figure 6–1. Six of the ten deaths occurred during the first six months of treatment. Causes of death were: two cerebrovascular accidents, one myocardial infarction, one cardiac arrythmia, one hypoglycemia, one hyperkalemia, three cachexia and one suicide.

Most complications occurred in the same patients: the overall duration of hospitalization in the nine patients who died accounted for 32% of their entire survival period. Six patients experienced pericarditis, with pericardial drainage being necessary in four.

Development of visual problems was as follows: Among the 20 patients in whom vision was more or less preserved at the start of treatment, worsening of the visual status occurred in only one following hemorrhage of the vitreous. Improvement of vision occurred in four patients, whereas it remained unchanged in 15. Visual status improved markedly in one patient within a few weeks after transplantation with a related-donor kidney. Four patients underwent operations because of cataracts complicating vitreous hemorrhages, which existed prior to dialysis treatment in three cases. Three patients had enucleation of one eye because of the development of a neovascular glaucoma.

Evolution of peripheral neuropathy was as follows: Clinical

Fig. 6–1.— Actuarial survival rates in 31 insulin-dependent diabetics and in 75 nondiabetic controls treated by maintenance hemodialysis at La Pitié Hospital in Paris (1972–77).

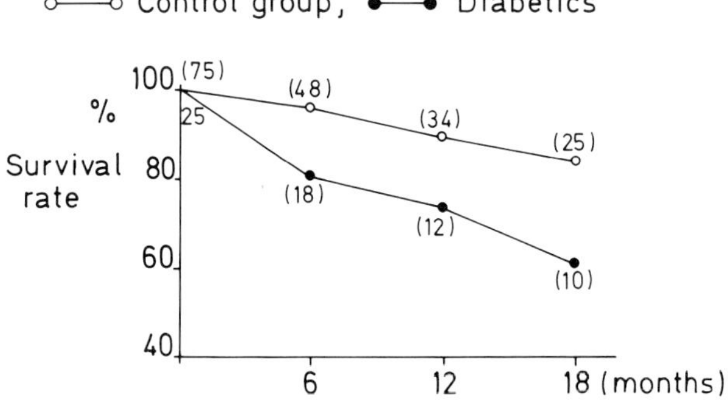

symptoms improved in nine patients and remained unchanged in 14. Motor and sensory alterations worsened in nine patients. Serial studies of motor nerve conduction velocity (MNCV) of the peroneal nerve were performed on 21 patients; stable figures were recorded in eight patients, MNCV decreased in seven patients and disappeared in five. Improvement of MNCV was seen in only one patient after 14 months of hemodialysis treatment.

Rehabilitation in dialysis patients is largely dependent on their previous clinical status. Professional occupations could be maintained in 11 patients until the final stage of their renal disease. Three of them were able to continue working while being treated by hemodialysis. Partial rehabilitation could be achieved by three more patients. Eighteen patients (64%) needed permanent assistance to carry out the basic acts of daily life, 13 because they were bilaterally blind and three because of severe motor neuropathy.

Three of the five transplanted patients are currently active with normal renal function, the longest follow-up period being seven months. Two transplantations have failed. In one case a vascular operative complication led to immediate removal of the graft. In the other patient, hemodialysis had to be resumed ten days after transplantation because of irreversible rejection. No urologic, infectious or metabolic complications related to the diabetic state have been recorded. A significant improvement of vision was observed in one patient who was able to resume her work six months after transplantation, after having been obliged to stay idle during the 15 months of dialysis treatment that preceded renal transplantation.

Requirements and Difficulties

Epidemiologic Aspects

According to several surveys carried out in the United States during the last 15 years, which were recently confirmed by Palumbo et al.,[54] the overall incidence of diabetes in the general population is 1.6%. The yearly incidence of insulin-dependent diabetes is 14 per 100,000 in the population group aged 6–18 years.[35, 42, 54] The prevalence of renal disease in diabetes is variously estimated according to the clinical or pathologic criteria adopted by different authors. Clinical diagnosis of diabetic nephropathy was made in 8% of the 30,000 patients admitted to the New England Deaconess Hospital in Boston between 1958 and 1965. The mortality attributed to renal disease in the 6,800 diabetic patients who were followed at the Joslin Clinic and died between 1956 and 1964 was 6%. Renal disease is responsible for 50% of all deaths in patients in whom diabetes is diagnosed before the age of 20.[3]

Extrapolating these data, it is estimated that there are approximately 800,000 diabetics in France, of whom at least 70,000 are insulin-dependent, with 7,000 new juvenile insulin-dependent diabetics each year. Close to 200 new patients reach the final stage of chronic renal failure each year and thus are eligible for dialysis and/or renal transplantation. They account for almost 8% of all new patients with end-stage renal failure seen each year. Mortality from renal disease in maturity-onset diabetics is much lower, but no precise figures are presently available. Because the increment of facilities permits a wider extension of the treatment of end-stage renal disease, the systematic exclusion of insulin-dependent diabetics from dialysis therapy and/or renal transplantation can no longer be justified. Such an attitude must be replaced by a meticulous analysis of the risk factors in each patient, in order to select the most appropriate strategy of treatment.

RISK FACTORS

Insulin-dependent diabetic patients with end-stage renal failure are always "high-risk" patients because of the numerous visceral lesions generally associated with the renal disease. The vascular risk related to the extension of micro- and macroangiopathy is the most prominent.

Almost all patients are hypertensive, some very severely. Adequate treatment of hypertension is often very difficult; renal failure increases the risk of overdoses of antihypertensive drugs and more frequent side effects, particularly from α-methyldopa and clonidine. Beta-blockers are contraindicated because of their interference with glucose metabolism.[61] Hydralazine may worsen clinical symptoms of coronary insufficiency. Hemodynamic instability is often present and may worsen during dialysis sessions. The variability in blood pressure levels often plays a part in rapid loss of vision and favors cerebrovascular or cardiac disorders. Left ventricular failure secondary to hypertension and to extended coronary lesions may render hemodialysis unsuitable and make peritoneal dialysis a better choice.

Visual impairment is the result of multiple causes: diabetic and hypertensive lesions of the retina, alterations of the lens and, especially, hemorrhages of the vitreous. Rapid deterioration of vision often occurs during the terminal phase of renal failure. Bilateral blindness is already established in almost one third of the diabetic patients considered for dialysis or transplantation. Loss of vision is the most dramatic complication directly related to poor control of diabetes and/or blood pressure.

Extended arterial atheroma, particularly when affecting the limbs or the abdominal vessels, may interfere with the treatment of renal failure. Creation of vascular access for hemodialysis may be impossible, efficiency of peritoneal dialysis may be limited[50] and vascular anastomoses required in renal transplantation may be difficult to perform. Ischemic lesions in the lower limbs may sometimes be more disabling than neuropathy, and amputations have to be performed frequently.[47, 48, 77]

Neurologic manifestations are common. Discrimination between diabetes and uremia in the genesis of peripheral neuropathy is often difficult. Decrease or loss of deep-tendon reflexes is often associated with superficial or deep sensory alterations. Values of MNCV (usually tested in the common peroneal nerve) are decreased in almost all patients, or MNCV may not be detectable at all.[5, 8]

Involvement of the autonomic nervous system is very frequent and must be checked routinely. The responses to the Valsalva maneuver and to the sustained handgrip test, as described by Ewing,[18] were found to be significantly lower in 13 diabetics compared with 26 nondiabetic patients treated by maintenance hemodialysis in the same center. Autonomous neuropathy is partly responsible for the hemodynamic instability as well as for alterations in urodynamics. Incomplete emptying and distension of the bladder may be initially very insidious. Stagnation of infected urine in the bladder may lead to life-threatening complications. Careful investigation of bladder function is mandatory, especially for renal transplantation candidates; diagnosis is best established by cystometry and a voiding cystogram. These investigations may lead to complications and should not be performed unless adequate urologic facilities are available.

Malnutrition, often present in diabetic patients, increases with the progression of renal failure. The loss in dry weight is often masked by overhydration. Malnutrition is of multiple origin.[11, 53] Loss of appetite is frequent. Too often, however, rigid dietary regimens prescribed to minimize biolipidemia and hyperazotemia result in inadequate caloric intake. A reduction of the daily requirements of insulin during reduced caloric intake may be misinterpreted as a favorable event. Urinary protein loss secondary to renal disease and autonomic enteropathy may both contribute to the decrease of plasma protein levels.

The multiple restraints of severe renal failure also increase the psychologic burdens and social handicaps of patients with diabetes. The progressive or abrupt occurrence of numerous complications, particularly loss of vision, may interfere with professional activities and social life. Rebellion against prescriptions or depressive reactions expressed by refusal of treatment or of dietary restrictions increase the risk of major complications and make dialysis treatment or transplantation more difficult.

The multiple risk factors of diabetes emphasize the importance of performing the necessary investigations in an early phase, before the occurrence of acute complications. The ophthalmologist, neurologist, psychiatrist, cardiologist, urologist and others should be consulted in order to have all possible ancillary complications adequately investigated. Close coordination for complementary investigations is required, since some may be potentially dangerous, such as exploration of the lower urinary tract or coronary angiography.[16, 36]

The psychosocial history of the patient and family should be known by the physician, since the success or failure of future treatments often depends on the patient's psychologic and material environment.

Exclusion from dialysis treatment should be exceptional if facilities are available. Such a decision was made only four times among the 36 patients who were referred to our department. In our mind, refusal of treatment can be justified only if the diabetic complications are incompatible with the prolongation of life in the near future, or if the social context will doom the patient to complete solitude.

Methods of Therapy

MAINTENANCE HEMODIALYSIS

SURVIVAL. — The regular improvement in the results obtained with dialysis techniques in insulin-dependent diabetics contrasts favorably with the dismal figures published some years ago.[59] In Avram's group, the one-year survival rate of diabetic patients increased from 50% to 72% between 1966 and 1976.[1] A similar trend is noted by Comty et al.[10] The best results reported to date are those by Ma and co-workers, with a one-year survival rate of 86% in 18 patients.[40] One should be cautious in drawing conclusions from the comparison of the results obtained in different series because of possible disparities in age, in the severity of diabetes and in techniques of treatment. For example, an increase in mortality may result from pretransplantation surgical procedures that are performed routinely by some groups.[48, 63]

In spite of the improved results, the increased mortality related to diabetics as compared with other hemodialysis patients persists. This fact is well illustrated in our own series. The one-year survival rate of dialyzed diabetics is 73.6% as compared with 88% in a control group of patients matched for sex and age and treated in the same center (see Fig. 6 – 1). A similar difference was noted at one year and two years after the start of dialysis in the latest statistics available from the European Dialysis and Transplant Association Report.[24] These disparities in survival rate are nevertheless moderate, and do not justify the exclusion of diabetic patients from dialysis programs.

CAUSES OF DEATH. — Causes do not differ markedly from those recorded in nondiabetic patients. In several reports, cardiovascular accidents account for 40 – 60% of the deaths.[10, 59, 63] Mortality from infections (15 – 25%) is lessening as septicemia secondary to infections of vascular access sites becomes less frequent.[10] Metabolic deaths (hyperkalemia or hypoglycemia) are not unusual. Irreversible cachexia may result from malnutrition, which is usually already present before dialysis treatment has begun. Extremely poor overall clinical status may lead some patients to suicide, either by discontinuing dialysis or by committing massive dietary abuses.[31]

Morbidity remains high. Prolonged periods of hospitalization may be necessary for some patients: for example, one of our patients has spent his whole time of survival (259 days) in the hospital because of numerous complications, mainly ischemic lesions of the lower limbs!

COMPLICATIONS. — Complications at vascular access sites have become less frequent since arteriovenous fistulas are created more proximally. Improved longevity of vascular accesses may be obtained with the use of prostheses of animal or industrial origin.[10] Pericarditis occurs with increased frequency in diabetics, and our experience is in accordance with the data reported by Ma *et al.* and Comty *et al.*[10, 40] Overhydration and malnutrition are the two factors most commonly involved in the origin of this complication.

Preservation of visual status is essential to the quality of life of the diabetic patient. The detrimental influence on vision of hemodynamic instability and of the heparin administration required for hemodialysis are among the strongest arguments for preferring renal transplantation[44, 66] or peritoneal dialysis[60, 72] to hemodialysis in treating diabetic patients. Our experience, however, seems to indicate that the loss of vision during hemodialysis treatment is far from inevitable. Stabilization or even improvement of vision may be obtained with hemodialysis associated with adequate control of blood pressure. The detrimental role of heparin, often emphasized to explain the outburst of vitreous hemorrhages, is questionable; indeed, prevention of these hemorrhagic complications has been obtained with subcutaneous injections of heparin.[58] Heparin and platelet aggregation inhibitors may have a positive action against the intravascular coagulation phenomena that occur in the eye and may be responsible for bleeding.

Peripheral neuropathy of diabetic and/or renal origin is almost invariably present in patients at the beginning of dialysis treatment; and worsening of neuropathy during dialysis is frequently reported.[5, 47] On the other hand, clinical improvement of neuropathy may be seen, even with persistently low or even undetectable values of MNCV. Improvement of neuropathy usually accompanies an amelioration of the overall clinical status. The precise reasons for the improvement of neuropathy remain unclear. In our experience, improvement of nerve conduction velocities or of clinical symptoms of neuropathy cannot be related solely to an increase of weekly dialysis time or to the use of dialysis membranes, such as polyacrylonitrile, which are highly permeable to middle-molecular-weight substances.

PREREQUISITES FOR IMPROVEMENT OF RESULTS.—The increase in survival and the reduction in morbidity recorded during the last years are encouraging. A critical analysis of the complications associated with renal failure emphasizes the factors that should be managed with special care in diabetic patients.

In vascular access, careful preoperative evaluation is necessary to select the site and technique most appropriate to insure adequate blood flow in spite of diffuse atheromatous lesions. Surgery should be performed at an early stage, since adequate enlargement of the veins may take place slowly. Vessels of the lower limbs should not be considered for vascular access. Arteriovenous fistulas should be created, as a rule more proximally than for nondiabetic patients, either with the radial or the ulnar artery at the upper part of the forearm. The lower segment of the brachial artery should be used with caution because of the danger of distal ischemia.

End-to-end or end-to-side vascular anastomoses should be performed by ligation of the arterial segment distal to the fistula in order to avoid an arterial "steal" syndrome and ischemic accidents, with possible gangrene of the fingers.[7] Detection of vascular calcification should be noted prior to surgery with soft tissue radiography. Angiography of arteries and veins may be necessary to select the proper operative site and procedure. Preoperative detection of hypercoagulability is mandatory; if present, surgery is performed while the patient is treated with small doses of heparin. If emergency dialysis is required and there is no time for a vascular access to develop adequately, peritoneal dialysis is preferable to the insertion of arteriovenous cannulas, which carry a high risk of infection and/or thrombosis.

Adequate preoperative and operative management assures successful arteriovenous fistulas in 50% of cases. In contrast, if this first attempt turns out to be a failure, it is often the initial phase of a long story of misfortunes.[57, 71, 73]

The dialysis session is often complicated by incidents, mainly sharp decreases in blood pressure, which occur more frequently in diabetic than in nondiabetic patients.[14] The increased risk of hypertension related to the use of large-surface-area dialyzers must be taken into account when selecting the type of dialyzer for the diabetic patient. Capillary fiber dialyzers should not be considered the best choice if one wishes to reduce to a minimum the doses of heparin infused during dialysis. Ultrafiltration should be smooth and progressive. Continuous recording of the volume of fluid ultrafiltrated from the patient or the monitoring of body weight with a bed scale is most useful.

The blood glucose level should remain stable and close to normal on dialysis days in order to avoid acute osmolar shifts, which contribute to hemodynamic instability. The glucose content of the dialysis fluid varies according to different groups: we provide 1.2 gm/L, but higher concentrations (2 – 2.50 gm/L) are preferred by others.[63, 73, 74] Conversely, some groups use glucose-free dialysate,[40, 57, 71] which increases the loss of amino acids through the dialysis membrane.[11] Continuous recording of blood glucose levels during dialysis shows that in a closed-circuit system 80 – 100 gm glucose is lost during a dialysis session; this amount is even greater when an open circuit is used. This loss of glucose during dialysis may induce acute variations in the blood glucose level of the patient, increasing the risk of hypoglycemia in spite of the oral glucose usually supplied during dialysis.

Dietary and insulin prescriptions must be tailored to the glucose content of the dialysate. The blood glucose level must be checked before, if necessary during, and after dialysis with a miniature apparatus (Eyetone). Should severe hyperglycemia be present at the start of dialysis (74 gm/L), the infusion of a hypertonic solution of mannitol may be necessary to avoid a dysequilibrium syndrome, with intracellular overhydration and drop of blood pressure.[63] The potassium content of the dialysate has to be adjusted to the patient's plasma potassium and glucose levels at the start of dialysis. These numerous precautionary measures illustrate the "personalized" dialysis technique necessary for each diabetic patient.

Dialysis modifies the hormonal and metabolic balance of the patient.[26, 49] Determinations of the plasma insulin level at the arterial and venous sites of the dialyzer suggest that some insulin crosses the dialysis membrane. The usually high level of plasma growth hormone falls during dialysis and returns to its predialysis value within about two hours after the end of treatment. The decrease in the amount of plasma triglycerides during dialysis is followed by a return to predialysis values a few hours after completion of dialysis; these variations are attributed to the activation of lipoprotein-lipase by the heparin infused during dialysis.[1]

A thrice-weekly dialysis schedule allows better control of homeostasis and a larger protein intake. The choice between home and hospital dialysis varies according to the patient. Except for one case, all our patients have been treated in the hospital. Some authors, however, advocate home dialysis; almost 10% of patients in the large series reported by Comty *et al.*[10] and by Slifkin *et al.*[68] were dialyzed at home, with no increase in mortality compared with hospital dialysis patients. These data demonstrate that home dialysis in the diabetic patient is feasible, provided adequate selection is made.

Dietary regimens to be followed during interdialytic intervals must be very accurately formulated. Daily protein intake should never be less than 1 gm/kg body weight, with a daily caloric intake ranging between 35 and 40 calories/kg body weight. In order to attain this goal, a daily ration of 300–350 gm carbohydrate is recommended by some groups.[11] Our patients usually ingest 200 gm carbohydrate per day. A considerable increase in insulin requirement usually becomes necessary because of the increased food intake made possible by adequate dialysis. The daily dose of insulin is usually administered by two injections of intermediate-acting insulin.

The diabetic patient treated by dialysis is exposed to two major metabolic hazards: overhydration secondary to thirst induced by severe hyperglycemia and acute hyperkalemia which may be associated with acute hyperglycemia, the latter remaining clinically undetected in the absence of polyuria.[23, 31]

The most effective prevention of the numerous complications that appear and rapidly worsen during the last months or weeks before the beginning of dialysis treatment is initiation of dialysis at a sufficiently early phase. Dialysis should be commenced in diabetic patients when creatinine clearance is about 10 ml/minute. Dialysis is often the only way to improve the patient's nutritional status and achieve an efficient control of blood pressure.

PERITONEAL DIALYSIS

The improvements introduced by Tenckhoff[6, 19, 46, 60, 70] to the technique of chronic peritoneal dialysis have extended its applicability to a wider selection of patients, including some with diabetes. The technique currently used is identical with the one carried out in nondiabetic patients. We prefer a fully automatic system that provides dialysis fluid by mixing proportions of a concentrate of electrolytes and tap water processed by a reverse osmosis unit. The weekly dialysis schedule is usually three sessions, lasting 12 hours each. Standard dialysate contains 15 gm glucose/L; 5 – 15 gm/L may be added to increase the removal of water. Forty to 50 L dialysate is necessary for each session. The replacement of glucose by fructose or sorbitol has been proposed. Sorbitol has not proved satisfactory because of alterations in the patients' state of consciousness.[6] Advantages of using fructose have not thus far been clearly demonstrated.[55]

Peritoneal clearance rates usually permit patients to keep an adequate nitrogen and electrolyte balance. Results may become unsatisfactory if widespread atherosclerotic lesions interfere with peritoneal transfer capacity[50] or if alterations in peritoneal permeability occur after a prolonged period of treatment. Conversely, the clearances of urea, creatinine and phosphorus may significantly increase with the use of drugs, such as platelet aggregation inhibitors taken orally[41] or vasodilators administered intraperitoneally.[51] Adequate control of the blood glucose level during peritoneal dialysis may be difficult to achieve. The glucose load transferred into the patient is high but variable, depending on the permeability of the peritoneal membrane to glucose, which is different in each patient. According to Crossley and Kjellstrand,[13] several authors add insulin to the dialysate; errors in insulin dosage, infection at the injection site and severe hypoglycemic reactions occurring a few hours after completion of dialysis have been encountered with this procedure. In accordance with Huang et al.[28] and White et al,[74] we prefer to give the patient a supplementary subcutaneous injection of regular insulin during dialysis. The additional amount of insulin required is usually 50% of the morning dose; adjustment of the insulin dose is made according to the level of serial blood glucose determinations. The use of an artificial pancreas during dialysis has been advocated.[37, 74]

Food intake is often poor during dialysis sessions, in part because of increased intra-abdominal tension. Protein requirements are, on the other hand, increased by the obligatory loss of albumin (1 gm/L on the average) in the dialysis fluid. Supplementation of amino acids via the oral or parenteral route may be necessary.

The results obtained to date from chronic peritoneal dialysis in diabetic patients encompass only a small series.[59, 60] The absence of acute hemodynamic fluctuations during dialysis and the absence of heparin administration may account for the better preservation of vision reported in patients treated by chronic peritoneal dialysis, at least over a short period of observations.[60, 72] Electromyographic and clinical symptoms of neuropathy may worsen.[60] A close follow-up of the usual parameters is necessary for early detection of "underdialysis."

The incidence of peritonitis is comparable in diabetic and nondiabetic patients treated with chronic peritoneal dialysis, ranging from 0.27% to 1.14%. If present, the clinical course of peritonitis is usually very severe and the death rate is high.[46] The overall mortality of diabetics treated with chronic peritoneal dialysis remains high: 25% after one year in the 12 patients reported by Rubin *et al.*[60] Five of the ten patients who died in the series of Blumenkrantz *et al.* died within the first six months after the start of treatment.[6]

These results must be interpreted with the cognizance that most diabetic patients treated with peritoneal dialysis have been relatively elderly, poor-risk subjects, who were often excluded from hemodialysis and transplantation programs because of major complications. Improvement in the results obtained with peritoneal dialysis may be anticipated by earlier commencement of treatment.

RENAL TRANSPLANTATION

The experience accumulated during the last decade by several transplantation groups, especially Najarian *et al.*, illustrates the efficacy of renal transplantation as a treatment of end-stage renal failure in diabetic patients.[22, 25, 32, 38, 39, 47, 48, 56, 76] Fears of the deleterious effects of prolonged high-dose steroid therapy in the management of diabetes have not been confirmed. The higher rate of complications, especially infections, noted in transplanted diabetic patients does not militate against this method of treatment, which often turns out to be the best.

SELECTION OF THE DONOR. — More than 70% of transplantations reported in the largest series were performed with living related-donor kidneys.[48, 77] This choice is influenced by the desire to do the transplant in the diabetic patient as rapidly as possible and under the best technical conditions. Early transplantation is advocated to prevent deterioration of the clinical status, particularly vision, which may take place during chronic dialysis treatment. The mean interval between the first dialysis and transplantation has been only three months in 111 patients transplanted by Najarian's group.[48] Twenty-one patients underwent renal transplantation without preliminary dialysis treatment.

The choice of a living donor to provide an organ for transplantation into an insulin-dependent diabetic patient may be difficult ethically. Is it suitable to submit a healthy subject to the physical and moral risks related to the removal of an organ to benefit a patient whose life expectancy is presently at best 50% after five years? Conversely, is one allowed to deny the voluntary gift of an organ which offers the best chances of prolonged and comfortable survival to the diabetic patient? In our group, we accept the gift of a kidney from an HL-A identical sibling, and also from parents for their offspring. Presently, most of our diabetic patients are registered on the waiting list for a cadaver-donor kidney.

SURGERY AND THERAPY. — The operative procedure is identical with the one used for nondiabetic patients. In case of extensive atheromatous lesions, endarterectomy of the iliac artery may be necessary prior to the insertion of the graft.[64]

The regimen of immunosuppressive therapy for the recipient is the same as for other transplanted patients, including rejection crises. The high doses of steroids necessary during the first days after transplantation and to reverse rejection episodes may cause acute changes in blood glucose concentration or even ketosis. Hyperglycemia may simulate rejection crises and lead to erroneous therapeutic measures.[43] Intravenous infusion of insulin may be required at times to insure adequate control of the blood glucose level. The temporary use of an external artificial pancreas can keep blood glucose levels within normal limits with low doses of insulin. Continuous normal blood glucose levels may thus be obtained during and after transplantation.

Except during emergencies, as previously mentioned, diabetes may be managed without major difficulties. More effective control of diabetes after transplantation is associated with more liberal food intake and the return to normal of insulin metabolism.[53, 77] Close control of diet is necessary to avoid obesity, with polyphagia being a side effect of steroid therapy. Daily requirements of insulin are commonly 50–60% higher than those during the period of dialysis treatment.

QUALITY OF RESULTS. — The survival rates are always lower in diabetics than in nondiabetic patients. The increase in mortality reported, however, remains small. The survival rate in the patients transplanted by Najarian and co-workers was 89% after one year for HL-A-identical living-donor kidney recipients, 78% for nonidentical living-donor graft recipients, and 68% for patients transplanted with cadaver-donor kidneys.[48] The respective survival rates after three years are 73%, 69% and 58%. Similar figures are reported in the series of Mitchell[47] and Zincke *et al.*[77] Mortality increases with age in all kidney recipients, except those transplanted with HL-A-identical kidneys. Infections and vascular accidents account for the increase in mortality: 27% of deaths in the series reported by Najarian *et al.*[48] and 50% of the patients of Zincke *et al.*[77] are of cardiac or cerebrovascular origin.

Failure of the graft is more frequent in diabetics than in other transplant recipients during the first two years after transplantation. This disparity seems to become less apparent afterward. In the patients reported by Zincke *et al.*,[77] 72% of the living-donor grafts and 40% of the cadaver-donor grafts were functioning three years after transplantation. These positive results are in contrast to those reported by other groups who have had less experience in renal transplantation in diabetics; graft survival rate was 31% at one year and 25% at two years in 118 diabetic patients who had received kidney grafts in various transplantation centers in Europe prior to 1976.[24]

The quality of life offered by transplantation also deserves consideration. Periods of hospitalization are short. After an average postoperative hospitalization period ranging from 19 to 35 days, the mean duration of hospitalization during the first two years after transplantation was 15 days per year.[66] Socioprofessional rehabilitation better than that which existed prior to transplantation may be achieved in more than 70% of the diabetics who have a functioning transplant. Full-time or part-time employment, however, was possible in only 30–40% of patients.[27, 65] Clinical improvement of peripheral neuropathy is often striking,[29, 47, 48, 75] and walking may become possible again for patients who were unable to do so previously. Visual status may also be improved after transplantation, provided the transplant was performed before irreversible lesions occurred. Improvement of vision is recorded in 15–25% of patients; stabilization is more frequent. Deterioration of vision related to the development of cataracts may be managed efficiently by appropriate surgery.

COMPLICATIONS. — Various complications may occur. Those related to the surgical procedure are often severe; ureteral necrosis, bladder leaks and wound infections are recorded with a higher frequency than in nondiabetics.[47, 66] Vascular complications, myocardial infarctions and cerebrovascular accidents account for the increase in morbidity compared with nondiabetic patients. Extension of peripheral vascular lesions may lead to amputation in 20–50% of the patients who survive more than one year after transplantation.[47, 48, 71, 77] Complications are similar to those recorded during dialysis treatment, and are more often related to preexisting vascular lesions than to the consequences of operation or immunosuppressive drugs.

The recurrence of lesions of diabetic nephropathy in patients with transplanted kidneys has been demonstrated in recent studies. Arteriolar hyalinosis in the afferent and efferent glomerular vessels is found as soon as one year after transplantation and is almost invariably present after three years. No detrimental effect on kidney function has been attributed so far to these vascular lesions. Development of typical nodular glomerulosclerosis is, however, exceptional.[44] Immunopathologic studies demonstrate the development shortly after transplantation of linear staining of IgG and albumin on glomerular and tubular basement membranes, as well as on Bowman's capsules. Typical pathologic lesions of diabetic nephropathy have been shown to occur in a graft inserted into a patient who was not diabetic prior to transplantation and in whom steroid-induced diabetes mellitus developed after transplantation.[15]

Transplantation is an experimental model of great interest for the investigation of the pathogenesis and the early aspects of diabetic nephropathy. The clinical incidence of histologic recurrence may be considered so far as negligible for the patient, and should not interfere with the decision of treating diabetic patients with renal transplantation.

The Choice Between Dialysis and Transplantation

The decision whether or not transplantation is suitable for the patient should result from extensive investigations carried out when creatinine clearance is about 15 ml/minute.

Are there major contraindications to renal transplantation? We, as a rule, adopt the following attitude. The operative mortality is higher when the recipient is more than 50 years old, except if transplantation is performed with an HL-A-identical kidney. Moreover, the benefits from transplantation are less evident in older patients than in those in the younger age groups. All other factors that may increase the risks of mortality or morbidity should also be considered, e.g., abnormalities of the urinary tract, infections and other complications.

In the absence of contraindications, transplantation without preliminary dialysis treatment is the best choice. However, we were able to follow this strategy only once in our group of patients.

Related living-donor kidney transplantation offers the best chance of good results and provides the best conditions for adequate planning. For ethical, logistic and immunologic reasons, this choice is only rarely possible.

Results obtained with cadaver-donor transplantation are comparable to those with chronic hemodialysis or peritoneal dialysis. Both methods of treatment yield a higher mortality in diabetic than in nondiabetic patients. A better quality of life and a frequent striking improvement of neurologic and visual symptoms are the prominent factors in favor of transplantation. However, dialysis treatment is often the only possible therapy because of the persistent shortage of cadaver kidneys. Registration on the waiting list for cadaver-kidney transplantation should be discussed with the patient at regular intervals, and decisions should be modified according to the results obtained with dialysis treatment.

Conclusions

Insofar as facilities are available, the exclusion of insulin-dependent diabetic patients with end-stage renal failure from dialysis therapy and/or renal transplantation is no longer acceptable. In Europe, as in the United States, loss of renal function occurs in four new insulin-dependent patients per million population each year. Thorough analysis of each case is mandatory in order to select the most appropriate among well-defined strategies of treatment.

Steady improvement has been obtained in the results of treatment of end-stage renal failure in diabetic patients. This trend should continue with more effective prevention of visual, neurologic and vascular complications. These are often the result of a negative attitude taken toward the patient during the development of renal failure secondary to diabetes. Multidisciplinary cooperation involving diabetologist, nephrologist and ophthalmologist is mandatory as soon as creatinine clearance is down to 30 ml/minute. The entire future strategy of treatment should be considered from this stage, with special emphasis on the nutritional status and adequate control of blood glucose and blood pressure levels. Progression of renal impairment is often rapid, with complete loss of renal function usually occurring within one year.

Chronic dialysis should be started or renal transplantation carried out when creatinine clearance is about 10 ml/minute, before irreversible complications, mainly visual, occur. All available techniques should be considered: living- or cadaver-donor kidney transplantation, center or home hemodialysis or peritoneal dialysis. The medical and social context of each patient, as well as the logistics in a given country, have to be taken into account for the ultimate choice between the various methods of treatment.

The best chances of prolonged survival and the best quality of life are offered by living related-donor kidney transplantation performed at an early stage, thus obviating the necessity for dialysis treatment. This scheme is realized much less frequently in Europe than in the United States, and only cadaver-donor transplantation may actually be considered for many patients. The complications, especially vascular, that occur during the prolonged waiting periods necessary to obtain a compatible organ may seriously interfere with the results of transplantation, once it has been performed.

Treatment by hemodialysis or peritoneal dialysis may offer long periods of survival and an acceptable quality of life. The conditions of successful treatment are well defined. No exceptional technology is required, but a very close follow-up of the clinical and metabolic status of the patients and great care in the technical aspects of treatment are mandatory.

The treatment of insulin-dependent diabetic patients contributes to the improvement in the quality of the medical care provided to the whole population of patients with end-stage renal failure.

Acknowledgments

We express our thanks to the medical team and to the nurses of the Dialysis and Transplantation Units of La Pitié Hospital who care for the diabetic patients, to Doctor El Shahat for collecting many documents, and also to Doctor Merouani and Mrs. Delage who monitored the blood glucose control of many patients with the artificial pancreas. We are deeply indebted to Mrs. Debrun for preparing the manuscript.

References

1. Avram, M. M., Lipner, M. I., Sadiquali, R., Lancu, M., and Gan, A. C.: Metabolic changes in diabetic uremic patients on hemodialysis, Trans. Am. Soc. Artif. Intern. Organs 22:412, 1976.
2. Bale, G. S., and Antmacher, P. S.: Estimated life expectancy of diabetics, Diabetes 26:437, 1977.
3. Balodimos, M. C.: Diabetic nephropathy, in Marble, A., White, P., Bradley, R. F., and Krall, L. P. (eds.): *Joslin's Diabetes Mellitus* (Philadelphia: Lea & Febiger, 1971), pp. 526–61.
4. Blagg, C. R.: Visual and vascular problems in diabetic dialyzed patients, Kidney Int. 6:S27, 1974.
5. Blagg, C. R., Tenckhoff, H., and Scribner, B. H.: Neuropathy in diabetic dialyzed patients, Kidney Int. 6: S86, 1974.
6. Blumenkrantz, M. J., Shapiro, D. J., Mimura, N., Oreopoulos, D. G., Friedler, R. M., Levin, S., Tenckhoff, H., and Coburn, J. W.: Maintenance peritoneal dialysis as an alternative in the patient with diabetic mellitus and end-stage uremia, Kidney Int. 6:S108, 1974.
7. Buselmeier, T. J., Najarian, J. S., Simmons, R. L., Ratazzi, L. C., von Hartitzsch, B., Callender, C. O., Goetz, F. C., and Kjellstrand, C. M.: A. V. Fistulas and the diabetic: ischemia and gangrene may result in the amputation, Trans. Am. Soc. Artif. Intern. Organs 19:49, 1973.
8. Castaigne, P., Cathala, H. P., Beaussart-Boulanger, L., and Petrover, M.: Effect of ischemia on peripheral nerve function in patients with chronic renal failure undergoing dialysis treatment, J. Neurol. Neurosurg. Psychiatry 35:631, 1972.
9. Chazan, B. T., Pees, S. B., Balodimos, M. C., Younger, D., and Ferguson, B. D.: Dialysis in diabetics. A review of 44 patients, J.A.M.A. 209:2026, 1969.
10. Comty, C. M., Kjellsen, D., and Shapiro, F. L.: A reassessment of the prognosis of diabetic patients treated by chronic hemodialysis therapy, Trans. Am. Soc. Artif. Intern. Organs 22:404, 1976.

11. Comty, C. M., Leonard, A., and Shapiro, F. L.: Nutritional problems in the dialyzed patients with diabetes mellitus, Kidney Int. 6:S51, 1974.

12. Comty, C. M., Leonard, A., and Shapiro, F. L.: Psychosocial problems in dialyzed diabetic patients, Kidney Int. 6:S 144, 1974.

13. Crossley, K., and Kjellstrand, C. M.: Intraperitoneal insulin for control of blood sugar in diabetic patients during peritoneal dialysis, Br. Med. J. 1:269, 1970.

14. Degoulet, P., Rojas, P., Boukari, M., Aime, F., and Reach, I.: Accident hypotensif de la séance d'hémodialyse. Etude épidémiologique et recherche des facteurs de risque, in Küss, R., and Legrain, M. (eds.): *Séminaires d'Uro-Nephrologie Pitié-Salpétrière* (Paris: Masson), in press.

15. Doud, R., Lee, D. B. N., Waisman, J., and Bergstein, J. M.: Development of a lesion resembling diabetic nephropathy in a renal homograft, Arch. Intern. Med. 137:945, 1977.

16. Draskoczy, S. P., Leland O. S., and Bradley, R. F.: Aortocoronary by-pass in the diabetic patient, Kidney Int. 6:S 37, 1974.

17. Ellenberg, M.: Neuropathy in long standing insulin dependent diabetic patients, Kidney Int. 6:S 77, 1974.

18. Ewing, D. J., Burt, A. A., Williams, I. R., Campbell, I. W., and Clarke, B. F.: Peripheral motor nerve function in diabetic autonomic neuropathy, J. Neurol. Neurosurg. Psychiatry 39:453, 1976.

19. Finkelstein, F. O., Kliger, A. S., Bastl, C., Yap, P., and Goffinet, J.: Chronic peritoneal dialysis in diabetic patients with end-stage renal failure, Proc. Clin. Dial. Transplant Forum 5:142, 1975.

20. Funck-Brentano, J. L., Sausse, A., Man, N. K., Granger, A., Rondon-Nucette, M., Zingraff, J., and Jungers, P.: Une nouvelle méthode d'hémodialyse associant une membrane à haute perméabilité pour les moyennes molécules et un bain de dialyse en circuit fermé, Proc. Eur. Dial. Transplant Assoc. 9:55, 1972.

21. Ghavamian, M., Gutch, C. F., Kopp, K. F., and Kolff, W. J.: The sad truth about hemodialysis in diabetic nephropathy, J.A.M.A. 222:1386, 1974.

22. Ghosh, P., and Evans, D. B.: Renal transplantation in patients with insulin-dependent diabetes, Lancet 2:208, 1974.

23. Goldfarb, S., Cox, M., Singer, I., and Golberg, M.: Acute hyperkalemia induced by hyperglycemia: hormonal mechanisms, Ann. Intern. Med. 84:426, 1976.

24. Gurland, H. J., Brunner, F. P., Chantler, C., Jacobs, C., Schärer, K., Selwood, N. H., Spies, B., and Wing, A. J.: Combined report on regular dialysis and transplantation in Europe, Proc. Eur. Dial. Transplant Assoc. 12:3, 1976.

25. Habal, M. B., Birtch, A. G., Kountz, S. L., Stephans, B., and Murray, J. E.: Renal allografting in the patients with juvenile diabetes mellitus, Am. J. Surg. 124:682, 1972.

26. Hampers, C. L., Soeldner, J. S., Doak, P. B., and Merrill, J. P.: Effect of chronic renal failure and hemodialysis on carbohydrate metabolism, J. Clin. Invest. 45:1719, 1966.

27. Haymond, M. R., Recker, L. A., and Willmert, J. G.: Vocational rehabilitation status of 125 diabetic transplant recipients, Dial. Transplant. 6:52, 1977.

28. Huang, C., Del Greco, F., Ivanovich, P., Krumlovski, F. A., Roguska, J., Simon, N. M., and Hano, J.: Maintenance dialysis for diabetic nephropathy with uremia, J. Chronic Dis. 28:365, 1975.

29. Ibrahim, M. M., Crosland, J. M., Honigs-Berger, L., Barnes, A. D., Dawson-Edwards, P., and Newman, C. E.: Effects of renal transplantation on uremic neuropathy, Lancet 2:739, 1974.

30. Jacobs, C., Brunner, F. P., Chantler, C., Donckerwolcke, R., Gurland, H. J., Hathway, R., Selwood, N. H., and Wing, A. J.: Combined report on regular dialysis and transplantation in Europe, Proc. Eur. Dial. Transplant Assoc., in press.

31. Jacobs, C., Rottembourg, J., and Legrain, M.: La dialyse itérative et la transplantation rénale chez les diabétiques, Diabete Metab. 3:59, 1977.
32. Johnson, W. J.: End-stage renal disease in the diabetic, Mayo Clin. Proc. 52:335, 1977.
33. Kjellstrand, C. M., Simmons, R. L., Goetz, F. C., Kline, M. B., Buselmeier, T. J., and Najarian, J. S.: Mortality and morbidity in diabetic patients accepted for renal transplantation, Kidney Int. 6:S 15, 1974.
34. Kjellstrand, C. M., and Buselmeier, T. J.: A simple method for anticoagulation during pre- and post-operative hemodialysis, avoiding rebound phenomenon, Surgery 72:630, 1972.
35. Knowles, H. C., Jr.: Magnitude of the renal failure problem in diabetic patients, Kidney Int. 6:S2, 1974.
36. Kuhenel, D., Lundh, H., Bennet, W., and Porter, G.: Aortocoronary bypass surgery in patients with end-stage renal disease, Trans. Am. Soc. Artif. Intern. Organs 22: 14, 1976.
37. Lambert, A. E., Buysschaert, M., Marchand, E., Pierard, M., Wojciz, S., and Lambotte, L.: Insulin requirements and blood glucose control in brittle diabetics before and after connection with an artificial pancreas, Diabetologia 13:411, 1977.
38. Larson, O., Brynger, H., Bengtsson, U., Ewald, J., and Gelin, L. E.: Kidney transplantation in patients with diabetic nephropathy, Scand. J. Urol. Nephrol. 38:105, 1977.
39. Lillehei, R. C., Simmons, R. L., Najarian, J. S., Weil, R., Uchida, M., Ruiz, J. O., Kjellstrand, C. M., and Goetz, F. C.: Pancreatic duodenal allotransplantation: experimental and clinical experience, Ann. Surg. 172:405, 1970.
40. Ma, K. W., Masler, D. S., and Brown, D. C.: Hemodialysis in diabetic patients with renal failure, Ann. Intern. Med. 83:215, 1975.
41. Maher, J. F., Hirszel, P., and Galen, A.: Enhanced peritoneal transport with dipyridamole, Trans. Am. Soc. Artif. Intern. Organs 23:1977, in press.
42. Marble, A.: Late complications of diabetes. A continuing challenge, Diabetologia 12: 193, 1976.
43. Matas, A. J., Simmons, R. L., Goetz, F. C., Kjellstrand, C. M., Buselmeier, T. J., Sutherland, D. E. R., and Najarian, J. S.: Hyperglycemic pseudo-rejection in the diabetic transplant patient, Surgery 79:132, 1976.
44. Mauer, S. M., Barbosa, J., Vernier, R. L., Kjellstrand, C. M., Buselmeier, T. J., Simmons, R. L., Najarian, J. S., and Goetz, F. C.: Development of diabetic vascular lesions in normal kidneys transplanted into patients with diabetes mellitus, N. Engl. J. Med. 295:916, 1976.
45. Mauer, S. M., Miller, K., Goetz, F. C., Barbosa, J., Simmons, R. L., Najarian, J. S., and Michael, A. F.: Immunopathology of renal extracellular membranes in kidneys transplanted into patients with diabetes mellitus, Diabetes 25:709, 1976.
46. Mion, Ch., and Slingenyer, A.: La dialyse péritonéale à domicile, traitement au long cours de l'urémie au stade ultime, in Küss R., and Legrain, M. (eds.): *Séminaires d'Uro-Néphrologie Pitié-Salpétrière* (Paris: Masson, 1977), pp. 119–130.
47. Mitchell, J. C.: End-stage renal failure in juvenile diabetes mellitus: a 5 year follow-up of treatment, Mayo Clin. Proc. 52:281, 1977.
48. Najarian, J. S., Sutherland, D. E. R., Simmons, R. L., Howard, R. J., Kjellstrand, C. M., Mauer, S. M., Kennedy, W., Ramsay, R., Barbosa, J., and Goetz, F. C.: Kidney transplantation for uremic diabetic patients, Surg. Gynecol. Obstet. 144:682, 1977.
49. Navalesi, R., Pilo, A., Lenzi, S., and Donato, L.: Insulin metabolism in chronic uremia and in the anephric state. Effect of the dialytic treatment, J. Clin. Endocrinol. Metab. 40:70, 1975.
50. Nolph, K. D., Stolz, M. L., and Maher, J. F.: Altered peritoneal permeability in patients with systemic vasculitis, Ann. Intern. Med. 75:753, 1971.
51. Nolph, K. D., Ghods, A. J., Van Stone, J., and Brown, P. A.: The effect of intraperito-

neal vasodilators on peritoneal clearances, Trans. Am. Soc. Artif. Intern. Organs 22: 586, 1976.

52. Nolph, K. D., Rosenfeldt, P. S., Powell, J. T., and Danforth, E.: Peritoneal glucose transport and hyperglycemia during peritoneal dialysis, Am. J. Med. Sci. 259:272, 1970.

53. Palumbo, P. J., Woods, J. E., Johnson, W. J., and John Service, F.: Metabolic problems in diabetic patients undergoing renal transplantation, Kidney Int. 6:S58, 1974.

54. Palumbo, P. J., Elverback, L. R., Chu Pin Chu, M. S., Connolly, D. C., and Kurland, L. T.: Diabetes mellitus; incidence, prevalence, survivorship and causes of death in Rochester, Minnesota, 1945–1970, Diabetes 25:566, 1976.

55. Raja, R. M., Kramer, M. S., Manchanda, R., Lazaro, N., and Rosenbaum, J. M.: Peritoneal dialysis with fructose dialysate. Prevention of hyperglycemia and hyperosmolality, Ann. Intern. Med. 79:511, 1973.

56. Rao, K. W., Sutherland, D., Kjellstrand, C. M., and Shapiro, F. L.: Comparative results between dialysis and transplantation in diabetic patients, Trans. Am. Soc. Artif. Intern. Organs 23:1977, in press.

57. Robinson, R. R.: Technical aspects of dialysis in diabetics: discussion, Kidney Int. 6:S 115, 1974.

58. Rousselie, F.: Personal communication.

59. Rubin, J. E., and Friedman, E. A.: Dialysis and transplantation of diabetics in the United States, Nephron 18:309, 1977.

60. Rubin, J., Oreopoulos, D. G., Gordon-Blair, R. D., Chisholm, L. D. J., Meema, H. E., and Veber, G. A. de: Chronic peritoneal dialysis in the management of diabetics with renal failure, Nephron 19:265, 1977.

61. Samiik, L. Ciancioni, C., Rottembourg, J., Bisseliches, F., and Jacobs, C.: Severe hypoglycemia due to propranolol in two regular dialysis patients, Lancet 1:545, 1977.

62. Schupak, E., Neff, M. S., Slifkin, R., and Baez, A.: Hemodialysis and diabetic nephropathy, J.A.M.A. 223:1157, 1974.

63. Shideman, J. R., Buselmeier, T. J., and Kjellstrand, C. M.: Hemodialysis in diabetics, Arch. Intern. Med. 136:1126, 1976.

64. Simmons, R. L., Kjellstrand, C. M., Kyriankydes, G. K., Ratazzi, L. C., Spanos, P. K., Casali, R., and Najarian, J. S.: Surgical aspects of transplantation in diabetic patients, Kidney Int. 6:S129, 1974.

65. Simmons, R. L., and Schilling, K. J.: Social and psychological rehabilitation of the diabetic transplant patient, Kidney Int. 6:S152, 1974.

66. Simmons, R. L., Merino, G. E., Tersigni, R., Kjellstrand, C. M., and Najarian, J. S.: Renal transplantation in diabetic patients, in Küss, R., and Legrain, M. (eds.): *Séminaires d'Uro-Néphrologie Pitié-Salpétrière* (Paris: Masson, 1976), pp. 189–98.

67. Slama, G., Klein, J. C., Tardieu, M. C., and Tchobroutsky, G.: Normalisation de la glycémie par pancréas artificiel non miniaturisé, Nouv. Presse Med. 6:2309, 1977.

68. Slifkin, R. F., Neff, M. S., Baez, A., Gupta, S., Mattoo, N., and Haimov, M.: Maintenance dialysis in diabetic patients, Proc. Eur. Dial. Transplant Assoc. 13:377, 1976.

69. Tenckhoff, H.: Peritoneal dialysis to-day: a new look, Nephron 12:420, 1974.

70. Tenckhoff, H.: Advantages and shortcomings of peritoneal dialysis in the management of chronic renal failure, in Küss, R., and Legrain, M. (eds.): *Séminaires d'Uro-néphrologie Pitié-Salpétrière* (Paris: Masson, 1977), pp. 107–18.

71. Thayssen, R., Roed Petersen, K., Nielsen, F. U., Svendsen, V., and Kemp, E.: The treatment of end-stage renal failure in insulin-dependent diabetic patients, Acta Med. Scand. 201:469, 1977.

72. Von Hartitzsch, B., and Medlock, T. R.: Chronic peritoneal dialysis. A regime comparable to conventional hemodialysis, Trans. Am. Soc. Artif. Intern. Organs 22:595, 1976.

73. Watkins, P. J., Parsons, V., and Bewick, M.: The prognosis and management of diabetic nephropathy, Clin. Nephrol. 7:243, 1977.

74. White, N., Snowden, S. A., Parsons, V., Sheldon, J., and Bewick, M.: The management of terminal renal failure in diabetic patients by regular dialysis therapy, Nephron 11:261, 1973.
75. Wilson, R. E., Goldman, M. H., Yen, M. C., Kassissieh, S. D., Strom, T., and Kahn, C. B.: Neuropathy in transplanted diabetic patients, Kidney Int. 6:S90, 1974.
76. Woods, J. E., Johnson, W. J., Anderson, C. F., Leary, F. J., Palumbo, P. J., Frohnert, P. P., Donadio, J. V., Jr., and Deweerd, J. M.: Renal transplantation in patients with diabetes mellitus, Lancet 2:795, 1972.
77. Zincke, H., Woods, J. E., Palumbo, P. J., Leary, F. J., and Johnson, W. J.: Renal transplantation in patients with insulin-dependent diabetes mellitus, J.A.M.A. 237:1103, 1977.

7

Pancreatic Transplantation in Cases of Diabetes Complicated by Renal Insufficiency

J. TRAEGER, M.D., J. M. DUBERNARD, M.D.,
J. L. TOURAINE, M.D., P. NEYRA, M.D.,
D. TRANCHANT, M.D., AND M. C. MALIK, M.D.

Cliniques Universitaires de Néphrologie et d'Urologie, and INSERM U 80,
Hôpital Edouard Herriot, Lyon, France

The apparently inexorable increase in cardiovascular and microangiopathic complications of diabetes with increased duration of this disorder, despite insulin therapy,[10, 57] had led to the development of new forms of treatment aimed at better physiologic control of blood glucose levels. Current studies involve four modalities: electromechanical artificial pancreas, transplantation of the islets of Langerhans, bioartificial pancreas or hybrid pancreas (islets of Langerhans cultured on a prosthesis) and total pancreas transplantation.

In this chapter, we will describe each of these modalities of treatment and will elaborate on our own experiences with transplantation of the pancreas in dogs and humans.

Electromechanical Artificial Pancreas

The electromechanical artificial pancreas consists of an analyzer for continuous measurement of blood glucose levels; a ser-

127

0084-5957/79/080127-23$3.75
© 1979, Year Book Medical Publishers, Inc.

vo-command unit, with or without a computer, to transform this information to insulin requirements; and a pump to inject the necessary amount of insulin. Clinically, this type of artificial pancreas has permitted better therapy for acute pancreatic insufficiency, diabetic coma and other acute disorders. Serial analyses of insulin requirements in patients with insulin-dependent diabetes mellitus facilitates more physiologic control of blood glucose levels[47, 56] and may be even more useful in those with diabetes complicated by renal insufficiency. Future development of this type of artificial pancreas awaits the design of implantable, tissue-compatible materials and a long-term source of energy.[9, 25]

Transplantation of Islets of Langerhans

The transplantation of islets of Langerhans, isolated after digestion by collagenase,[32] separated on a Ficoll gradient[61] and then injected into the portal vein of diabetic rats, has resulted in the cure of experimental diabetes for periods of up to 18 months.[27] With similar techniques, it has been possible to isolate and partially extract the active material from the islets of Langerhans in dogs,[54] pigs,[64] monkeys[62] and humans.[49, 63] The pancreases of newborn infants or fetuses contain few exocrine enzymes and a fairly large percentage of endocrine parenchyma,[34] which are isolated more easily after simple digestion by collagenase. Their use might represent a better qualitative and quantitative approach and may eventually result in the possibility of a single donor for treating a recipient.

Although different transplant sites are possible, e.g., intraperitoneal or intramuscular, it would appear more physiologic to administer the material from the islets of Langerhans by intraportal,[23] intrasplenic[30, 46] or renal subcapsular[5] routes, or possibly via reniportal-venous anastomoses. A major difficulty that remains is long-term preservation of the islets of Langerhans. Simple refrigeration to 4 C permits only limited survival,[17, 29] as does freezing, where results are still uncertain.[16] Tissue culture risks both cytologic and functional modifications of the cells.[2, 31] Islets of Langerhans prepared from neonatal pancreases appear to tolerate ischemia and preserve their function when removed as long as 3 hours after death or when refrigerated for up to 63 hours.[41]

The most serious remaining problem with this technique is

the immunologic modification of the allografts of the islets of Langerhans. Although the administration of antilymphocyte serum prolongs the allografts between rats of similar genetic background[39, 59] and a specific tolerance can be induced in rats and mice,[50, 51, 55] antilymphocyte serum or conventional immunosuppressive therapy becomes relatively inefficient as soon as strong histocompatibility antigens intervene;[59] and islet allografts appear very sensitive to cellular or humoral components of the immune response.[50]

Bioartificial Pancreas

Beta cells are cultured in a cylindrical or circular container in a culture medium. The container is crossed by a network of semipermeable capillaries with extremities that can be connected to vessels. The capillary membrane has a permeability threshold for substances with a molecular weight of 50,000, allowing transport of insulin and glucose while remaining impermeable to antibodies and lymphocytes. When grafted arterio-arterially in the neck of a pancreatectomized dog[54] or extra-corporeally in a diabetic rat,[7] the membrane has had short-term but encouraging results.[69] The principal advantage is the absence of immunologic reaction against the β-cells; the main disadvantages are preparation of viable cells and capillary thromboses.

Total Organ Transplantation

In contrast to experimental renal, hepatic or cardiac transplants, it has been difficult to find a valid experimental animal model for pancreatic transplantation. Pancreatic autografts in dogs have been largely unsuccessful, regardless of the technique used.[66] Allografts have been complicated by frequent vascular thromboses, pancreatitis or enzymatic digestion of the recipient tissue,[35] which have prevented appropriate studies of organ rejection. The necessity for replacement of the exocrine function of the pancreas is another complication of this technique.

Transplantation of a segment of the pancreas following simple ligation of the duct of Wirsung has yielded variable results in rats,[52, 70] but when grafted in diabetic animals the secretion of insulin may be controlled and normal growth observed.[52] In other species, different methods used to immunologically modify the pancreatic tissue have been unsuccessful, e.g., irradiation of the graft and treatment of the recipient with 5-fluorouracil,[6, 44] glucagon and methylprednisolone.[28]

Various methods for the administration of pancreatic secretions have been explored. These include: pancreatico-duodenal transplantation with duodeno-ileal anastomosis or cutaneous duodenostomy;[35] total pancreas transplant, preserving a duodenal collarette to simplify the digestive anastomosis;[3] graft of a pancreatic segment of which a section is anastomosed to a previously prepared ileal loop in a retroperitoneal Y;[11] and anastomosis between the canal of Wirsung of a pancreas left in place in the host and the ureter.[19-21] Technical obstacles are still very frequent, but studies in surviving animals have led to better understanding of graft function. There appears to be little preference between portal or systemic venous drainage, as judged by blood glucose levels.[60] Rejection is accompanied by fairly rapid alterations in blood glucose levels, associated with increased serum amylase levels, and seems to affect endocrine and exocrine parenchyma simultaneously.[3, 60]

The last publication of the ACS–NIH Transplant Registry reported 57 pancreatic transplants in humans.[72] If one excludes the five cases in our group, the transplantation techniques used were: 26 pancreatico-duodenal transplantations, 25 transplantations of subtotal pancreas (body and tail) and one whole pancreas. No successes were reported after a pancreatic segment graft and simple ligature of the principal pancreatic canal. A pancreatico-duodenal graft carried out by Lillehei in 1971 functioned for 12 months until the unrelated death of the patient.[36] Other cases had secondary complications, such as pancreatic fistulas, local and generalized infections and duodenal or pancreatic rejection.[33] Fistulas and rejections largely account for the poor results of transplantation of an anastomosed pancreatic segment onto a retroperitoneal Y loop.[24] The technique of releasing pancreatic juice into the ureter of the recipient, which necessitates leaving a catheter in place, is not without complications,[20] although it has resulted in the longest surviving human registrant (47 months).

Because of these difficulties, we explored the possibility of suppressing the exocrine function of a transplanted pancreas by injecting neoprene into the principal pancreatic canal of dogs, prior to applying this method to humans.

Animal Experiments

Neoprene is a synthetic rubber, liquid in its natural state, and made up of an aqueous suspension of chloroprene, which has the chemical characteristic of flocculation when its pH is modified by pancreatic juice, which has a pH (8 or 9) that is less basic than that of neoprene (12 to 14). The viscosity is relatively weak (70 units). In these experiments, the principal pancreatic canal was isolated at the duodenal level and a polyethylene catheter (no. 16 or 18) was inserted. After gentle aspiration of the pancreatic juice, 1 – 6 ml neoprene was injected, followed immediately by the injection of 0.2 ml acetic acid, to accelerate polymerization and obtain complete obstruction of the canal.

Twenty-seven dogs were used in these experiments. After an observation period of several weeks, they were weighed and their serum was analyzed for glucose, amylase, urea and serum electrolytes. The dogs received no food for 24 hours prior to operation, and received intramuscular injections of atropine (0.25 mg) 12, 6 and 1 hour before the operation. The animals were separated into three groups: Group I: Seven dogs received an injection of 2 – 3 ml neoprene with ligature of the principal pancreatic canal and accessory canals. Group II: Six dogs received an injection of 2 – 3 ml neoprene with ligature of the pancreatic and accessory canals. Lyophilized pancreatic extracts and medium-chain triglycerides were added to their basic diet. Group III: Fourteen dogs underwent cephalic pancreatectomy after injection of 1.5 – 6 ml neoprene, leaving the left part of the pancreas vascularized by the upper mesenteric splenic artery.

During the postoperative course, the animals were weighed regularly and blood samples were taken twice a week. Glycosuria was checked each day. Oral or intravenous glucose tolerance tests and serial measurements of insulin (Amersham Kit) and glucagon were carried out at regular intervals.

RESULTS

GROUP I. – Two animals died in the first few hours following intervention; autopsies performed the following day revealed necrotic pancreases. The five other dogs in the series were killed after three to five weeks. None was diabetic (normal blood glucose levels, glucose tolerance and no glycosuria). They all had pancreatic exocrine insufficiency with cachexia (20 – 30% weight loss), copious stools containing undigested meat and numerous oily globules (Sudan III stain) and steatorrhea, with increased excretion of fats and proteins.

GROUP II. – The six animals survived in good condition until the day they were killed, confirming the efficacy of added dietary ingredients. As in group I, serum amylase levels were normal and none of the dogs was diabetic. Five were killed three months after intervention and the sixth after 14 months. The pancreases were atrophied, and histologic examination showed severe parenchymal fibrosis with survival of normal endocrine cells. At 14 months, the fibrosis was extremely dense, and only subnormal islets of Langerhans could be identified (Fig. 7 – 1).

GROUP III. – Four technical complications were observed (three duodenal necroses and one biliary peritonitis). One animal died of intercurrent infection after three months, with normal endocrine function. One of the dogs had diabetes after the second postoperative week, which worsened progressively; it was killed during the 15th week. The pancreas was even more

Fig. 7–1. – Canine pancreas 14 months after injection of neoprene (low magnification). Normal islets are seen in a dense fibrosis.

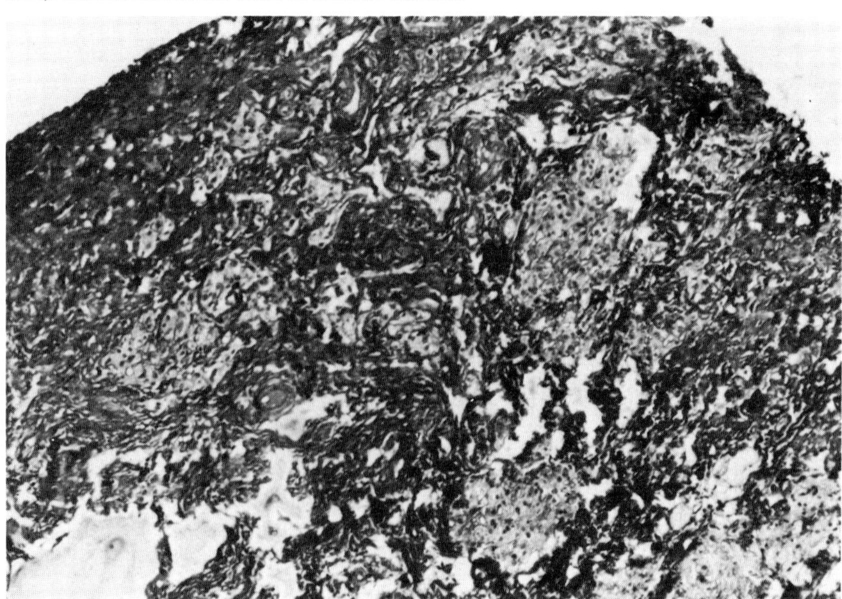

atrophied than those in the animals of Group II, and it was very difficult to find normal islets on histologic examination.

The eight other dogs survived in generally good condition, with normal levels of blood glucose, insulin and glucagon, and without glycosuria. Glucose tolerance curves were also within normal limits. A moderate increase in the serum amylase levels was noted in all animals during the first 15 postoperative days, with subsequent normalization. Four dogs were kept alive for between 7 and 19 months after intervention for further studies.

Thus, in animals the injection of neoprene does not cause acute pancreatitis, necrosis or lysis of the pancreas, as one might have expected with this caustic substance. The two cases of necrosis in group I dogs are doubtlessly explained by cadaveric lysis, since the autopsies were performed 18–24 hours after death. The high pH of neoprene is a possible explanation for the absence of acute pancreatic reaction and represents one of the reasons for the choice of this substance. The method we describe appears to be a simple and efficient means of suppressing the exocrine function of the pancreas (group I). A diet rich in medium-chain triglycerides and extracts of lyophilized pancreas easily compensated for the absence of this secretion (groups II and III) for periods of up to 20 months (length of survival of the oldest animals in group III).

The technique of cephalic pancreatectomy, leaving the left part of the pancreas in place, appeared to constitute a better experimental approach than the autograft grafted in dogs, which presented numerous technical complications. No drainage was necessary, and no fistulas or pancreatic pseudocysts were observed in dogs in this series.

The moderate increase of serum amylase levels noted during the first two postoperative weeks in group II animals bore no relation to the quantity of neoprene injected, since the two dogs in this group that received 6 ml neoprene did not show higher levels of amylase than the other dogs.

Since the exocrine parenchyma represents more than 95% of the pancreatic tissue, the presence of slowly progressive fibrosis is not surprising. After a year, only the islets of Langerhans and vessels were unaffected. The only dog that became diabetic had more marked pancreatic atrophy, perhaps due to transverse ligature of the pancreatic artery in this animal. Since the two longest-surviving animals in group III still had perfectly normal endocrine function, it would appear that islet function may remain intact despite severe parenchymal fibrosis.

Similar histologic aspects were described after injection of a cyanoacrylic gum into the pancreases of dogs and humans in the treatment of chronic pancreatitis.[37] During preliminary experiments we used an equivalent substance, but abandoned it because of injection difficulties linked with the rapidity of solidification. The mechanism of neoprene action is not precise: doubtless it causes mechanical obstruction in the small branches of the pancreatic canals and a chemical reaction demonstrated indirectly by polymerization of the substance.

In conclusion, in animals the injection of neoprene appears to be a simple and efficient way to suppress the exocrine function of the pancreas. It causes a fibrous atrophy around the islets of Langerhans, which continues for up to 20 months. These results led us to try this technique in humans, since the release of pancreatic juice, which complicates the surgical process, caused the failure of most previous attempts.

Human Pancreatic Transplantation

The surgical techniques of harvesting the cadaver donor pancreas and transplanting it into a live recipient have been described in detail in a prior publication.[68]

With regard to removal of the pancreas, it is important to note that chilled Collins solution is used for retrograde washing in situ via the splenic artery. Neoprene is introduced slowly through a polyethylene catheter in the canal of Wirsung, and completed by injection of 0.5 ml acetic acid, which accelerates its flocculation.

The vessels of the graft organ are connected to the external iliac vessels and the graft is implanted in the left or right iliac fossa. In our experience with five human transplants and 16 mock transplantations in cadavers, no cases were observed in which the splenic artery did not irrigate the body and tail of the pancreas satisfactorily, in contrast to the findings of Mellière.[43]

CASE REPORTS

PATIENT 1.—This patient was a 40-year-old man with known insulin-dependent diabetes since the age of 20. His history included myocardial infarction, episodes of left ventricular insufficiency, peripheral polyneuritis of the lower extremities, severe diabetic retinopathy and chronic renal insufficiency secondary to diabetic nephropathy. He was on chronic hemodialysis for several years prior to the pancreas transplant, during which time he had multiple episodes of hypo- and hyperglycemia. Anti-insulin antibodies were present.

The donor was a young person with a diagnosis of cerebral death. As shown in Table 7 – 1, there was an ABO compatibility between the donor and recipient, but no HL-A compatibility. Despite prior transfusion of 37 units of blood, the recipient did not develop cytotoxic anti-HL-A antibodies, and the crossmatch between the serum of the recipient and the lymphocytes of the donor was negative.

Following the transplant, the patient received parenteral nutrition for three days, after which time oral feeding was resumed. Immunosuppressive therapy consisted of azathioprine at an initial dose of 150 mg/day, rapidly reduced to 0 – 75 mg/day, depending on the white blood cell count (Fig. 7 – 2), and prednisolone in an initial dose of 40 mg/day for ten days, followed by 20 mg/day.

Despite a transitory increase in serum amylase levels following transplantation, there was no evidence of pancreatitis. Aprotinine, a trypsin inhibitor, 800,000 units/day, was administered intravenously during the first 14 days following transplantation. A fistula developed in the scar tissue with leakage of an amylase-rich fluid and superinfection by *Klebsiella pneumonia*, which was resistant to local antiseptics and generalized

TABLE 7 – 1. – PRINCIPAL IMMUNOLOGIC
CHARACTERISTICS OF THE RECIPIENT
(PATIENT 1) AND DONORS*

SUBJECT	ERYTHROCYTIC GROUPS	HL-A GROUPS
Recipient (patient 1)	O Rh+	A 11, A 29, B 18, Bw 35
Donor of pancreas	O Rh+	A 2, A 9, B 8, B 7
Donor of kidney	O Rh+	A 2, A 9, B 12, B 7

*The recipient received a total of at least 37 units of blood (leukocyte-poor red blood cells). No cytotoxic anti-HL-A antibodies were detected until May 1977, at which time antibodies developed against lymphocytes of 15% of the donors. The crossmatch between the serum of the recipient and lymphocytes of the donors was negative.

TRAEGER ET AL.

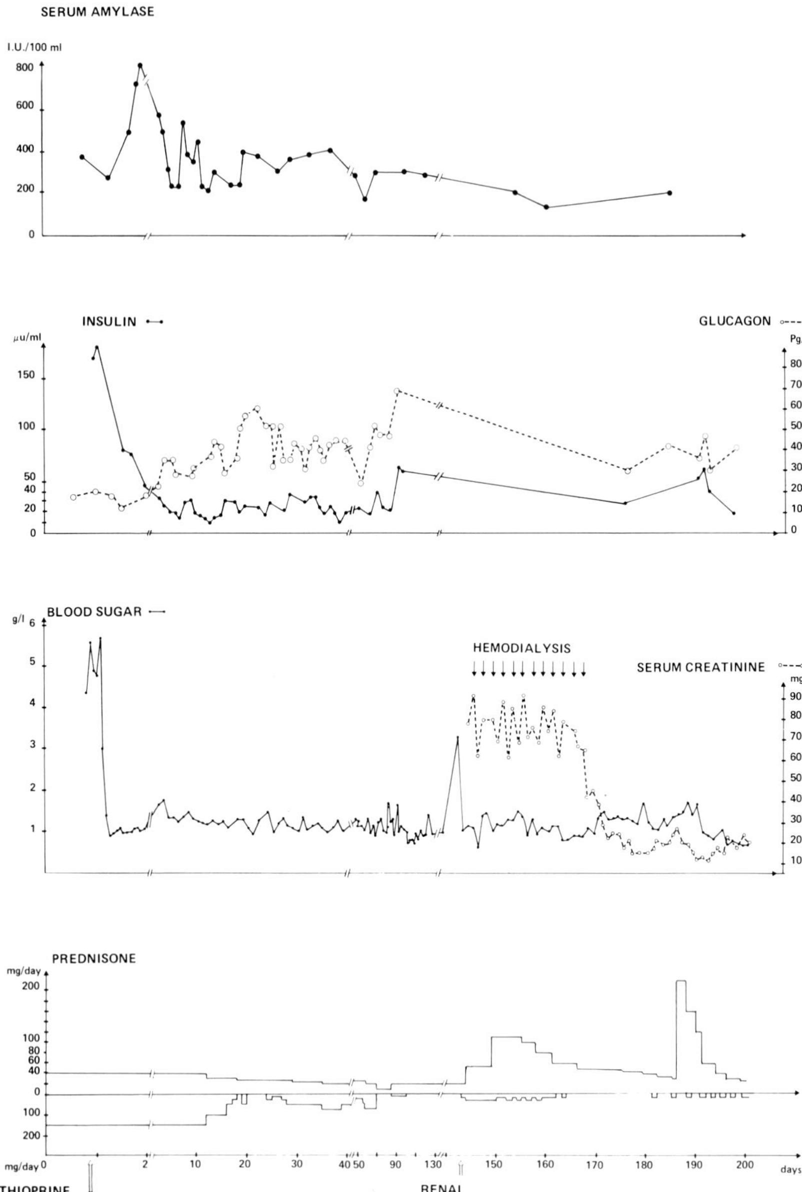

Fig. 7–2.—Pancreatic and renal function after transplantation and adaptation to immunosuppressive treatment.

antibiotic therapy; this infected fistula persisted until the patient's death one year after the pancreas transplantation.

Various complications included an episode of left ventricular failure, azathioprine-induced leukopenia, multiple infections with various types of bacteria and transitory facial paralysis.

As shown in Figure 7–2, the severe hyperglycemia present just prior to unclamping the vascular anastomoses of the graft decreased to normal values within eight hours and remained normal thereafter. High insulin levels decreased rapidly within the first 15 hours and normalized by the second day (see Fig. 7–2). Serial oral or intravenous glucose tolerance tests demonstrated normal responses of blood glucose and circulating insulin levels. The circulating glucagon level (radioimmunoassay) was 180 μu/ml prior to the pancreas transplant (normal basal level: 153 ± 27 μu/ml), and increased progressively after the third day to levels of between 300 and 800 pg/ml (see Fig. 7–2).

There were no indications of rejection of the pancreatic transplant at any time. Arteriographic studies verified satisfactory arterial and venous perfusion of the graft.

Nearly five months after the pancreatic transplant, a renal transplant was performed, utilizing a cadaver kidney. There was ABO compatibility, but no HL-A compatibility with the recipient. The crossmatch between the serum of the recipient and the lymphocytes of the donor was negative. It should be noted that the kidney and pancreas donors had three HL-A antigens in common (see Table 7–1). Following an initial episode of acute renal failure, renal function steadily improved, creatinine clearance decreased to near normal levels and hemodialysis was discontinued (see Fig. 7–2). There was a temporary glucose intolerance, which became normal 21 days after renal transplantation. With further improvement of renal function, however, mild hyperglycemia and glycosuria occurred. An oral antidiabetic agent (gliclazide, one tablet per day) was given between the 46th and 52d days after renal transplant (189th to 195th days following pancreatic transplant). Thereafter blood sugar levels remained within normal limits. On the 210th day following pancreatic transplantation, while the patient was receiving 55 mg prednisolone, the glucose tolerance test results were mildly abnormal, both with regard to blood glucose levels and radioimmunoassays of insulin (Fig. 7–3). The basal levels of insulin and glucagon, however, were similar to those observed before renal transplantation.

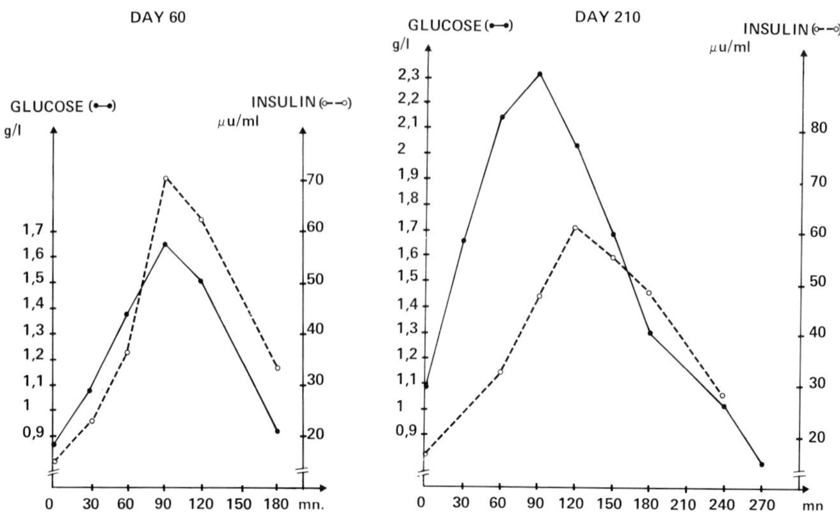

Fig. 7–3. – Oral glucose tolerance tests after pancreatic transplant only *(left)*, and after pancreatic and renal transplant *(right)*.

During the next few months the main complications consisted of various localized and generalized infections with *Pseudomonas, Candida* and cytomegalovirus, necessitating antibiotic therapy. Several rejection episodes were treated with increased doses of glucocorticoids.

Eleven months after pancreatic transplantation, renal function was stable with a serum creatinine clearance of 2.4 mg/100 ml and a blood urea level of 0.8 gm/L. Blood glucose levels were also within normal limits without therapy. However, anorexia, nausea, dehydration and general deterioration occurred in conjunction with azathioprine-induced leukopenia and major infections. The patient died of these secondary complications approximately six months following the renal transplant and nearly one year after the pancreatic transplant.

PATIENT 2. – This 41-year-old man had a history of insulin-dependent diabetes since the age of nine. Complications of diabetes included numerous episodes of hypoglycemic coma, complete blindness, peripheral polyneuritis and terminal renal failure secondary to diabetic nephropathy. The patient had been on chronic hemodialysis approximately one year prior to the pancreatic transplant, during which time the diabetes was extremely difficult to control.

The patient had the HL-A phenotype 2, 29, 5 and 12, and the pancreatic transplant was carried out with ABO compatibility, two HL-A identities and a negative crossmatch. Anti-insulin antibodies were present. Severe hyperglycemia (425 mg/100 ml) at the time of pancreatic transplant became normal within several hours after transplantation. Serum amylase levels increased to 3,000 IU/L. Immunosuppressive therapy consisted of azathioprine, 100 mg/day, and prednisolone, 60 mg/day. In addition, the patient received 800,000 units of aprotinine per day. Forty-eight hours after transplantation, blood glucose levels increased rapidly to 800 mg/100 ml, necessitating therapy with intravenous insulin. Amylase levels decreased to 600 IU/L. Circulating insulin levels, which had increased to 440 μu/ml, decreased to 80 μu/ml. At this time the graft ceased to function due to thrombosis of the splenic vein of the graft, probably secondary to compression by a large hematoma in the iliac fossa.

PATIENT 3. – This 42-year-old man had known insulin-dependent diabetes since the age of 25. Complications included numerous episodes of hypoglycemia, diabetic retinopathy and complete blindness, severe arterial hypertension with an episode of hypertensive encephalopathy, peripheral and intestinal polyneuritis and terminal renal failure secondary to diabetic nephropathy requiring chronic hemodialysis.

The pancreatic transplant was carried out with ABO compatibility but without HL-A compatibility (recipient: 1, 2, 8 and 18; donor: 9, 10 and 12). The patient received two blood transfusions. Cytotoxic anti-HL-A antibodies were not present.

Immunosuppressive therapy consisted of azathioprine, 150 mg/day initially followed by 50 mg/day, and prednisolone, 60 mg/day and then decreased to 15 mg/day. Antilymphocyte serum was administered at a dose of 27 ampules of 5 ml each over 11 days. Aprotinine was given at a dose of 800,000 units per day for 17 days.

Complications consisted of initial digestive problems requiring prolonged parenteral feeding, a transitory extrapyramidal syndrome secondary to drug therapy, duodenal and esophageal ulcers with gastrointestinal hemorrhages and severe thrombopenia requiring concentrated platelet transfusions. In addition, a suppurative hematoma was evacuated, and *Staphylococcus* organisms were isolated from the discharge.

The blood glucose level was approximately 600 mg/100 ml

prior to transplantation and gradually decreased to normal levels over the following ten days. This slow development of satisfactory pancreatic endocrine function may have been secondary to a "shock pancreas," since a relatively prolonged period of 138 minutes of cold ischemia time had been necessary. Two and one-half months following pancreatic transplantation, blood glucose levels increased to 500 mg/100 ml, necessitating insulin therapy for the first time since the transplant. Thereafter, insulin was required at approximately the same doses as prior to transplantation. Blood insulin levels increased to 510 μu/L at the time of vascular clamping, and then stabilized at normal values between 20 and 50 μu/L. One month after transplantation insulin levels increased to 200 μu/L, followed by a progressive decrease to normal values just prior to the reappearance of insulin-dependent diabetes.

Four and one-half months following transplantation, the patient had pericarditis and a cutaneous *Staphylococcus* infection. He died during a hemodialysis session from a cardiac arrythmia.

PATIENT 4.—This patient was a 28-year-old woman with known insulin-dependent diabetes since the age of three. Her illness included severe retinopathy with partial blindness, peripheral polyneuritis, peripheral atherosclerosis requiring repeated amputations, pneumococcal septicemia, transitory hemiparesis and pericarditis, and diabetic nephropathy necessitating chronic hemodialysis two years before the pancreatic transplant. Her diabetes required 30 units of insulin daily during chronic hemodialysis.

The recipient had an HL-A phenotype 2, 12, W40; and the pancreatic transplant was carried out with ABO compatibility and two HL-A identities. The crossmatch was negative. The HBs antigen was positive. Immunosuppressive treatment consisted of azathioprine, 50 mg/day, prednisolone, 40 mg/day slowly decreased to 15 mg/day, and antilymphocytic serum, 27 ampules of 5 ml each over 16 days. Aprotinine was given at a dose of 800,000 units per day for nine days.

Serum amylase levels increased to 900 IU/L, and then stabilized at between 100 and 300 IU/L. The initial marked hyperglycemia normalized within 12 hours following transplantation. Forty-five days after transplantation, blood glucose levels suddenly increased to 1000 mg/100 ml, requiring insulin therapy.

At that time an abcess containing *Klebsiella* and *Staphylococcus* organisms was evacuated and antibiotics prescribed. Corticosteroids were slightly increased because of the possibility of rejection. Arteriography eliminated the possibility of vascular thrombosis. The most probable hypothesis was that of a non-immunologic necrosis of the transplant, with local infection.

After the pancreatic transplant, basal levels of radioimmunoactive insulin remained in the normal range of 20–60 μu/ml, and showed a normal response to glucose tolerance tests. It decreased to less than 20 μu/ml when the function of the transplant decreased.

The clinical condition of the patient is now comparable to what it was prior to the pancreatic transplant.

PATIENT 5.— This 33-year-old woman had known insulin-dependent diabetes since age 14. Her course included numerous episodes of hypoglycemia, renal insufficiency, diabetic retinopathy, arterial hypertension with left ventricular hypertrophy, peripheral polyneuritis and terminal renal failure requiring hemodialysis approximately two years prior to the transplant. Her diabetes required 60 units of insulin daily. Anti-insulin antibodies were not detected. The general condition of the patient was fair.

The recipient had an HL-A phenotype of 11, 8 and 18, and the pancreatic transplant was carried out with ABO compatibility but without HL-A compatibility. Cytotoxic anti-HL-A antibodies were detected, but the crossmatch was negative with relation to the donor. Transplantation was technically difficult because of severe atherosclerosis in the recipient.

Immunosuppressive therapy consisted of azathioprine, 50 mg/day, prednisolone, 50 mg/day and then decreased to 15 mg/day, and antilymphocyte serum, 27 ampules of 5 ml each for one month. Aprotinine was prescribed at a dose of 800,000 units per day for 29 days. The patient received no insulin therapy. Hyperglycemia of 640 mg/100 ml just prior to unclamping normalized after 12 hours and subsequently remained normal in the basal state, as well as following glucose tolerance tests. Serum amylase levels increased to between 1,000 and 3,000 and remained at between 350 and 400 IU/L for the three months following the transplant.

A fistula developed in the scar tissue with an amylase-rich exudate. The fistula persisted for four months following the transplant, but pancreatic endocrine function remained normal. Circulating insulin increased to 700 μu/ml, and then rapidly decreased to basal values of between 20 and 50 μu/ml, where it has remained ever since. Insulin response to oral glucose tolerance tests has been normal.

DISCUSSION

The methods of preparation for and transplantation of the pancreas considerably reduce the usual pancreatic exocrine difficulties linked with the other modes of transplantation of this organ.[68] The effect of the transplant on glucose metabolism is satisfactory and the duration of graft function is longer than that obtained by transplantation of the islets of Langerhans. Islet transplantation in humans has not eliminated the need for insulin and the improvement noted has been only transitory.[49] The method that we recommend in treating end-stage diabetes not only allows better diabetic control, but also may improve the clinical status sufficiently for a subsequent renal transplant. Insulin needs are variable after renal transplantation, and are dependent on medications, corticoid doses, the occurrence of possible immunologic or infectious complications, and other factors. When the control of diabetes is difficult before kidney transplantation, recourse to the artificial pancreas or to a pancreatic transplant appears justified.

Glucose Metabolism

In the five diabetics we treated by pancreatic transplantation, it was possible to interrupt insulin therapy at the end of the operation (Table 7–2). Graft function was sufficiently effective to decrease blood glucose levels to normal during the hours following transplantation, except in one case in which this process took ten days, perhaps due to a longer ischemia time.

In the four observations in which the graft function could be studied for a sufficient period of time, satisfactory diabetic control was achieved, allowing discontinuation of insulin. Fasting glucose levels and glucose tolerance tests were normal or near normal, as were glucagon and circulating insulin levels.

Long-term glucocorticoid therapy, hyperglucagonemia secondary to renal insufficiency[4] and/or corticoid treatment[38] and

TABLE 7-2.—GLUCOSE METABOLISM AFTER PANCREATIC TRANSPLANTS

PATIENTS	DURATION OF HYPERGLYCEMIA (HR)	BLOOD GLUCOSE LEVEL (FUNCTIONAL TRANSPLANT)	THERAPY		DURATION OF GRAFT FUNCTION (DAY)
			DIABETIC DIET	INSULIN	
1	8	Normal	0	Single dose of 16 units at 4 hr repeated at 10 months for several days	345 – death
2	7	Normal	0	Restarted at 48 hr	2 – interrupted function
3	240	Normal	0	Restarted at 75 day	75 – interrupted function
4	12	Normal	0	Restarted at 45 day	45 – interrupted function
5	12	Normal	0	0	125* – persisting function

*As of November 1, 1977.

the well-known insulin resistance in renal insufficiency[58] could explain the fasting glucose levels. Growth hormone cannot be incriminated, since its pre- and postoperative levels were always found to be normal (less than 2 μu/ml by radioimmunoassay).[71]

In the patient who underwent a renal transplantation after the pancreatic transplantation, the increase in blood glucose levels observed after the 171st day coincided with the recurrence of normal renal function after a period of acute tubular necrosis during the first three weeks following the renal transplant; this probably points to catabolism of insulin in a functional kidney.[58]

Basic hyperinsulinemia and that observed during induced hyperglycemia (glucose tolerance test) could precede both renal insufficiency and corticoid treatment.[38] A part of the radioimmunoassay of insulin is perhaps, in fact, proinsulin, and the precise fraction of active insulin in the serum of our patients is now being determined. Moreover, the insulin secreted by the graft is drained by the caval system and not by the physiologic portal system, and this could result in different levels of serum insulin and glucagon concentration, even if the effect on general glucose metabolism does not seem to be affected considerably.[1, 15, 26]

The presence of anti-insulin antibodies detected before transplantation in certain patients did not appear to be of any clinical importance, because these antibodies are not usually directed against human insulin.

Complications (Table 7–3)

A sudden cessation of pancreatic function was noted on the third and 55th days after transplantation in two patients, coinciding with a compressive hematoma during a hemodialysis session (patient 2) and a retroperitoneal abcess in the iliac fossa (patient 4). A pancreatectomy was carried out on the first case, since the evacuation and drainage of the abcess had not reestablished graft function in the second.

In spite of precautions taken in the donor to modify the pancreatic exocrine secretion at the time of its removal, either by gastric aspiration and injection of atropine or, conversely, by injection of chlocytokinine and pancreatozymine, the injected neoprene escaped from the pancreatic acini into the retroperito-

TABLE 7-3.—COMPLICATIONS AFTER
PANCREATIC TRANSPLANTATION

PATIENTS	VASCULAR COMPLICATION	LOCAL INFECTION	FISTULA	REJECTION
1	0	±	+	0
2	+	0	0	0
3	0	+ +	0	±
4	0	+ +	0	0
5	0	±	+	0

neal tissue of the recipient. In all patients small quantities of amylase-rich exudate escaped during the first few postoperative days. The chronic fistula observed in patient 1 was undoubtedly due to the insufficient quantity of neoprene injected (3 ml). In the other patients, 9–10 ml was used with good functional tolerance, and the amylase-rich exudate observed during the first six weeks in patient 5 can be explained by escape through a noninjected region of the pancreas. The viscosity of neoprene and the regulation of pressure at the time of injection play important roles. Minor drainage of aseptic pus, seen in two other patients, could be dependent on a local reaction to neoprene, or could be linked to the release of chlorine by this substance.

Rejections

In patient 3, a rapid increase in blood glucose levels occurred two and one-half months after transplantation, which may have been due to a partial rejection episode. Rejection could also explain the hyperglycemia and glycosuria observed in the tenth month in patient 1, who then required temporary insulin therapy. The general condition of this patient (leukopenia and thrombopenia) was a contraindication to increasing immunosuppressive therapy. The diagnosis of rejection is difficult to establish. Pancreatic rejections were rare, however, considering the absence of HL-A compatibility and in comparison with renal transplantation.

These preliminary results with pancreatic transplantation in humans are promising with regard to the control of diabetes, and in patients with terminal renal insufficiency may permit subsequent renal transplantation under better conditions than were hitherto possible. It is still too early to calculate the average duration of graft survival and function and whether earlier pancreatic transplantation might retard the development of vascular complications of diabetes mellitus. The partial reversibility of certain of these vascular lesions has been shown in diabetic animals after grafts of islets of Langerhans,[18, 42] but extrapolation to humans is difficult, particularly since prolonged therapy with glucocorticoids and immunosuppressive agents is invariably required.

Acknowledgments

We acknowledge with thanks the invaluable collaboration of Drs. J. F. Moskovtchenko, C. Meyer, N. Gignoux, S. Beorchia, H. Bétuel, J. P. Revillard, D. Mongin, S. Dahri, A. Ruitton, C. A. Bizollon, D. Lyonnet and A. Pinet.

References

1. Albisser, A. M., Leibel, B. S., Marliss, E. B., Zinman, B., Botz, C. K., Zingg, W., Murray, F. T., and Denoga, A.: Physiopathologie du diabète et pancréas endocine artificiel, in *J. Ann. Diabetol. Hôtel-Dieu* (Paris: Flammarion, 1976), p. 259.
2. Anderson, A., Borg, J., and Groth, C. G.: Survival of isolated human islets of Langerhans maintained in culture, J. Clin. Invest. 57:1295, 1976.
3. Aquino, C., Ruiz, J. O., Schultz, L. S., and Lillehei, R. C.: Pancreatic transplantation without duodenum in the dog, Am. J. Surg. 125:240, 1973.
4. Bilbrey, G. L., Faloona, G. R., White, M. G., Atkins, C., Hull, A. R., and Knochel, J. P.: Hyperglucagonemia in uremia: reversal by renal transplantation, Ann. Intern. Med. 82:525, 1975.
5. Botz, C. K., Leibel, A. S., Zingg, W., Gander, R. I., and Albisser, A. M.: Comparison of peripheral and portal routes of insulin infusion by a computer-controlled insulin infusion system, Diabetes 25:691, 1976.
6. Castellanos, J., Manifacio, G., Toledo-Pereyra, L. M., and Lillehei, R. C.: Consistent protection from pancreatitis in canine pancreas allografts treated with 5 fluorouracil, J. Surg. Res. 18:305, 1975.
7. Chick, W. L., Like, A. A., and Lauris, V.: Beta cell culture on synthetic capillaries. An artificial endocrine pancreas, Science 187:847, 1975.
8. Collins, G. M., Bravo-Shugerman, L., and Terasaki, P. I.: Kidney preservation for transportation, Lancet 2:1219, 1969
9. Cough, D. A., Aisenberg, S., Colton, C. R., Giner, J., and Soeldner, J. S.: The status of electrochemical sensors for in vivo glucose monitoring, in *Proceedings of the Workshop Conference, Freiburg 1976*, pp. 10–22.
10. Crofford, O. B.: Report of the National Commission on Diabetes to the Congress of the United States. U.S. Department of Health, Education and Welfare, Publication No. 76, 1018 (Washington, D.C.: U.S. Government Printing Office, 1975).
11. Dickerman, R. M., Twiest, M. W., Crudup, J. W., and Turcotfe, J. G.: Transplantation of the pancreas into a retroperitoneal jejunal loop, Am. J. Surg. 129:48, 1975.
12. Dubernard, J. M., Pin, J., Gignoux, N., and Perrin, J.: Utilisation de l'artère épigastrique en transplantation rénale, J. Urol. Nephrol. 82:469, 1976.

13. Dubernard, J. M., Traeger, J., and Neyra, P.: Suppression of the exocrine function in view of segmental pancreatic transplantation in dogs, Biomedicine 27:172, 1977.

14. Dubernard, J. M., Traeger, J., Neyra, P., Blanc-Brunat, N., and Ruitton, A.: Une nouvelle méthode de transplantation pancréatique. I. Effet sur le pancréas du chien de l'injection intracanalaire de néoprène, Nouv. Presse Med., in press.

15. Erwald, R., Hed, R., Nygren, A., Rojdmark, S., and Wiechel, K. L.: Comparison of the effect of intraportal and intravenous infusion of insulin on blood glucose and free fatty acids in peripheral venous blood of man, Acta Med. Scand. 195:351, 1974.

16. Ferguson, J., Allsopp, R. M., Taylor, R. M., and Johnston, I. D.: Isolation and long term preservation of pancreatic islets from mouse, rat and guinea pigs, Diabetologia 12:115, 1976.

17. Frankel, B. J., Gylfe, E., Hellman, B., and Idahl, L. A.: Maintenance of insulin release from pancreatic islets stored in the cold for up to 5 weeks, J. Clin. Invest. 57:47, 1976.

18. Gabbay, K. H.: The sorbitol pathway and the complications of diabetes, N. Engl. J. Med. 288:831, 1973.

19. Gliedman, M. L., Tellis, V., Sobermar, R., Rifkin, H., Freed, S. C., and Veith, F. J.: Pancreatic transplantation, Transplant. Proc. 7:729, 1975.

20. Gliedman, M. L., Tellis, V., Rifkin, H., Freed, S. Z., and Veith, F. J.: Segmental pancreatic transplantation, in Touraine, J. L., Traeger, J., Revillard, J. P., Bétuel, H., Dubernard, J. M., and Triau, R. (eds.): *Transplantation et Immunologie Clinique, Lyon 1975,* (Villeurbanne: Simep-Editions, 1976), pp. 178–85.

21. Gold, M., Wittaker, J. R., Veith, F. J., and Gliedman, M. L.: Evaluation of ureteral drainage for pancreatic exocrine secretion, Surg. Forum 23:375, 1972.

22. Gregoir, W.: Traitement chirurgical du reflux congenital et du megauretere primaire, Urol. Int. 24:502, 1969.

23. Grenier, J. F., Haffen, K., Kedinger, M., Daulmel, J., and Eloy, R.: Implantation intrahepatique d'îlots endocrines de pancreas. Son efficacité dans le traitement du diabète expérimental, Chirurgie 102:256, 1976.

24. Groth, C. G., Lundgren, G., and Arner, P.: Rejection of isolated pancreatic allografts in patients with diabetes, Surg. Gynecol. Obstet. 143:933, 1976.

25. Guyton, J. R., Chang, R. W., Aisenberg, S., and Soeldner, J. S.: Activity of various endogenous compounds and pharmacologic agents at a glucose-oxidizing platinum electrode, Med. Instrum. 9:227, 1975.

26. Holdsworth, C. D., Nye, L., and King, E.: The effect of portacaval anastomosis on oral carbohydrate tolerance and on plasma insulin levels, Gut 13:58, 1972.

27. Kemp, C., Knight, M., Scharp, D., Ballinger, W., and Lacy, P.: Effect of transplantation site on results of pancreatic islet isografts in diabetic rats, Diabetologia 9:486, 1973.

28. Kiriakides, G. K., Arora, V. K., Lifton, J., Nuttal, F., and Miller, J.: Porcine pancreatic transplantation. Autotransplantation of duct ligated pancreatic segments, J. Surg. Res. 20:451, 1976.

29. Knight, M. J., Scharp, D. W., Kemp, C. B., Ballinger, W. F., and Lacy, P. E.: Effects of cold storage on the function of isolated pancreatic islets, Cryobiology 10:89, 1973.

30. Koncz, L., Zimmerman, C. E., De Leuis, R. A., and Davidoff, F.: Transplantation of pancreatic islets into the spleen of diabetic rats and subsequent splenectomy, Transplantation 21:427, 1976.

31. Kostianovsky, M., Lacy, P. E., Greider, M. H., and Still, M. F.: Long term (15 days) incubation of islets of Langerhans maintained in tissue culture, Lab. Invest. 27:53, 1972.

32. Lacy, P. E., and Kostianovsky, M.: Method for the isolation of intact islets of Langerhans from the rat pancreas, Diabetes 16:35, 1967.

33. Largiader, F., Uhlschmid, G., Binswanger, V., and Zaruba, K.: Pancreas rejection in combined pancreatico-duodenal and renal allotransplantation in man, Transplantation 19:185, 1975.

34. Lazarow, A., Weus, L., Carpenter, A., Hegre, O., and Leonard, R.: Islet differentiation, organ culture and transplantation, Diabetes 22:877, 1973.
35. Lillehei, R. C., Simmons, R. L., Najarian, J. S., Weil, R., Uchida, H., Ruiz, J. O., Kjellstrand, C. M., and Goetz, F. C.: Pancreaticoduodenal allotransplantation. Experimental and clinical experience, Ann. Surg. 172:405, 1970.
36. Lillehei, R. C., Simmons, R. L., Najarian, J. S., Kjellstrand, C. M., and Goetz, F. C.: Current state of pancreatic allotransplantation, Transplant. Proc. 3:318, 1971.
37. Little, J. M., Laver, C., and Hogg, J.: Pancreatic duct obstruction with an acrylate glue: a new method for producing pancreatic exocrine atrophy, Surgery 81:243, 1977.
38. Marco, J., Calle, C., Roman, D., Diaz-Fierros, M., Villanueva, M. L., and Valverde, I.: Hyperglucagonism induced by glucocorticoid treatment in man, N. Engl. J. Med. 288:128, 1973.
39. Marquet, R. L., and Heyster, G. A.: The effect of immunosuppressive treatment on the survival of allogeneic islets of Langerhans in rats, Transplantation 20:428, 1975.
40. Matas, A. J., Sutherland, D. E. R., and Najarian, J. S.: Current status of islet and pancreas transplantation in diabetes, Diabetes 25:785, 1976.
41. Matas, A. J., and Sutherland, D. E.: Pancreas and islet transplantation world, J. Surg. 1:189, 1977.
42. Mauer, S. M., Sutherland, D. E. R., Steffes, M. W., Leonard, R. J., Najarian, J. S., Michael, A. F., and Brown, D. M.: Pancreatic islet transplantation. Effects on the glomerular lesions of experimental diabetes in the rat, Diabetes 23:748, 1974.
43. Mellière, D.: Variations des artères hépatiques et du carrefour pancreatique, J. Chir. 95:5, 1968.
44. Merkel, R. K., Kelly, W. D., Goetz, F. C., and Maney, J. W.: Irradiated heterotopic segmental canine pancreatic allografts, Surgery 63:291, 1968.
45. Miogley, A. R., Rebar, R. W., and Niswender, G. D.: Radioimmuno-assays employing double antibody techniques, Acta Endocrinol. 142(Suppl.):247, 1969.
46. Mirkovich, V., and Campiche, M.: Successful intrasplenic autotransplantation of pancreatic tissue in totally depancreatized dogs. Transplantation 21:265, 1976.
47. Mirouze, J., Selam, J. L., and Pham, T. L.: Le pancreas artificiel extracorporel: applications en clinique et en recherche diabetologique, Nouv. Presse Med. 6:1837, 1977.
48. Mirouze, J., Selam, J. L., Pham, T. C., and Orsetti, A.: Le pancreas artificiel extra corporel: nouvelle orientation du traitement insulinique, in XIV Congr. Internat. Therap. Montpellier (Paris: Expansion Scientifique, 1977), pp. 79–91.
49. Najarian, J., Sutherland, D., and Steffes, M.: Isolation of human islets of Langerhans for transplantation, Transplant, Proc. 7(Suppl.):611, 1975.
50. Naji, A., Reckard, C. R., Ziegler, M. M., and Barker, C. F.: Vulnerability of pancreatic islets to immune cells and serum, Transplantation 26:459, 1975.
51. Nelken, D., Morse, S. I., Beyer, M. M., and Friedman, E. A.: Prolonged survival of allotransplanted islet of Langerhans cells in the rat, Transplantation 22:74, 1976.
52. Orloff, M. F., Lee, S., Charters, A. C., Grambort, D. E., Storck, G., and Knox, D.: Long term studies of pancreas transplantation in experimental diabetes mellitus, Ann. Surg. 182:198, 1973.
53. Orsetti, A., Puech, A. M., Zouari, N., Guy, C., and Passebois, F.: Isolement d'îlots de Langerhans intacts au moyen de chambres de digestion-filtration: leur utilisation chez le chien totalement dépancréaté, J. Ann. Diabetol. Hôtel-Dieu (Paris: Flammarion, 1977), pp. 66–75.
54. Orsetti, A., Zouari, N., Guy, Ch., Hagelsteen, Ch., and Puech, A. M.: Mise en place d'un distributeur bio-artificiel d'insuline chez le chien totalement dépancreaté, in XIV Congr. Internat. Therap. Montpellier (Paris: Expansion Scientifique, 1977), pp. 93–103.
55. Panijayamond, P., and Monaco, A. P.: Enhancement of pancreatic islet allograft survival with ALS and donor bone marrow, Surg. Forum 25:379, 1974.

56. Pfeiffer, E. F., Kerner, W., and Beischer, W.: The artificial endocrine pancreas: experimental research and clinical application, in XIV Congr. Internat. Therap. Montpellier (Paris: Expansion Scientifique, 1977), pp. 59–78.

57. Pirart, J.: Rigueur du traitement du diabète et complications rétiniennes, *Journées de Diabétologie Hôtel-Dieu* (Paris: Flammarion, 1977), pp. 282–96.

58. Reavew, G. M., Weisinger, J. R., and Swenson, R. S.: Insulin and glucose metabolism in renal insufficiency, Kidney Int. 6(Suppl.):63, 1974.

59. Reckard, C. R., Ziegler, M. M., and Barker, C. F.: Physiological and immunological consequences of transplanting isolated pancreatic islet, Surgery 74:91, 1973.

60. Ruiz, J. O., Uchida, J., Schultz, L. S., and Lillehei, R. C.: Function studies after auto and allotransplantation and denervation of pancreatico-duodenal segment in dogs, Am. J. Surg. 123:236, 1972.

61. Scharp, D. W., Kemp, C. B., Knight, M. J., Ballinger, W. F., and Lacy, P. E.: The use of Ficoll in the preparation of viable islets of Langerhans from the rat pancreas, Transplantation 6:686, 1973.

62. Scharp, D. W., Murphy, J. J., Newton, W. T., Ballinger, W. F., and Lacy, P. E.: Application of an improved isolation technique for islet transplantation in primates and rats, Transplant. Proc. 7(Suppl. 1):739, 1975.

63. Shibata, A., Ludvigsen, C., Naber, S., McDaniel, M., and Lacy, P. E.: Standardization of a digestion-filtration method for isolation of pancreatic islets, Diabetes 25: 667, 1976.

64. Sutherland, D. E., Steffes, M. W., Bauer, G. E., McManus, D., and Najarian, J. S.: Isolation of human and porcine islets of Langerhans and islet transplantation in pigs, J. Surg. Res. 16:102, 1974.

65. Sutherland, D. E., Matas, A. J., and Najarian, J. S.: Pancreas and islet transplantation, World J. Surg. 1:185, 1977.

66. Toledo-Pereyra, L. H., Castellanos, J., and Lampe, E. W.: Comparative evaluation of pancreas transplantation technics, Ann. Surg. 182:567, 1975.

67. Traeger, J., Dubernard, J. M., Touraine, J. L., Tranchant, D., and Neyra, P.: Une nouvelle méthode de transplantation pancreatique. II. Double transplantation pancreatique et rénale chez un diabétique en insuffisance rénale, Nouv. Presse Med., in press.

68. Traeger, J., Dubernard, J. M., Touraine, J. L., Neyra, P., Tranchant, D., and Malik, M. C.: Transplantation pancréatique dans le diabète compliqué d'insuffisance rénale, in *Actualités Néphrologiques* (Paris: Flammarion, in press).

69. Tze, W., Wong, F., Chen, Z., and O'Young, S.: Implantable artificial endocrine pancreas unit used to restore normoglycemia in diabetic rat, Nature 264:466, 1976.

70. Weil, R., Nozawa, M., Koss, M., Weber, C., Reemisma, K. B., and McIntosh, R.: Pancreatic transplantation in diabetic rats: renal function, morphology, ultrastructure and immuno histology, Surgery 78:142, 1975.

71. Wright, A. D., Lowy, C., Fraser, T. R., Spitz, I. M., Rubenstein, A. H., and Bersohn, I.: Serum growth-hormone and glucose tolerance in renal failure, Lancet 2:798, 1968.

72. ACS–NIH Organ Transplant Registry, Chicago, June 30, 1977.

Part II

THE KIDNEY, VITAMIN D AND RENAL OSTEODYSTROPHY

8

The Role of the Kidney in Vitamin D Metabolism

IAIN MacINTYRE, MB., Ch.B., Ph.D., D.Sc.

*Endocrine Unit, Royal Postgraduate Medical School,
University of London, London, England*

There has been an explosive increase in the knowledge of vitamin D metabolism during the past few years. We now know that the vitamin is the prohormone of the extremely potent secosteroid secreted by the kidney. This is the main hormone regulating the absorption of calcium and phosphorus from the intestine and its existence makes it easy to understand the central role of the kidney in calcium metabolism. Although it is now much easier to understand the occurrence of disturbances of calcium metabolism in cases of severe renal disease, we are still uncertain of exactly how the production of this new hormone by the kidney is regulated. But the major regulatory factors are probably known, at least in outline, and in this chapter I shall try to summarize the present state of knowledge.

Chemistry and Metabolism

Cholecalciferol (vitamin D_3) is a steroid derivative. Figure 8–1 shows the structure of 5α-cholestane, the parent saturated hydrocarbon of the particular steroid class from which vitamin D_3 and its congeners are derived. It is a tetracyclic structure

153

0084-5957/79/080153-11$3.75

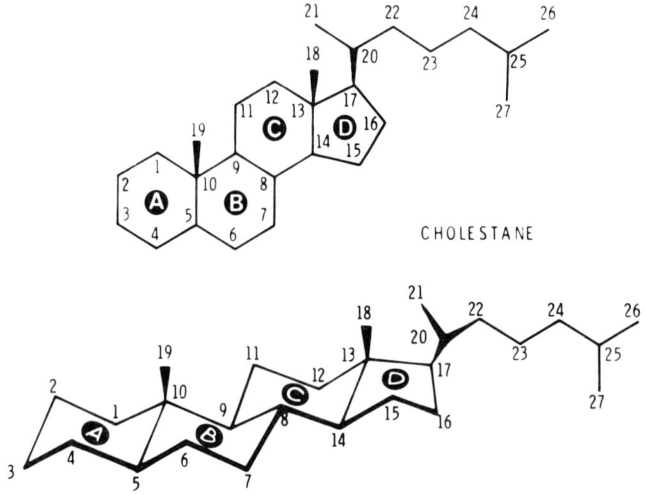

Fig. 8–1.—The conventional formula of 5α-cholestane, parent hydrocarbon of vitamin D₃ *(top)*. The perspective formula of the same hydrocarbon *(bottom)*.

made up by the *trans*-fusion of three cyclohexane rings A, B and C and one cyclopentane ring D. Attached to ring D at position 17 is an eight-carbon side chain, and at positions 10 and 13, respectively, there are two so-called angular methyl groups.

By convention (IUPAC-IUB Commission, 1967) the steroid ring system is always represented as shown in Figure 8 – 1, A: a top view with ring A at the lower left and ring D at the top right. When viewed in this way, the angular methyl groups and the side chain project above the plane of the rings; this is called the β-configuration. Substituents that project below the plane of the rings (e.g., the hydrogen atom at position 5 in 5α-cholestane) are designated as having the α-configuration. Conventionally, β-bonds are represented by heavy lines and α-bonds by broken lines. The spatial arrangement of the cholestane molecule is shown more clearly in the perspective view in Figure 8 – 1, B. Vitamin D₃ is normally synthesized in the skin from its precursor, 7-dehydrocholesterol, under the influence of sunlight. This compound differs from the parent cholestane in that it contains a 3β-hydroxyl group and two conjugated double bonds at positions 5 and 7 (Fig. 8 – 2). The 9 – 10 bond of this compound is broken by ultraviolet irradiation, thus disrupting ring B. Ring A then rotates 180 degrees around the 6 – 7 single bond to assume

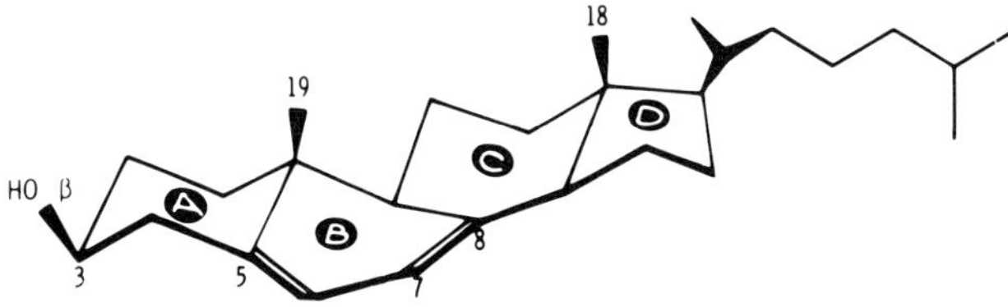

Fig. 8–2. – The conventional *(top)* and perspective *(bottom)* formulas of 7-dehydrocholesterol, the precursor of vitamin D_3.

Fig. 8–3. – Formation of vitamin D_3 (cholecalciferol) from its precursor 7-dehydrocholesterol, which occurs with ultraviolet irradiation.

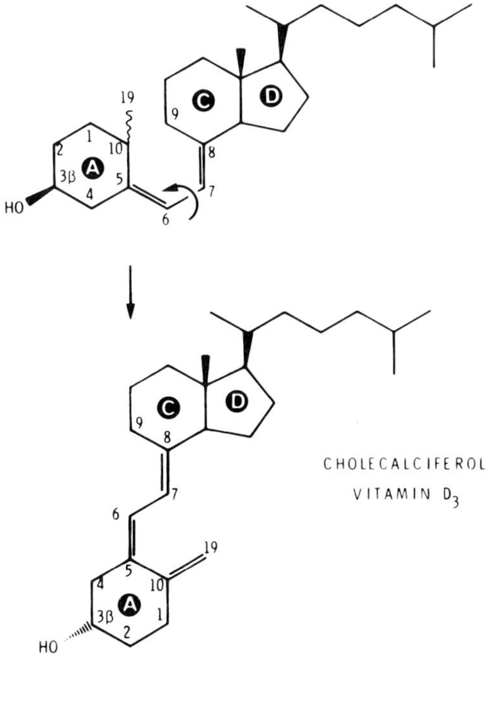

the stable conformation shown in Figure 8–3. This is cholecalciferol or vitamin D_3. Surprisingly, it seems that the major vitamin D source is synthesis in the skin rather than absorption from the diet. This is true even in people living in countries like Britain where the amount of sunlight is limited.

But vitamin D itself has very low activity. It must be transformed by two metabolic steps before exerting its characteristic effects. The first step involves the addition of a hydroxyl group at position 25, which converts vitamin D_3 to its major circulating form, 25-hydroxycholecalciferol $(25(OH)D_3)$ (Fig. 8–4). This step occurs in the liver and gut and is subject to only slight regulation. 25-Hydroxycholecalciferol was once thought to be the final active form of the vitamin and, in sufficient concentration, it does have biologic activity; but a further and crucial hydroxylation takes place in the kidney, converting $25(OH)D_3$ to $1\alpha,25$-dihydroxycholecalciferol $(1\alpha,25(OH)_2D_3)$. This latter compound should be regarded as an extremely potent steroid hormone secreted by the kidney: it is the most important humoral agent involved in the regulation of calcium metabolism (Fig. 8–5). This final hydroxylation is under extremely precise metabolic regulation, which adjusts the secretion of $1\alpha,25(OH)_2D_3$ to the calcium and phosphate needs of the organism.

The Regulation of Vitamin D Metabolism

$1\alpha,25$-Dihydroxycholecalciferol is the most potent single hormonal agent affecting calcium metabolism. Regulation of its

Fig. 8–4.—Formation of 25-hydroxycholecalciferol from cholecalciferol.

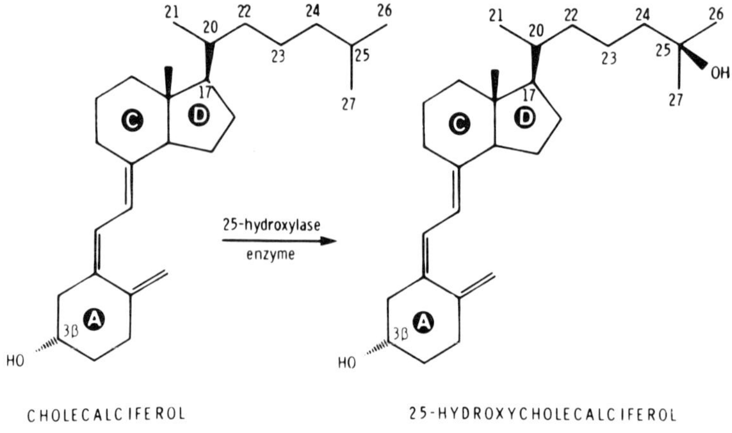

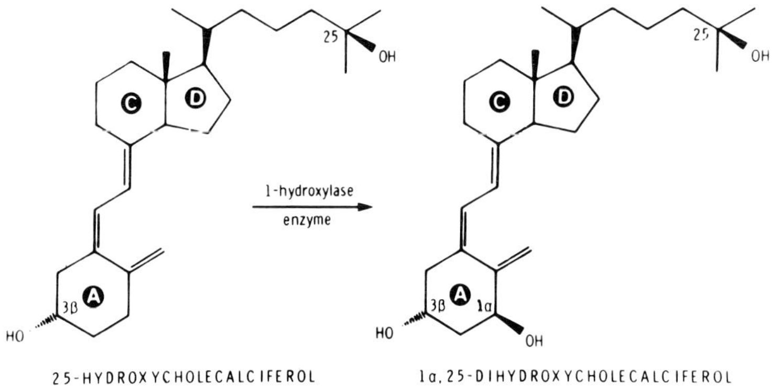

1-hydroxylase enzyme

25-HYDROXYCHOLECALCIFEROL   1α,25-DIHYDROXYCHOLECALCIFEROL

Fig. 8–5.—Formation of 1α,25-dihydroxycholecalciferol from 25-hydroxycholecalciferol.

secretion by the kidney must therefore be responsive to changing physiologic needs in order to achieve precise homeostasis of calcium and phosphorus metabolism. The question is: How is this achieved? The answers have been several and often hotly disputed. However, a number of regulatory factors are now known and generally accepted. These are: $1\alpha,25(OH)_2D_3$ itself,[7, 17] the calcium and phosphorus content of the diet[2, 6, 8] and parathyroid hormone.[3] But important as these factors are, they do not provide a satisfactory explanation for the major changes in calcium and phosphorus absorption that occur during growth, pregnancy and lactation. In each of these situations the plasma level of $1\alpha,25(OH)_2D_3$ is increased,[11] suggesting that this hormone is the physiologic agent of the changes. None of the known factors discussed above is fully adequate to account for the increases in plasma $1\alpha,25(OH)_2D_3$ levels in these situations.[9] Thus, for example, parathyroid hormone is clearly necessary in some circumstances for normal vitamin D metabolism, and may be responsible, at least in part, for adaptation to some of the extreme variations in calcium and phosphorus content of diets produced in the laboratory. But these manipulations are no model of the marked changes in calcium and phosphorus metabolism in the physiologic situations mentioned above. We regard parathyroid hormone and the other factors cited above as important permissive elements, rather than the primary agents of physiologic regulation of vitamin D metabolism in health.

I believe that the more important physiologic regulators are prolactin and growth hormone, and I shall now summarize the recent evidence supporting this view.

PROLACTIN

Prolactin has a striking effect in enhancing the production of $1\alpha,25(OH)_2D_3$ in the chick,[14, 16] but the many different actions of prolactin in various species make it difficult to·extrapolate from one to the other. However, there are two sets of experiments showing that prolactin is also of importance in mammals. The first reported a fourfold increase in $1\alpha,25(OH)_2D_3$ levels during lactation in the rat.[1] Although consistent with the effect of prolactin, such an increase might have been caused by stimulation of $1\alpha,25(OH)_2D_3$ production by the calcium loss produced by lactation, rather than by a more direct involvement of prolactin.

For this reason a second set of experiments was carried out.[15] Prolactin secretion was suppressed suddenly by the administration of bromocryptine to female rats one day after delivery of their litters. At this stage lactation was just being established

Fig. 8–6. – The design of the experiment to assess the importance of prolactin on plasma $1\alpha,25(OH)_2D_3$ levels after delivery. The rats were maintained on a diet of 0.2% calcium, 0.9% phosphorus and 2 IU vitamin D_3/gm for 30 days. Bromocryptine was given to the indicated groups one day after delivery. This complete experiment was carried out twice.

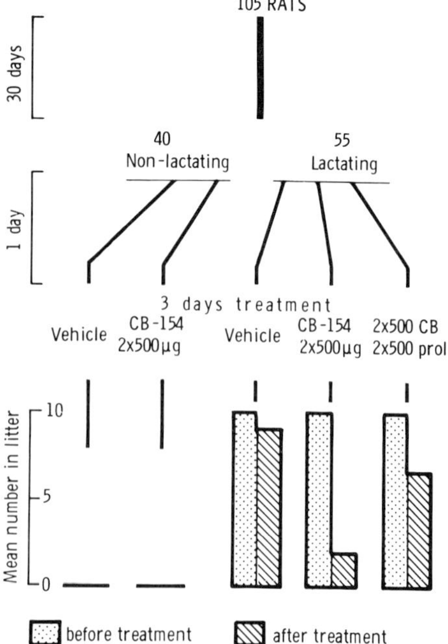

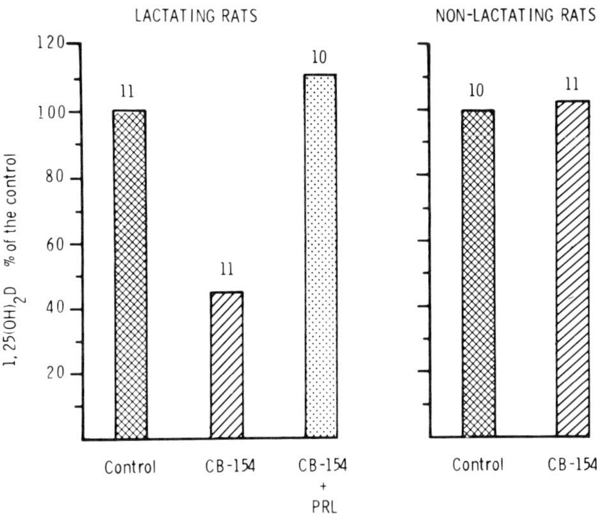

Fig. 8–7. — Results of experiment described in Figure 8–6. Prolactin affects the level of plasma $1\alpha,25(OH)_2D_3$ in certain physiologic settings.

and the calcium drain must have been minimal and much less than in the later stages of established lactation. The design of the experiment is illustrated in Figure 8–6; the results are shown in Figure 8–7. They are very striking. Inhibition of the secretion of prolactin halved the plasma $1\alpha,25(OH)_2D_3$ level; and this effect of bromocryptine was reversed by the administration of ovine prolactin. It can be seen that bromocryptine had no effect on the normal lactating control rats. This experiment shows conclusively that prolactin has an effect on plasma $1\alpha,25(OH)_2D_3$ levels, but that it acts only in the correct physiologic setting. It is not certain, however, that the effect of prolactin is a direct one. It remains conceivable that these changes are produced by the alterations in calcium metabolism produced by lactation. But there can be no question that prolactin does act in mammals, and that its action is of major physiologic importance. I shall discuss below one possible mechanism of this effect.

GROWTH HORMONE

The similarities in the sequence of prolactin and growth hormone naturally suggest that the effects of prolactin just described might also be found in growth hormone, thus explaining the increased calcium and phosphorus retention during growth. This hypothesis was tested experimentally and will be reported in detail elsewhere.[13] The essential results are shown in Figures 8–8 and 8–9. Hypophysectomy in rats produces a dramatic decrease in the plasma $1\alpha,25(OH)_2D_3$ levels, and this decrease is completely restored by the administration of growth hormone. Of great interest was the additional observation, not shown in the figure, that ovine prolactin was quite ineffective in elevating the depressed levels of $1\alpha,25(OH)_2D_3$ produced by hypophysectomy. This emphasizes and confirms the conclusions from the prolactin experiment reported above: prolactin is active in mammals in increasing $1\alpha,25(OH)_2D_3$ production but only in concert with other factors and in the appropriate physiologic setting.

Fig. 8–8.—The design of the experiment to assess the effect of growth hormone on hypophysectomized rats. Male Wistar rats were maintained on a diet containing 1.0% calcium, 0.9% phosphorus and 2 IU vitamin D_3/gm for four weeks after weaning. After hypophysectomy or sham-operation and a further equilibration period of eight days on the same diet, highly purified human growth hormone or ovine prolactin was given to the groups as indicated.

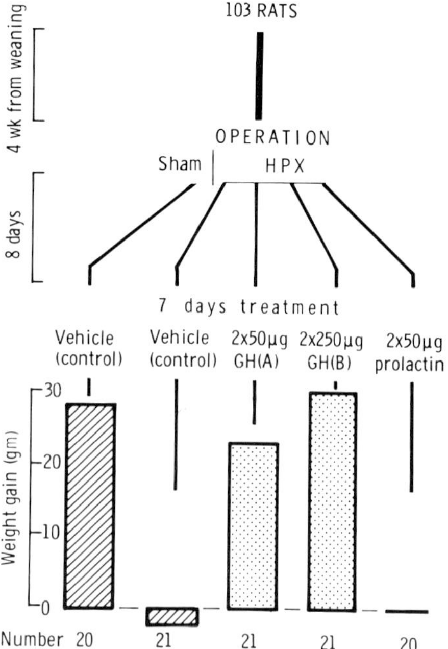

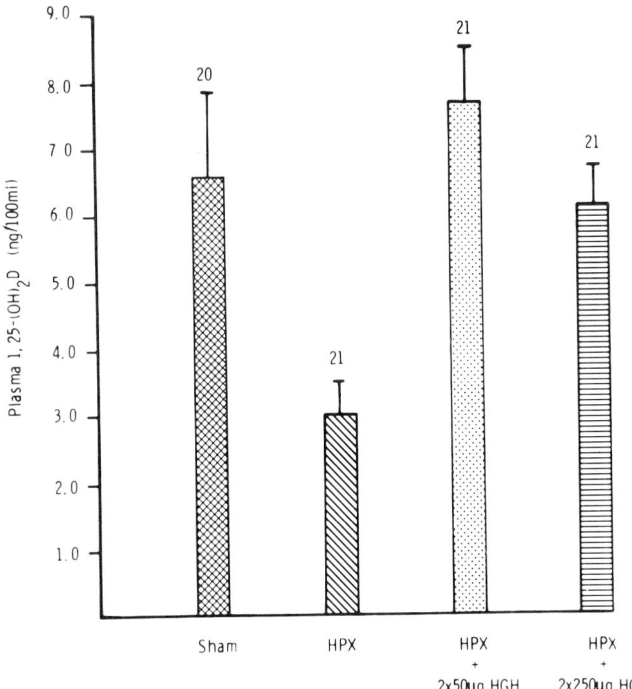

Fig. 8–9.—Results of experiment described in Figure 8–9. Hypophysectomized rats showed a decrease in the level of plasma $1\alpha,25(OH)_2D_3$, which returned to normal after the administration of growth hormone.

The demonstrated action of growth hormone needs little qualification. It completely accounts for the enhanced alimentary absorption of calcium and phosphorus during growth and indicates that it is due to stimulation of $1\alpha,25(OH)_2D_3$ production by growth hormone, with a consequent increase in plasma levels. This effect is probably also the basis of the known disturbances of calcium and phosphorus metabolism seen in patients with acromegaly.[4]

MECHANISM OF ACTION OF PROLACTIN AND GROWTH HORMONE

The mechanism of action is still unknown. One cannot rule out the possibility that these hormones act via the known regulators of vitamin D metabolism discussed at the beginning of this chapter, but this is rather unlikely. Thus, for example, the administration of growth hormone to hypophysectomized rats increased the plasma calcium and phosphorus levels only slightly, changes which in themselves would have tended to depress $1\alpha,25(OH)_2D_3$ production.[8] A much more attractive hypothesis is that both growth hormone and prolactin act via somatomedin. This is supported by the observation that insulin can increase the levels of plasma $1\alpha,25(OH)_2D_3$,[5] since somatomedin and insulin are known to be closely related in structure.[10, 12]

Whether or not this turns out to be true, there is now no reasonable doubt that the pituitary gland plays a dominant role in regulating vitamin D metabolism in healthy subjects.

Summary

The kidney should be regarded as an organ of central importance in the regulation of calcium metabolism. Its secretion product, $1\alpha,25(OH)_2D_3$, is regulated by several factors, including the calcium and phosphorus content of the diet, parathyroid hormone and the level of $1\alpha,25(OH)_2D_3$ itself. The main occasions in health where $1\alpha,25(OH)_2D_3$ secretion is enhanced are during growth and reproduction. In these situations the secretion of this new renal hormone is under at least partial control of growth hormone and prolactin.

Acknowledgments

Much of the work reported here was supported in part by grants from the Wellcome Trust and Medical Research Council.

References

1. Boass, A., Toverud, S. U., McCain, T. A., Pike, J. W., and Haussler, M. R.: Elevated serum levels of 1α,25-dihydroxycholecalciferol in lactating rats, Nature 267:630, 1977.
2. Boyle, I. T., Gray, R. W., and DeLuca, H. F.: Regulation by calcium of *in vivo* synthesis of 1,25-dihydroxycholecalciferol and 21,25-dihydroxycholecalciferol, Proc. Natl. Acad. Sci. USA 58:2131, 1971.
3. Garabedian, M., Holick, M. F., DeLuca, H. F., and Boyle, I. T.: Control of 25-hydroxycholecalciferol metabolism by parathyroid glands, Proc. Natl. Acad. Sci. USA 69:1673, 1972.
4. Hanna, S., MacIntyre, I., Harrison, M. T., and Fraser, R.: Effects of growth hormone on calcium and magnesium metabolism, Br. Med. J. 2:12, 1961.
5. Haussler, M. R.: Personal communication.
6. Haussler, M. R., Baylink, D. J., Hughes, M. R., Brumbaugh, P. F., Wergedal, J. W.,

Shen, F. H., Nielsen, R. L., Counts, S. J., Bursac, K. M., and McCain, T. A.: The assay of 1α,25-dihydroxyvitamin D$_3$: physiologic and pathologic modulation of circulating hormone levels, Clin. Endocrinol. 5(Suppl.):151, 1976.

7. Larkins, R. G., Macauley, S. J., and MacIntyre, I.: Feedback control of vitamin D metabolism by a nuclear action of 1,25-dihydroxycholecalciferol on the kidney, Nature, 252:412, 1974.

8. Larkins, R. G., Macauley, S. J., Colston, K. W., Evans, I. M. A., Galante, L. S., and MacIntyre, I.: Regulation of vitamin D metabolism without parathyroid hormone, Lancet 2:289, 1973.

9. Leader: Lancet 1:840, 1977.

10. Niall, H.: The evolution of peptide hormones: relaxin and insulin as growth regulatory peptides, in MacIntyre, I., and Szelke, M. (eds.): *Proceedings of the Sixth International Conference on Endocrinology.* Amsterdam: Elsevier/North Holland, in press.

11. Pike, J. W., Toverud, S., Boass, A., McCain, T., and Haussler, M. R.: Circulating 1α,25(OH)$_2$D$_3$ during physiological states of calcium stress, in Norman, A. W., Schaefer, K., Coburn, J. W., Deluca, H. F., Fraser, D., Grigoleit, H. G., and Herrath, D. V. (eds.): *Vitamin D, Biochemical, Chemical and Clinical Aspects Related to Calcium Metabolism* (New York: Walter de Gruyter, 1977), pp. 187–89.

12. Shields, R.: Growth hormones and serum factors, Nature 267:308, 1977.

13. Spanos, E., Barrett, D., MacIntyre, I., Pike, J. W., Safilian, E., and Haussler, M. R.: Nature, in press.

14. Spanos, E., Colston, K. W., Evans, I. M. A., Galante, L. S., Macauley, S. J., and MacIntyre, I.: Effect of prolactin on vitamin D metabolism, Mol. Cell. Endocrinol. 5:163, 1976.

15. Spanos, E., Colston, K. W., Robinson, C. J., MacIntyre, I., Pike, J. W., McCain, T. A., and Haussler, M. R.: Unpublished data.

16. Spanos, E., Pike, J. W., Haussler, M. R., Colston, K. W., Evans, I. M. A., Goldner, A. M., McCain, T. A., and MacIntyre, I.: Circulation of 1α,25-dihydroxyvitamin D in the chick: Enhancement by injection of prolactin and during egg-laying, Life Sci. 19:1751, 1976.

17. Tanaka, Y., and DeLuca, H. F.: Stimulation of 24,25-dihydroxyvitamin D$_3$ production by 1α,25-dihydroxyvitamin D$_3$, Science, 183:1198, 1974.

9

Metabolic and Cellular
Activity of Vitamin D

M. GARABEDIAN, M.D., AND A. ULMANN, M.D.

Hôpital Necker, Enfants Malades, Paris, France

Vitamin D_3 (cholecalciferol) exerts its tissue effects via its hydroxylated metabolites, among them $1\alpha,25$-dihydroxyvitamin D_3 [1,25(OH)$_2$D$_3$] and possibly 25-hydroxyvitamin D_3 [25(OH)D$_3$] and 24,25-dihydroxyvitamin D_3 [24,25(OH)$_2$D$_3$].[23, 39, 47, 56] The fact that they were only recently discovered explains why their respective biologic activities are not yet fully understood.

First, we shall review our knowledge regarding the effect of these metabolites on vitamin D target organs. Then we shall review their cellular mechanisms of action.

Tissue Effects of Vitamin D and Its Metabolites

INTESTINAL EFFECT

Vitamin D influences intestinal calcium absorption.[54] This absorption is the result of passive and active phenomena. Vitamin D may increase passive calcium absorption, since it modifies the lipid composition of the microvilli.[29] Vitamin D also stimulates active calcium absorption through the brush border of duodenal and jejunal cells. The active metabolite for this vitamin D effect seems to be 1,25(OH)$_2$D$_3$, since in vivo it has been

165

shown that $1,25(OH)_2D_3$ stimulates calcium absorption faster than do the other D_3 metabolites[25] and that its effect persists in nephrectomized animals.[7]

Vitamin D also stimulates the calcium-independent phosphorus absorption process.[33] Its active form is also $1,25(OH)_2D_3$.[16]

BONE EFFECT

It has been known for a long time that vitamin D enhances bone mineralization. This effect is used as a test of biologic activity for vitamin D metabolites. After administration of the metabolite studied, its biologic activity in vitamin D-deficient animals can be quantified[6, 8, 49, 68] by weighing mineral ashes from tibia or femur,[6, 49, 68] studying bone biopsies[8] or using the line test.[68] In all these systems, $1,25(OH)_2D_3$ is equally if not more potent than $25(OH)D_3$ when administered daily. However, $24,25(OH)_2D_3$ is less potent than $25(OH)D_3$.[6] There is no evidence for a direct effect of vitamin D or its metabolites on bone mineralization. Until now, the antirachitic effect of vitamin D was thought to be due to the $1,25(OH)_2D_3$-enhanced intestinal absorption of calcium and phosphorus and mobilization from bone. Calcium and phosphorus mobilization from deep bone constitutes the only direct proven effect of vitamin D on bone. The vitamin D metabolite responsible for this action is $1,25(OH)_2D_3$. In vivo, its injection into calcium- and vitamin D-deprived animals is followed by an increase in both serum calcium and phosphorus concentrations. In nephrectomized animals, $1,25(OH)_2D_3$ is still active, whereas $25(OH)D_3$ and some other metabolites [$24,25(OH)_2D_3$ and 25,26-dihydroxy-vitamin D_3 ($25,26(OH)_2D_3$)] are not.[23, 59] Higher potency of $1,25(OH)_2D_3$ has also been demonstrated in vitro: $1,25(OH)_2D_3$ permits calcium liberation from fetal bone at a lower concentration than other vitamin D metabolites.[48, 66, 67] Similarly, parathyroid hormone (PTH), vitamin A and molecules such as heparin can "mobilize" calcium and phosphorus. The interaction sites between such substances and $1,25(OH)_2D_3$ are still unknown.

Recent work has shown that vitamin D may have bone effects other than calcium and phosphorus mobilization and that such effects may be mediated by vitamin D metabolite(s) other than $1,25(OH)_2D_3$. Thus, there have been instances of in vitro calcium transport into cells from fetal bone, which is modified by 25(OH)-D_3 or 24,25$(OH)_2D_3$, but not by 1,25$(OH)_2D_3$.[24] In addition, the resorbing effect of substances such as PTH, vitamin A and heparin is inhibited in vitro by low concentrations of 24,25$(OH)_2D_3$ but not by 1,25$(OII)_2D_3$.[45] In vivo, results from histologic bone studies performed in rats[52] and in anephric patients[5] support the hypothesis of a bone action of vitamin D metabolites other than 1,25$(OH)_2D_3$.

Finally, vitamin D or one of its metabolites may control collagen synthesis,[50] thus modifying bone composition.

Renal Effects

Controversy still exists as to whether or not vitamin D has an effect on the urinary elimination of calcium and phosphorus. A fortiori, the vitamin D metabolite responsible for this action remains unknown. Some workers think that vitamin D decreases urinary elimination of calcium by increasing its tubular reabsorption. Others have found that 1,25$(OH)_2D_3$ does not change the urinary calcium excretion of rats whether they are thyroparathyroidectomized or not.[38] At a low dose, 25(OH)D_3 has no effect on urinary phosphorus excretion of either vitamin D-deficient[63] or normal[60] thyroparathyroidectomized rats, whereas it lowers phosphaturia when perfused at a higher concentration[62, 63] or in the presence of small amounts of PTH.[60, 63] Popovtzer *et al.* even suggested that 25(OH)D_3 decreases the PTH- and calcitonin-dependent renal cyclic adenosine monophosphate (cAMP) content, thus decreasing urinary phosphorus elimination.[60, 61] On the contrary, 25(OH)D_3 or one of its metabolites has been shown to have a "permissive" effect on the phosphaturic action of PTH.[63] Moreover, physiologic doses of 1,25$(OH)_2D_3$ can correct the decrease in urinary phosphorus excretion in subjects following thyroparathyroidectomy.[4]

Thus, the renal actions of vitamin D do not appear to be well defined. Similarly, relations between PTH and vitamin D are unclear, since PTH itself influences the 25(OH)D_3 metabolism into its active forms.[23] It is conceivable that in thyroparathyroidectomized rats the decrease in 1,25$(OH)_2D_3$ synthesis unmasks an antiphosphaturic effect of 25(OH)D_3 or of its other metabolites. In addition, we have shown that 1,25$(OH)_2D_3$ itself may control blood phosphorus homeostasis[28] by correcting both

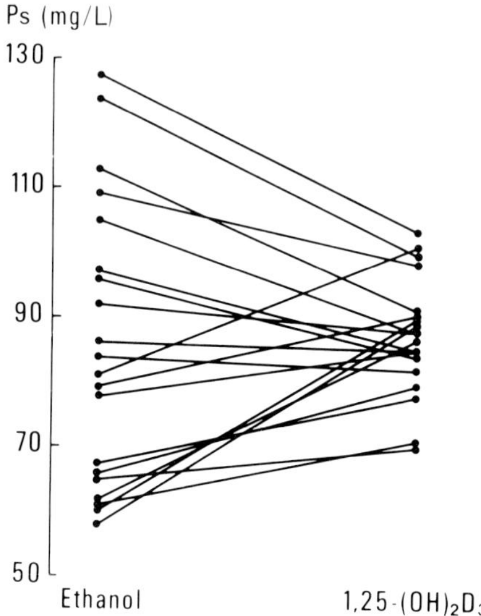

Fig. 9–1. — Serum phosphorus concentration *(Ps)* in mg/L of growing rats 24 hours after the last of one or five daily injections of 130 pM 1,25(OH)$_2$D$_3$ *(right)* or its ethanol solvent *(left)*. Each symbol represents the mean of five to ten rats. Diets used to obtain group of rats with different Ps are detailed in reference 28.

hypophosphatemia and hyperphosphatemia in growing rats (Fig. 9–1). The mechanism of this effect remains unknown. Were it at the renal level, a given dosage of 1,25(OH)$_2$D$_3$ should have either a "phosphaturic" effect or an "antiphosphaturic" effect, depending on the phosphorus and calcium balance at the time of the experiment.

Effects on Parathyroid Glands

As to a possible direct action of vitamin D on parathyroid glands, opinions vary and depend on the metabolite studied. It seems that 1,25(OH)$_2$D$_3$ decreases PTH secretion both in vivo and in vitro.[19] This action may be an indirect one, as other workers have observed an increase in PTH secretion at the beginning of 1,25(OH)$_2$D$_3$ administration.[15, 46] Such a discrepancy may be explained by the recent work of Oldham *et al.*, which suggests that 1,25(OH)$_2$D$_3$ could "sensitize" parathyroid glands to changes in extracellular calcium concentration.[58] Conversely,

24,25$(OH)_2D_3$ administration decreases PTH secretion.[14, 15] It has been suggested that changes in PTH secretion require the presence of both 1,25$(OH)_2D_3$ and 24,25$(OH)_2D_3$.[36]

EFFECTS ON MUSCLE

In vitro, 25$(OH)D_3$ increases the protein synthesis and the adenosine triphosphate (ATP) content of muscle cells and stimulates inorganic phosphate incorporation into these cells.[3] The muscular asthenia observed in vitamin D-deficient subjects might be related to this effect.

EFFECTS ON GROWTH AND CARTILAGE

These effects may be secondary to the role of vitamin D in bone mineralization. The possibility of a direct effect of vitamin D on growth has not been proved in vivo.[65] However, an interaction between vitamin D and growth plate cartilage has been demonstrated recently in vitro. Radioactive sulfur incorporation into proteoglycan from cultured chondrocytes is enhanced by 25$(OH)D_3$, and even more by its 1- and 24-hydroxylated metabolites.[22] Moreover, in vitro, cartilage metabolizes 25$(OH)D_3$ into 24,25$(OH)_2D_3$.[27] This transformation was thought until recently to occur only in the kidney. The existence of extrarenal 25$(OH)D_3$-24-hydroxylase could account for the low but detectable concentrations of 24,25$(OH)_2D_3$ found in binephrectomized patients.[26]

Cellular Actions of Vitamin D Metabolites

Cellular action of 1,25$(OH)_2D_3$ initiates protein synthesis in its target cells. An agent blocking the DNA transcription, actinomycin D, inhibits the intestinal effects of 1,25$(OH)_2D_3$ both in vivo[55] and in vitro.[21] It is to be noted, however, that this effect has not been found by all authors.[69] Experiments in chicks strongly suggest a 1,25$(OH)_2D_3$ action via protein synthesis. Administration of 1,25$(OH)_2D_3$ increases both in vivo and in vitro chick intestinal chromatin template activity toward *Escherichia coli* RNA polymerase; i.e., RNA polymerase activity decreases in chick intestinal nuclei after vitamin D treatment.[76]

This effect might be nonspecific, however, and related to the calcium ion.[43] One of the $1,25(OH)_2D_3$-dependent proteins is the calcium-binding protein (CaBP), described by Wasserman *et al.*[74] Intestine from vitamin D-deficient chicks contains no CaBP, but CaBP appears in the intestine several hours after vitamin D administration. The lack of intestinal CaBP therefore appears to be suitable evidence of vitamin D deficiency. Using a cell-free system, Lawson and Emtage have shown that only polysomes from vitamin D-treated chicks were able to initiate de novo synthesis of an immunoprecipitable CaBP.[43] Polysomes from vitamin D-deficient and nontreated chicks were incapable of such action.

The $1,25(OH)_2D_3$-dependent synthesis of new proteins may involve a cellular mechanism of action identical to that described for steroid hormones. The $1,25(OH)_2D_3$ migrates through the cell membrane, and binds with a high affinity to a cytoplasmic protein or "receptor" with low maximal binding capacity. In the intestinal cell cytoplasm of the chick[41, 70] and rat,[18, 40, 71] these receptors are present in embryos more than 15 days old. This observation correlates well with the fact that CaBP synthesis also occurs in chick embryos after the 15th day.[57] Inside chick intestine the $1,25(OH)_2D_3$ complex migrates to the nucleus via a temperature-dependent process.[13, 44] It binds to nuclear chromatin in a specific and saturable manner.[9, 12] This finding was used in making the first $1,25(OH)_2D_3$ radioreceptor assay.[11] A similar process has been observed in duodenal cells from vitamin D-deficient rats (Table 9–1).[2]

The exact role of CaBP in calcium absorption remains unknown. It is a widespread protein found also in tissues other

TABLE 9–1.—TRITIATED $1,25(OH)_2D_3$ (^{3}H-$1,25(OH)_2D_3$) NUCLEAR UPTAKE BY DUODENAL MUCOSA CELL NUCLEI FROM VITAMIN D-DEFICIENT RATS

STEROLS IN INCUBATION MEDIUM	RADIOACTIVE STEROL FOUND IN NUCLEI* (pM/mg DNA)	
^{3}H-$1,25(OH)_2D_3$ (8 nM) alone	1.40 + 0.43	(No.† = 3)
^{3}H-$1,25(OH)_2D_3$ (8 nM) + $1,25(OH)_2D_3$ (8 μM)	0.65 + 0.24	(No. = 3)
^{3}H-$1,25(OH)_2D_3$ (8 nM) + $1\alpha(OH)_2D_3$ (8 μM)	1.21 + 0.30	(No. = 3)
^{3}H-$1,25(OH)_2D_3$ (8 nM) + $25(OH)D_3$ (8 μM)	1.51 + 0.23	(No. = 3)

*Nuclei were prepared as described in reference 2.
†Number of experiments.

than intestine.[73] In addition, Spencer *et al.* have shown that $1,25(OH)_2D_3$ injection into rachitic chicks is followed first by an increase in intestinal calcium absorption, then by the appearance of messenger RNA coding for CaBP, increasing to a maximal level after 24 hours.[64] After about four hours, CaBP becomes detectable. Its intestinal concentration reaches a plateau after 16 hours and stays maximum for 48 hours. Thus calcium absorption *precedes* the CaBP synthesis in this system. Such results have led workers to look for some other vitamin D-dependent protein(s), the synthesis of which takes place earlier than that of CaBP. Indeed, Wilson and Lawson have shown that two proteins (MW 45,000 and 85,000) are synthesized in chick intestinal brush border within four hours after $1,25(OH)_2D_3$ administration.[75] The role of such proteins in calcium transport is not yet defined.

The presence of $1,25(OH)_2D_3$ also stimulates the activity of some enzymes, among which are a calcium-dependent ATPase and an alkaline phosphatase.[34, 51] A single protein could possess both activities.[34] The activation of alkaline phosphatase occurs soon after $1,25(OH)_2D_3$ administration. This activation is probably the consequence of the fixation of a sialic acid molecule on the inactive form of the enzyme. The administration of $1,25(OH)_2$-D_3 stimulates sialic acid fixation.[53] Enzyme activation could be secondary to a direct effect of $1,25(OH)_2D_3$ on cellular membranes. Its role in calcium intestinal absorption has not been defined.

Among $1,25(OH)_2D_3$ structural analogues, 1α-hydroxyvitamin D_3 ($1\alpha(OH)D_3$) is nearly as potent as $1,25(OH)_2D_3$. We have shown that $1\alpha(OH)D_3$ cannot prevent $1,25(OH)_2D_3$ from migrating to the nuclei of rat duodenal mucosa cells (Table 9–1).[2] Such a finding is in agreement with results of physiologic experiments showing that in rats the biologic activity of $1\alpha(OH)D_3$ occurs only after 25-hydroxylation.[37]

Intestinal mucosa cells are not the sole target cells of $1,25(OH)_2D_3$. For instance, some workers have looked for a possible direct action of $1,25(OH)_2D_3$ on parathyroid cells. Henry and Norman have shown that radioactive $1,25(OH)_2D_3$ produced after parenteral administration of radioactive vitamin D to rachitic chicks is concentrated in the parathyroid glands.[35] Brumbaugh *et al.* have demonstrated the existence inside chick parathyroid cells of nuclear and cytoplasmic components with a high affinity for $1,25(OH)_2D_3$.[10] Our group has shown that $1,25(OH)_2D_3$ binding receptors exist in porcine parathyroid cell cytosol,[20] and that $1,25(OH)_2D_3$ migrates to the nucleus (Fig. 9–2).

Nothing is known about the cellular action of $1,25(OH)_2D_3$ in bone. In kidney, $1,25(OH)_2D_3$ stimulates tritiated uridine incorporation into nuclear RNA.[17]

Some experiments suggest that $25(OH)D_3$ has a cellular action independent from its metabolism into $1,25(OH)_2D_3$. Cultured cells from chick intestinal mucosa synthesize CaBP and transport calcium in the presence of $25(OH)D_3$, which in this system cannot be transformed into $1,25(OH)_2D_3$.[21] As noted above, Birge and Haddad have shown that $25(OH)D_3$ increases the ATP and protein content of cultured rat muscle cells, whereas $1,25(OH)_2D_3$ has no effect in this system.[3]

Several workers have described cytoplasmic proteins having a

Fig. 9–2.—Nuclear uptake at 37 C of radioactive $1,25(OH)_2D_3$ inside porcine parathyroid cells (nuclei were prepared as indicated in reference 20). The difference between migration inside cells incubated with ^3H-$1,25(OH)_2D_3$ alone *(left)* or in the presence of a large excess of unlabeled $1,25(OH)_2D_3$ *(right)* represents the saturable nuclear uptake.

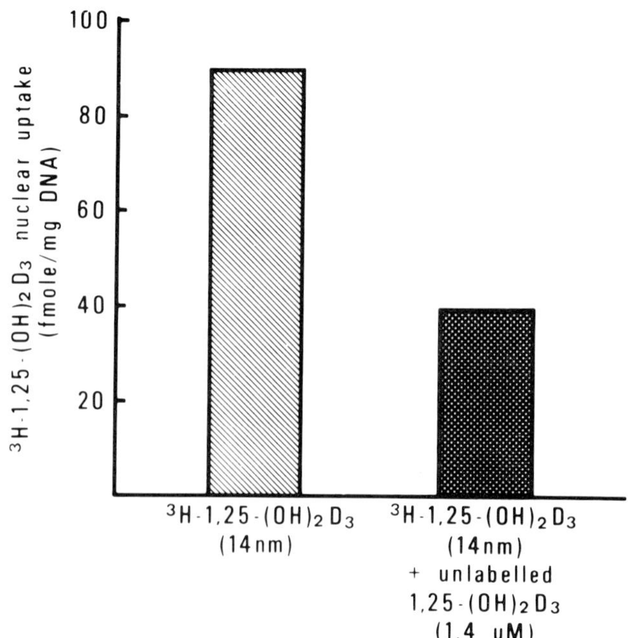

high affinity for $25(OH)D_3$ with biochemical features differing from those of $1,25(OH)_2D_3$.[30, 32, 42, 71] Such proteins have a widespread distribution; they have been found in the cytoplasm of all nucleated cells.[30, 43] Their functional role is still unknown. They surely are not functional "receptors" because, for example, we never found a $25(OH)D_3$-specific nuclear uptake inside rat intestinal mucosa cells.[2] It has been recently proposed that such $25(OH)D_3$ binders may result from an aggregation between plasma $25(OH)D_3$ binder and a cytoplasmic protein having no affinity for $25(OH)D_3$. This aggregation may be the result of an artifact.[72] Whatever its functional role, $25(OH)D_3$ binding protein is used in some $25(OH)D_3$ assay processes.[31]

The cellular action of other vitamin D metabolites is unknown. However, work is in progress to discover the $24,25(OH)_2$-D_3 cellular mechanism of action in rabbit growth plate cartilage.

Summary

Most of the effects of vitamin D on calcium and phosphorus homeostasis result from an increase in intestinal absorption of calcium and phosphorus and from bone mobilization. These effects are due to $1,25(OH)_2D_3$, one of the renal vitamin D metabolites. Besides ionic mobilization, vitamin D may exert additional effects on bone which depend on metabolites other than $1,25(OH)_2D_3$. Kidneys, parathyroid glands and muscle are probably target organs for vitamin D. The metabolite(s) responsible for these actions remain unknown.

References

1. Au, W. Y. W., and Bukowski, A.: Inhibition of PTH secretion by vitamin D metabolites in organ cultures of rat parathyroids, Fed. Proc. 35:530, 1976.
2. Bachelet, M., Ulmann, A., Cloix, J. F., and Funck-Brentano, J. L.: Nuclear uptake of cholecalciferol metabolites in rat duodenal mucosa, J. Steroid Biochem. 8:1047, 1977.
3. Birge, S. J., and Haddad, J. G.: 25-hydroxycholecalciferol stimulation of muscle metabolism, J. Clin. Invest. 56:1100, 1975.
4. Bonjour, J. P., Preston, C., and Fleisch, H.: Role of 1,25-dihydroxyvitamin D_3 (1,25-$(OH)_2D_3$) in the renal handling of inorganic phosphate (Pi) in rats, Experientia 33:777, 1977 (Abstract).
5. Bordier, P. J., Tun Chot, S., Eastwood, J. B., Fournier, A., and De Wardener, H. E.: Lack of histological evidence of vitamin D abnormality in the bones of anephric patients, Clin. Sci. Mol. Med. 44:33, 1973.

6. Boris, A., Hurley, J. F., and Trmal, T.: Relative activities of some metabolites and analogs of cholecalciferol in stimulation of tibia ash weight in chicks otherwise deprived of vitamin D, J. Nutr. 107:194, 1977.

7. Boyle, I. T., Miravet, L., Gray, R. W., Holick, M. F., and DeLuca, H. F.: The response of intestinal calcium transport to 25-hydroxy and 1,25-dihydroxyvitamin D in nephrectomized rats, Endocrinology 90:605, 1972.

8. Brickman, A. S., Reddy, C. R., Coburn, J. W., Passaro, E. P., Jowsey, J., and Norman, A. W.: Biologic action of 1,25-dihydroxyvitamin D_3 in the rachitic dog, Endocrinology 92:728, 1973.

9. Brumbaugh, P. F., and Haussler, M. R.: Specific binding of 1α,25-dihydroxycholecalciferol to nuclear components of chick intestine, J. Biol. Chem. 250:1588, 1975.

10. Brumbaugh, P. F., Hugues, M. R., and Haussler, M. R.: Cytoplasmic and nuclear binding components for 1α,25-dihydroxyvitamin D_3 in chick parathyroid glands, Proc. Natl. Acad. Sci. USA 72:4871, 1975.

11. Brumbaugh, P. F., Haussler, D. H., Bursac, K. M., and Haussler, M. R.: Radioreceptor assay for 1α,25-dihydroxyvitamin D_3, Science 183:1089, 1974.

12. Brumbaugh, P. F., and Haussler, M. R.: 1α,25-dihydroxycholecalciferol receptors in intestine. I. Association of 1α,25-dihydroxycholecalciferol with intestinal mucosa chromatin, J. Biol. Chem. 249:1251, 1974.

13. Brumbaugh, P. F., and Haussler, M. R.: 1α-dihydroxycholecalciferol receptor in intestine. II. Temperature dependent transfer of the hormone to chromatin via a specific cytosol receptor, J. Biol. Chem. 249:1258, 1974.

14. Canterbury, J. M., and Reiss, E.: Predominance of suppressive effects of D metabolites on PTH secretion, Sixth Parathyroid Conference, Vancouver, Canada, June 12–17, 1977, (Abstract), in press.

15. Care, A. D., Bates, R. F. L., Pickard, D. W., Peacock, M., Tomlinson, S., O'Riordan, J. C. H., Mawer, E. B., Taylor, C. M., DeLuca, H. F., and Norman A. W.: The effects of vitamin D metabolites and their analogues on the secretion of parathyroid hormone, in *Proceedings of the 11th European Symposium on Calcified Tissue* (Copenhagen: FADL Publishing Co., 1975), p. 142.

16. Chen, T. C., Castillo, L., Korycka-Dahl, M., and DeLuca, H. F.: Role of vitamin D metabolites in phosphate transport of rat intestine, J. Nutr. 104:1056, 1974.

17. Chen, T. C., and DeLuca, H. F.: Stimulation of [^{3}H]-uridine incorporation into nuclear RNA of rat kidney by vitamin D metabolites, Arch. Biochem. Biophys. 156:321, 1973.

18. Chen, T. C., and DeLuca, H. F.: Receptors of 1,25-dihydroxycholecalciferol in rat intestine, J. Biol. Chem. 248:4890, 1973.

19. Chertow, B. S., Baylink, D. J., Wergedal, J. E., and Norman, A. W.: Decrease in serum immunoreactive parathyroid hormone in rats and in parathyroid hormone secretion in vitro by 1,25-dihydroxycholecalciferol, J. Clin. Invest. 56:668, 1975.

20. Cloix, J. F., Ulmann, A., Bachelet, M., and Funck-Brentano, J. L.: Cholecalciferol metabolites binding in porcine parathyroid glands, Steroids 28:743, 1976.

21. Corradino, R. A.: Embryonic chick intestine in organ culture: response to vitamin D_3 and its metabolites, Science 179:402, 1973.

22. Corvol, M. T., Dumontier, M. F., Garabedian, M., and Rappaport, R.: Vitamin D and cartilage. II. Biological activity of 25-hydroxycholecalciferol, 24,25-dihydroxycholecalciferol and 1,25-dihydroxycholecalciferol in cultured growth plate chondrocytes, Endocrinology, in press.

23. DeLuca, H. F.: Recent advances in our understanding of the vitamin D endocrine system, J. Lab. Clin. Med. 7:87, 1976.

24. Dziak, R. M.: The effects of D_3 metabolites on bone cell calcium, Sixth Parathyroid Conference, Vancouver, Canada, June 12–17, 1977, (abstract), in press.

25. Frolick, C. A., and DeLuca, H. F.: 1,25-dihydroxycholecalciferol: the metabolite of

vitamin D responsible for increased intestinal calcium transport, Arch. Biochem. Biophys. 147:143, 1971.

26. Garabedian, M., Corvol, M. T., Nguyen, T. M., and Balsan, S.: Metabolisme et activité du 25-hydroxycholecalciferol dans les chondrocytes en culture, Ann. Biol. Anim. Biochim. Biophys. in press.

27. Garabedian, M., Bailly Du Bois, M., Corvol, M. T., Pezant, E., and Balsan, S.: Vitamin D and cartilage. I. In vitro conversion by cartilage of 25-hydroxycholecalciferol, Endocrinology, in press.

28. Garabedian, M., Pezant, E., Miravet, L., Fellot, C., and Balsan, S.: 1,25-dihydroxycholecalciferol effect on serum phosphorus homeostasis in rats, Endocrinology, 98: 794, 1976.

29. Goodman, D. B. P., Haussler, M. R., and Rasmussen, H.: Vitamin D_3-induced alteration of microvillar membrane lipid composition, Biochem. Biophys. Res. Commun. 46:80, 1972.

30. Haddad, J. G., and Birge, S. J.: Widespread, specific binding of 25-hydroxycholecalciferol in rat tissues, J. Biol. Chem. 250:299, 1975.

31. Haddad, J. G., and Chyu, K. J.: Competitive protein-binding radioassay for 25-hydroxycholecalciferol, J. Clin. Endocrinol. Metab. 38:1046, 1974.

32. Haddad, J. G., Hahn, T. J., and Birge, S. F.: Vitamin D metabolites specific binding by rat intestinal cytosol, Biochim. Biophys. Acta 329:93, 1973.

33. Harrison, H. E., and Harrison, H. C.: Intestinal transport of phosphate: action of vitamin D, calcium, and potassium, Am. J. Physiol. 201:1007, 1961.

34. Haussler, M. R., Nagode, L. A., and Rasmussen, H.: Induction of intestinal brush border alkaline phosphatase by vitamin D and identity with Ca-ATPase, Nature 228:1199, 1970.

35. Henry, H. L., and Norman, A. W.: Mechanism of action of calciferol VII, localization of 1,25-dihydroxyvitamin D_3 in chick parathyroid glands, Biochem. Biophys. Res. Commun. 62:781, 1975.

36. Henry, H. L., Taylor, A. N., Wecksler, W. R., and Norman, A. W.: Effect of vitamin D metabolites on parathyroid gland size, in Fifth International Congress of Endocrinology (Geisen: Brühlsche Universitätdruckerei, in press).

37. Holick, M. F., Tavela, T. E., Holick, S. A., Schnoes, H. K., DeLuca, H. F., and Gallagher, B. M.: Synthesis of 1α-hydroxy (6-^{3}H) vitamin D_3 and its metabolism to 1α-25-dihydroxy (6-^{3}H) vitamin D_3 in the rat, J. Biol. Chem. 251:1020, 1976.

38. Hugi, K., Preston, C., Fleisch, H., and Bonjour, J. P.: Role of 1,25-dihydroxyvitamin D_3 (1,25-$(OH)_2D_3$) in the renal handling of calcium in rats, Experientia 33:781, 1977 (Abstract).

39. Kodicek, E.: The story of vitamin D from vitamin to hormone, Lancet 1:325, 1974.

40. Kream, B. E., and DeLuca, H. F.: A specific binding protein for 1,25-dihydroxyvitamin D_3 in rat intestinal cytosol, Biochem. Biophys. Res. Commun. 76:735, 1977.

41. Kream, B. E., Reynolds, R. D., Knutson, J. C., Eisman, J. A., and DeLuca, H. F.: Intestinal cytosol binders of 1,25-dihydroxyvitamin D_3 and 25-hydroxyvitamin D_3, Arch. Biochem. Biophys. 176:779, 1976.

42. Lawson, D. E. M., Charman, M., Wilson, P. W., and Edelstein, S.: Some characteristics of new tissue binding proteins for metabolites of vitamin D other than 1,25-dihydroxyvitamin D, Biochim. Biophys. Acta 437:403, 1976.

43. Lawson, D. E. M., and Emtage, J. S.: Molecular action of vitamin D in the chick intestine, Vitam. Horm. 32:277, 1974.

44. Lawson, D. E. M., and Wilson, P. W.: Intranuclear localisation and receptor proteins for 1,25-dihydroxycholecalciferol in chick intestine, Biochem. J. 144:573, 1974.

45. Liebherrer, M., Garabedian, M., Guillozo, H., and Balsan, S.: Vitamin D_3 metabolites and parathyroid extract in vitro effects on bone phosphatases, Thirteenth European Symposium on Calcified Tissues, Noordwijkerhout, the Netherlands, September 1977, (Abstract), in press.

46. Llach, F., Coburn, J. W., Brickman, A. S., Kurokawa, K., Norman, A. W., Canterbury, J. M., and Reiss, E.: Acute actions of 1,25-dihydroxyvitamin D_3 in normal man: effect on calcium and parathyroid status, J. Clin. Endocrinol. Metab. 44:1054, 1977.
47. MacIntyre, I., Evans, I. M. A., and Larkins, R. G.: Vitamin D, Clin. Endocrinol. 6(1): 65, 1977.
48. Mahgoub, A., and Sheppard, H.: Effect of hydroxyvitamin D_3 derivatives on [45]Ca release from rat fetal bones in vitro, Endocrinology 100:629, 1977.
49. McNutt, K. W., and Haussler, M. R.: Nutritional effectiveness of 1,25-dihydroxycholecalciferol in preventing rickets in chicks, J. Nutr. 103:681, 1973.
50. Mechanic, G. L., Toverud, S. V., Ramp, W. K., and Gonnerman, W. A.: The effect of vitamin D on the structural crosslinks and maturation of chick bone collagen, Biochim. Biophys. Acta 393:419, 1975.
51. Melancon, M. J., Jr., and DeLuca, H. F.: Vitamin D stimulation of calcium dependent adenosine triphosphatase in chick intestinal brush borders, Biochemistry 9: 1658, 1970.
52. Miravet, L., Bordier, P. J., Queille, M. L., Carre, M., and Redel, J.: The effects on bone of 25-(OH)D_3; 1,25-(OH)$_2D_3$; 24,25-(OH)$_2D_3$ and 25,26-(OH)$_2D_3$ in vitamin D-deficient rats, Sixth Parathyroid Conference, Vancouver, Canada, June 12–17, 1977, (Abstract), in press.
53. Moriuchi, S., Yoshizawa, S., and Hosoya, N.: 1,25-dihydroxycholecalciferol and the multiple forms of alkaline phosphatase in chick duodenum, Sixth Parathyroid Conference, Vancouver, Canada, June 12–17, 1977, (Abstract), in press.
54. Nicolaysen, R.: The absorption of calcium, Acta Physiol. Scand. 6:201, 1943.
55. Norman, A. W.: Actinomycin D effect on lag in vitamin D-mediated calcium absorption in the chick, Am. J. Physiol. 211:829, 1966.
56. Norman, A. W., and Henry, H.: 1,25-dihydroxycholecalciferol; a hormonally active form of vitamin D, Recent Prog. Horm. Res. 30:431, 1974.
57. Oku, T., Shimura, F., Moriuchi, S., and Hosoya, N.: Development of 1,25-dihydroxycholecalciferol receptor in the duodenal cytosol of chick embryon, Endocrinol. Jpn. 23:375, 1976.
58. Oldham, S. B., Smith, R., Hartenbower, D. L., and Henry, H.: Effects of 1,25-dihyroxyvitamin D_3 on serum calcium and immunoreactive parathyroid hormone in the dog, Sixth Parathyroid Conference, Vancouver, Canada, June 12–17, 1977, (Abstract), in press.
59. Omdahl, J. L., and DeLuca, H. F.: Regulation of vitamin D metabolism and function, Physiol. Rev. 53:327, 1973.
60. Popovtzer, M. M., Robinette, J. B., DeLuca, H. F., and Holick, H. F.: The acute effect of 25-hydroxycholecalciferol on renal handling of phosphorus, J. Clin. Invest. 53: 913, 1974.
61. Popovtzer, M. M., Blum, M. S., and Flis, R. S.: Evidence for interference of 25-(OH) vitamin D_3 with phosphaturic action of calcitonin, Am. J. Physiol. 232:E515, 1977.
62. Puschett, J. B., Fernandez, P. C., Boyle, I. T., Gray, R. W., Omdahl, J. L., and DeLuca, H. F.: The acute renal tubular effects of 1,25-dihydroxycholecalciferol, Proc. Soc. Exp. Biol. Med. 141:379, 1972.
63. Puschett, J. B., Beck, W. S., Jr., and Jelonek, A.: Parathyroid hormone and 25-hydroxyvitamin D_3: synergistic and antagonistic effects on renal phosphate transport, Science 190:473, 1975.
64. Spencer, R., Charman, M., Wilson, P., and Lawson, E.: Vitamin D-stimulated intestinal calcium absorption may not involve calcium-binding directly, Nature 263:161, 1976.
65. Steenbock, H., and Herting, D. C.: Vitamin D and growth, J. Nutr. 57:449, 1955.
66. Stern, P. H., DeLuca, H. F., and Ikekawa, N.: Bone resorbing activities of 24-hydroxystereoisomers of 24-hydroxyvitamin D_3 and 24,25-dihydroxyvitamin D_3, Biochem. Biophys. Res. Commun. 67:965, 1975.

67. Stern, P. H., Trummel, C. L., Schnoes, H. K., and DeLuca, H. F.: Bone resorbing activity of vitamin D metabolites and congeners in vitro: influence of hydroxyl substituents in the A ring, Endocrinology 97:1552, 1975.

68. Tanaka, Y., and DeLuca, H. F.: Role of 1,25-dihydroxyvitamin D_3 in maintaining serum phosphorus and curing rickets, Proc. Natl. Acad. Sci. USA 71:1040, 1974.

69. Tanaka, Y., DeLuca, H. F., Omdahl, J., and Holick, M. F.: Mechanism of action of 1,25-dihydroxycholecalciferol on intestinal calcium transport, Proc. Natl. Acad. Sci. USA 68:1286, 1971.

70. Tsai, H. C., and Norman, A. W.: Studies on calciferol metabolism. VIII. Evidence for a cytoplasmic receptor for 1,25-dihydroxyvitamin D_3 in the intestinal mucosa, J. Biol. Chem. 248:5967, 1973.

71. Ulmann, A., Brami, M., Pezant, E., Garabedian, M., and Funck-Brentano, J. L.: Binding of cholecalciferol metabolites to rat duodenal mucosa cytosol, Acta Endocrinol. (Kbh.) 84:439, 1977.

72. Van Baelen, H., Bouillon, R., and DeMoor, P.: Binding of 25-hydroxycholecalciferol in tissues, J. Biol. Chem. 252:2515, 1977.

73. Wasserman, R. H., Corradino, R. A., Fullmer, C. S., and Taylor, A. N.: Some aspects of vitamin D action; calcium absorption and the vitamin D-dependent calcium-binding protein, Vitam. Horm. 32:299, 1974.

74. Wasserman, R. H., Taylor, A. N., and Corradino, R. A.: Vitamin D-dependent calcium-binding protein. Purification and some properties, J. Biol. Chem. 243:3978, 1968.

75. Wilson, P. W., and Lawson, D. E. M.: 1,25-dihydroxyvitamin D stimulation of specific membrane proteins in chick intestine, Biochim. Biophys. Acta 497:805, 1977.

76. Zerwekh, J. E., Lindell, T. J., and Haussler, M. R.: Increased intestinal chromatin template activity. Influence of 1α,25-dihydroxyvitamin D_3 and hormone-receptor complexes, J. Biol. Chem. 251:2388, 1976.

10

Disordered Divalent Ion Metabolism in Kidney Disease: Comments on Pathogenesis and Treatment

NACHMAN BRAUTBAR, M.D., AND
CHARLES R. KLEEMAN, M.D.

*Division of Nephrology, University of California at Los Angeles,
School of Medicine, Los Angeles, California*

Since the fundamental papers of Dent, Harper and Philpot,[31] Lichtwitz and Parlier,[64] Stanbury[105] and our earliest review,[60] we have witnessed an incredible increase in interest, research activity, publication, and progress in the area of divalent ion metabolism and osteodystrophy in chronic renal disease. The "breakthroughs" in radioimmunoassay of parathyroid hormone (PTH) and radioreceptor assays for vitamin D metabolites, and the availability of these metabolites for therapy have allowed us to build on the foundations of the work of Liu and Chu[65] and the earlier classic contributions.[31, 64, 105] This chapter will present, in brief, the state of the art as we see it and an update of our last review and formulation.[61]

We begin by emphasizing that the disturbance in divalent ion metabolism and the consequent bone abnormalities probably begin at a very early stage of chronic, bilateral, parenchymal renal disease. The overall process, when uninterrupted by appropriate therapy, continues in an inexorable manner to end-

179

0084-5957/79/080179-27$3.75

© 1979, Year Book Medical Publishers, Inc.

stage renal disease, often further worsening during dialysis and even, on occasion, after "successful" renal transplantation. Why some patients seem to go through the entire life-span of their disease with little or no overt clinical evidence or disability from disordered divalent ion metabolism, while others are almost totally incapacitated by it, remains one of the unanswered problems before us.

While we are dealing with a continuum from early to terminal renal failure and beyond, we believe, for purposes of analysis and discussion, that it is important to separate out an "early" preazotemic stage, i.e., less than 30% functional renal mass. During that stage and into chronic dialysis, the process may be qualitatively altered and/or accelerated by uremia per se.

Alteration in Vitamin D Metabolism, Vitamin D-Resistant State

In our previous review, we suggested that a disturbance in vitamin D metabolism was the major factor responsible for the early hypocalcemia and secondary hyperparathyroidism in patients with early renal disease. We continue to feel that this is so. This suggestion was made originally by Liu and Chu 30 years ago.[65] Patients with renal disease tend to have defective intestinal absorption of calcium, hypocalciuria, diminished calcemic response to endogenous or exogenous PTH and refractoriness to physiologic doses of vitamin D_3 in end-stage renal disease. This vitamin D resistance is not corrected by adequate hemodialysis,[21, 41, 79] but is corrected by renal transplantation. These observations have suggested that the vitamin D resistance has something to do with diffuse renal parenchymal injury or decreased functional renal mass. Today our knowledge of vitamin D metabolism has expanded and this subject has been reviewed elsewhere.[24, 30] However, the essence of this knowledge is that calciferol (vitamin D_3) undergoes a two-step obligatory metabolic transformation, first in the liver to 25-hydroxycholecalciferol [25(OH)D_3][51, 88] and subsequently in the kidney to 1,25-dihydroxycholecalciferol [1,25(OH)$_2$D$_3$], the biologically active form of this steroid.[37, 46, 80] It is accepted that the mitochondrial fraction of the renal cortical cells is the only site of 1α-hydroxylation of 25(OH)D_3.[37] The identification of the kidney as the major organ for 1,25(OH)$_2$D$_3$ production provides a reasonable framework for considering the early hormonal, osseous and divalent ion disturbances of chronic renal disease and the possibility that diffuse renal cortical pathology or renal cortical mass is responsible for defective 1,25(OH)$_2$D$_3$ production and the vitamin D$_3$-resistant state. Vitamin D "resistance" develops early in the course of chronic renal failure — glomerular filtration rate (GFR) 50–80%; and it has been shown to appear immediately with acute insults to the kidneys.[10] It is widely accepted that early in the course of renal failure there is skeletal resistance to the *calcemic* action of endogenous or exogenous PTH.[66, 71, 72] This is suggested by the mild hypocalcemia in patients with early renal failure,[25] blunted calcemic response to parathyroid extract[33, 71] shown to be greatly but not totally corrected by administration of 1,25(OH)$_2$D$_3$,[73] and impaired or hypoparathyroid-like response of the skeleton to standard hypocalcemic stimulus.[67]

In using the term "skeletal resistance to PTH," we must emphasize that we and others are referring to the action of the hormone on those bone cells that are responsible for the maintenance and elevation of serum calcium. Parfitt, in his recent review,[83] clearly separates this action of the hormone step from its control of the osteoclastic bone remodeling process. In patients with renal disease we see a definite dissociation between the normalcy of the latter and the inability of PTH to transport calcium from the bone to the extracellular fluid, i.e., its calcemic action. It is this step that may be critically dependent on vitamin D [1,25(OH)$_2$D$_3$]. Current data strongly suggest a role for 1,25(OH)$_2$D$_3$ in the transcellular transport of calcium.[48] Therefore, when bone is examined at any stage of chronic renal disease, we may see varying degrees of osteitis fibrosa, a sign of PTH-induced osteoclastic activity. This may or may not be associated with osteomalacia but, regardless, the presence of only osteitis fibrosa in a bone biopsy from a patient with early renal failure does not signify that early secondary hyperparathyroidism *preceded* any disturbance of vitamin D metabolism. The latter may impair the *calcemic* action of PTH without the presence of osteomalacia on bone biopsy. Obviously, the presence of excess osteoid covering metabolically active bone surfaces may contribute to the decreased calcemic response to PTH.[55]

Haussler and McCain found that the concentration of 1,25(OH)$_2$D$_3$ in the blood of patients with early renal failure may be normal.[47a] It is apparent that if at this stage there were no defects in the renal synthesis of this metabolite, we would expect high levels in the circulation because these patients have mild hypocalcemia and hypophosphatemia,[39, 89] hypocalciuria, increased phosphorus clearance and a significant elevation of PTH levels in the blood. This combination of biochemical changes should cause an *increased* synthesis of $1,25(OH)_2D_3$. Parenthetically, these are the classic changes observed in pure vitamin D deficiency. If, as seems to be the case, the secretion of PTH can be directly inhibited in a feedback homeostatic manner by $1,25(OH)_2D_3$,[54] the high level of PTH found in the blood of patients with early renal failure may in part be due to the decreased renal synthesis of $1,25(OH)_2D_3$, rather than solely the result of hypocalcemia.

In our discussion to this point, we have emphasized the defect in the synthesis of $1,25(OH)_2D_3$ in the chronically diseased kidney as the basic abnormality in vitamin D metabolism. However, several recent observations suggest that the picture may be much more complicated. Before discussing these observations, it is appropriate to review very briefly our understanding of the physiologic regulation of certain vitamin D metabolites.

The mitochondrial enzyme hydroxylases in the tubular cells of the renal cortex responsible for the hydroxylation of $25(OH)D_3$ are regulated in a homeostatic manner by the level of PTH. A rise in the latter, by low calcium intake and/or hypocalcemia, stimulates 1α-hydroxylation and inhibits 24-hydroxylation, whereas a fall in the PTH level, by high calcium intake and/or hypercalcemia, inhibits 1α- and stimulates 24-hydroxylation.[38, 81] Phosphorus deprivation will stimulate 1α-hydroxylation and will result in increased production of $1,25(OH)_2D_3$.[53]

There are also observations indicating that $1,25(OH)_2D_3$ is linked to $24,25(OH)_2D_3$ and both are related to inorganic phosphorus, calcium and parathyroid hormone.[16, 40] The role of the new metabolite, $24,25(OH)_2D_3$, has been recently studied. It has been shown that after parathyroidectomy, $24,25(OH)_2D_3$ levels are increased.[23] Fischer *et al.* found that during the treatment of patients with hypocalcemic rickets with intravenous infusions of calcium, the amount of PTH secretion was still high despite normocalcemia, whereas this is not the case with vitamin D-repleted subjects.[34] They speculated that a deficient vitamin D metabolite was responsible for the persistent secretion of PTH despite normocalcemia. Bates *et al.* found, in the goat, direct inhibition of PTH secretion by 24,25(OH)$_2$D$_3$.[9] Carr *et al.* proposed that 24,25(OH)$_2$D$_3$ may play an important role in the vitamin D-PTH feedback loop and that a defect in 24,25(OH)$_2$D$_3$ synthesis in patients with early renal failure could be as important as the defect in 1,25(OH)$_2$D$_3$ synthesis.[23] Kanis *et al.* administered doses of 24,25(OH)$_2$D$_3$, which they estimated to be at a physiologic level, to two patients with end-stage renal disease and compared their metabolic effects with those of patients given comparable doses of 1,25(OH)$_2$D$_3$.[57] They found that both equally enhanced the intestinal absorption of calcium, but only 1,25(OH)$_2$D$_3$ increased urinary excretion of calcium. In other words, the 24,25(OH)$_2$D$_3$ caused a more positive calcium balance and, supposedly, greater bone mineralization. Kanis, at the same conference, referred to unpublished observations by Bordier on advanced renal failure, which showed that 24,25(OH)$_2$D$_3$ caused a normal mineralization front in the osteoid, whereas 1,25(OH)$_2$-D$_3$ did not. The apparent hypercalcemic effect of 1,25(OH)$_2$D$_3$ in contrast to vitamin D$_3$, dihydrotachysterol (DHT), 25(OH)D$_3$ and 24,25(OH)$_2$D$_3$ in patients with chronic renal failure will be discussed in greater detail below.

From other clinical studies it may be possible to infer that a deficiency of 1,25(OH)$_2$D$_3$ may not be the only serious derangement of vitamin D metabolism in early renal failure. Bordier *et al.* compared the effects of vitamin D$_3$ and 25(OH)D$_3$ with 1,25(OH)$_2$D$_3$ and 1α(OH)D$_3$ in patients with vitamin D-deficient rickets.[14] Both vitamin D$_3$ and 25(OH)D$_3$ caused a significant increase in mineralization front, whereas 1,25(OH)$_2$D$_3$ and 1α(OH)D$_3$ had minimal, if any, effect. While vitamin D$_3$ and 25(OH)D$_3$ caused an increase in the level of serum phosphorus and a sustained fall in urinary calcium excretion as well as phosphorus, 1,25(OH)$_2$D$_3$ and 1α(OH)D$_3$ did not. On the basis of their observations, they suggested that 25(OH)$_2$D$_3$ or a further metabolite, possibly 24,25(OH)$_2$D$_3$, truly corrected the bone lesion of rickets, while 1,25(OH)$_2$D$_3$ did not. Eastwood *et al.* measured 25(OH)D$_3$ and 1,25(OH)$_2$D$_3$ levels in uremic patients and concluded that a deficiency of 25(OH)D$_3$ as well as of 1,25(OH)$_2$-D$_3$ was responsible for the renal osteodystrophy rather than 1,25(OH)$_2$D$_3$ deficiency alone.[32] The cause of this deficiency of 25(OH)D$_3$ in patients with chronic renal failure could be a deficient dietary intake of vitamin D$_3$ or an impaired conversion of vitamin D$_3$ to 25(OH)D$_3$ in the liver.

In light of the above discussion of vitamin D metabolism, we conclude that:

1. The major initiating factor in the disturbed divalent ion in patients with early renal failure and osteodystrophy is defective vitamin D metabolism.

2. This defective vitamin D metabolism of $1,25(OH)_2D_3$, $25(OH)D_3$ and $24,25(OH)_2D_3$ will cause skeletal resistance to the calcemic action of PTH.

3. This, in turn, will cause hypocalcemia and secondary hyperparathyroidism.

4. Deficiency in $1,25(OH)_2D_3$ and $24,25(OH)_2D_3$ will further contribute to secondary hyperparathyroidism by reducing the direct feedback inhibition of PTH secretion by these metabolites.

Finally, we should refer to an additional possible contributing factor to the blunted calcemic response to PTH in patients with early renal failure. This is the possible "exhaustion" of intracellular mechanisms due to prolonged overstimulation of the bone cells by PTH. Tomlinson *et al.* showed that prolonged stimulation of *renal* adenylate cyclase by PTH in normal subjects can produce refractoriness to the renal action of the hormone,[110] and recent studies have shown that in vitamin D-deficient rats, the resistance to the calcemic effect of PTH could be decreased by reducing the secondary hyperparathyroidism (without vitamin D replacement).[85] We feel that these mechanisms are not likely contributors because parathyroidectomy (removal of excess PTH) in uremic patients has not been found to reverse this resistance to exogenous PTH,[71] and the studies by Evanson in patients with primary hyperparathyroidism show that there is no decrease in calcemic response to PTH infusion despite chronic overstimulation of bone cells by PTH.[33]

The Role of Hyperphosphatemia, Retention of Phosphorus

Hyperphosphatemia, which may occur with the loss of renal function in patients with advanced renal disease, has been incriminated as the cause of secondary hyperparathyroidism in cases of early renal failure.[19] Slatopolsky *et al.* showed that in dogs the development of secondary hyperparathyroidism in renal failure is dependent on the magnitude of phosphate intake.[103] The levels of inorganic PTH correlated directly with dietary phosphorus intake. The fact that hyperphosphatemia will cause secondary hyperparathyroidism is well accepted; however, the role of phosphate retention in the initiation of the pathophysiologic events in early renal failure is still questionable. Bricker *et al.*[19] and Slatopolsky *et al.*[104] postulated that a postprandial transient and almost undetectable increase in the amount of serum phosphorus occurs in the course of early renal failure. Such increments in plasma phosphorus levels will cause decrements in the level of ionized calcium and in the stimulation of PTH secretion. As a result of this hyperparathyroidism, the renal clearance of phosphorus will increase and the serum phosphorus and calcium levels will return to normal. However, it is difficult to reconcile a number of facts with this information.

1. Skeletal resistance to the calcemic action of parathyroid hormone has been discussed previously. Massry *et al.* showed that in patients with early renal failure, this blunted calcemic response was not related to the degree of plasma phosphorus and occurred in normo- or hypophosphatemic patients.[73, 74] Recently, Llach *et al.* proposed that repeated postprandial hyperphosphatemia in cases of early renal failure (GFR at least 50% of normal) may induce renal intracellular hyperphosphatemia, decreased production of $1,25(OH)_2D_3$ and, as a result of the latter, skeletal resistance to the calcemic action of PTH.[66] In their study, they showed that restricting the amount of dietary phosphorus in proportion to the decreased renal function lowered the level of circulating PTH toward normal, improved intestinal absorption of calcium and improved the calcemic response to PTH. Urinary calcium levels rose in these subjects and urinary phosphorus levels dropped to extreme lows. It is possible that with the dietary phosphate restriction, a situaton called normophosphatemic phosphate depletion occurred.[17] This syndrome is characterized by marked hypophosphaturia and hypercalciuria, decreased levels of PTH, increased bone response to $1,25(OH)_2D_3$ and increased intestinal absorption of calcium. It is possible that at least in part, both the patients Llach *et al.* studied[66] and the dogs studied by Slatopolsky *et al.*[103, 104] (no balance studies were done on these animals) were in mild phosphorus depletion and this was responsible for the fall in the levels of circulating PTH, a possible rise in $1,25(OH)_2D_3$ and increased responsiveness of the skeleton to the calcemic action of PTH. However, it is clear that as renal failure progresses, for any given metabolic setting,

an abnormal rise in the concentration of inorganic phosphorus in the plasma will tend to decrease the free calcium ion concentration and stimulate PTH secretion. Furthermore, the evidence is overwhelming that the hyperphosphatemia plays an important role in the pathogenesis of renal osteodystrophy. In fact, as Parfitt suggested, in patients with end-stage kidney disease in dialysis treatment, hyperphosphatemia may be the single most important determinant of severe secondary hyperparathyroidism.[84]

2. Friis *et al.*,[39] Coburn *et al.*[25] and Llach *et al.*[66] showed that the mean levels of serum calcium *and* phosphorus in patients with early renal failure are significantly lower than those in normal controls, an observation unlikely to be due to simple phosphorus excess and secondary hyperparathyroidism.

3. Appropriate regulation of plasma phosphate and its renal clearance can take place in progressive experimental renal failure in parathyroidectomized dogs. Swenson *et al.* found that while the plasma calcium levels were maintained normal with calcium and vitamin D in these animals, they were normophosphatemic, and fractional excretion of phosphorus was appropriate to their phosphorus intake.[108] Similarly, Loreau *et al.* showed that animals with tubulo-interstitial nephritis and tubular resistance to PTH action maintained normal blood phosphorus levels and increased fractional excretion of phosphorus.

Magnesium

As the renal failure advances and absolute magnesium (Mg^{2+}) clearance decreases, magnesium retention and hypermagnesemia start to develop. It is possible that Mg^{2+} retention may play a role in the renal osteodystrophy of patients with advanced late renal failure. In early renal failure, the MG^{2+} clearance/creatinine clearance is significantly high, and patients at this stage may be hypomagnesemic.[75] In patients without renal disease, hypomagnesemia will cause hypocalcemia, which is due to both impaired release of PTH and its calcemic action on bone.[100] With replacement of magnesium salt acutely and chronically, both hypocalcemia and the functional hypoparathyroidism are corrected.[75] Chronic Mg^{2+} depletion, should it develop at any stage of renal failure, would be expected to show the same pathophysiology noted in patients without renal disease. The effects of Mg^{2+} depletion on vitamin D metabolism and action have been recently reported. Most investigators show that Mg^{2+} depletion causes increased intestinal absorption of calcium, but there is no interference with vitamin D metabolism.

The kidney plays the major role in regulating Mg^{2+} homeostasis. With reduction of renal function and the number of nephrons available to excrete Mg^{2+}, magnesium retention develops. The intestinal absorption of Mg^{2+} is normal in cases of advanced renal failure.[26] Although the amount of dietary Mg^{2+} is decreased in patients with advanced renal failure due to a decrease in protein intake, ingestion of Mg^{2+}-containing laxatives or antacids that contain magnesium will increase Mg^{2+} intake.[96] A major factor in the hypermagnesemia seen with terminal renal failure is dialysate concentration of magnesium. It has been shown that with dialysate solution containing 1.5 mEq/L Mg^{2+}, serum Mg^{2+} was 2.5–4.5 mEq/L.[22, 27] In our center, most of the patients on chronic hemodialysis have high serum Mg^{2+} concentrations—3.0–4.0 mEq/L. Acute elevations of serum Mg^{2+} have been shown to suppress PTH secretion;[76] however, this is not the case in chronic advanced renal failure and the reason is that the hypocalcemia is a more sensitive stimulus for PTH secretion.[47] Skeletal Mg^{2+} is increased with chronic hypermagnesemia,[3] and Alfrey *et al.* suggested that magnesium pyrophosphate, which is present in excess in the bones of uremic patients, will cause abnormal bone turnover.[4, 5] Recently, it has been shown in in vitro studies on bone preparation that intracellular Mg^{2+} is critical for the stabilization of amorphous calcium phosphate in the mitochondrial phase.[91] On the other hand, Raisz and Neimann, using bone culture preparations with different Mg^{2+} concentrations, could not show any significant effect of increased Mg^{2+} concentration on bone response to PTH or calcitonin.[95] Recently, Coburn *et al.* reported on hemodialysis patients with severe osteodystrophy in late advanced renal failure who were resistant to treatment with $1,25(OH)_2D_3$, high-dialysate calcium.[28] They suggested that chronic hypermagnesemia and increased bone content of Mg^{2+} might be factors in the bone disease of these patients. Further studies will be necessary to learn if excess bone Mg^{2+} is a factor in the bone disease of patients with end-stage renal failure or in those on maintenance hemodialysis.

Parathyroid Hormone, Nature of Secretion and Circulation

As early as 1935, Papenheimer and Willens showed increased parathyroid gland mass and hyperplasia in patients with renal failure.[82] The most common histologic abnormality is the chief cell hyperplasia and, in some patients, adenomatous formation. The theoretical causes for these changes have been stated before: (1) hypocalcemia due to defective vitamin D metabolism in early renal failure, and (2) lack of $1,25(OH)_2D_3$ and/or $24,25(OH)_2D_3$, which normally have an additional inhibiting effect on the secretion of PTH. The question of an autonomous hyperfunctioning gland has been discussed before,[60] and it still seems to us that this is a rare complication. Two mechanisms have been proposed to explain an apparent autonomous function of the parathyroid gland or so-called nonsuppressible levels of the hormone in the circulation after calcium loading: (1) increased cellular mass of hypersecreting cells,[45, 84] and (2) delayed inactivation or decreased degradation of circulating PTH. Massry *et al.* followed the disappearance of PTH from the circulation of seven uremic patients following parathyroidectomy.[77] The pattern suggested the presence of two forms of parathyroid hormone. Berson and Yalow reported the immunochemical characteristics of the circulating hormone.[11] They showed that in patients with hyperparathyroidism the circulating hormone was different from the glandular hormone. Recent development of radioimmunoassay techniques has helped to clarify the pathophysiology of PTH in uremic patients. The PTH secreted by the gland has a molecular weight of 9,500, with an amino acid chain (N-terminal) responsible for its activity. This is quickly degraded by both the kidney and liver to an inactive form with a molecular weight of 7,000, containing a carboxyl terminal (C-terminal).[52, 78] In end-stage renal failure, the liver may play a greater role than the kidney in PTH degradation, and it has been found that the main fraction of circulating PTH is C-terminal. The fact that a large amount of circulating PTH is inactive biologically but measured immunologically may be an important factor in the so-called nonsuppressibility of the parathyroid glands. It is difficult to interpret the available data from different laboratories, as the antiserum used widely is the one that also detects C-terminal chains. Thus, a high value of circulating PTH, despite increasing the ionized calcium levels in the plasma, does not necessarily mean that the gland is not being suppressed.[44] However, the question of the origin of the PTH C-terminal fragment is not settled. Potts *et al.* recently showed that all the PTH secreted by the gland is the native 1–84 amino acid hormone and that degradation to fragments takes place in the periphery by kidney and liver.[92, 101, 102] However, Arnaud *et al.*[7, 8] and Sherwood *et al.* showed that fragments may be secreted, at least, from parathyroid adenomas. Recently, Flueck *et al.* concluded that the hyperfunctioning gland may be a source of PTH fragments.[35] In any event, it is doubtful that the qualitative nature of the fragments is important in determining the presence or absence of osteitis fibrosa in patients with chronic renal disease.

The Nature of Renal Osteodystrophy

As we mentioned earlier, the nature of the osteodystrophy will depend, to a large extent, on the stage of renal failure. Bone changes during evolution of renal osteodystrophy have been difficult to study due to several factors.

1. Technical: What do we use for evaluating the bone disease?

2. Interpretation of biopsy specimens: One of the difficulties in interpretation of bone biopsy is the fact that the changes are not homogeneous, and a different response to the same stimulus may be found in different parts of the skeleton.[97]

3. Interpretation of studies from different countries and different patient populations: The nature of the bone histology in renal osteodystrophy in patients at various stages of chronic renal failure may well be determined by the geographic and socioeconomic conditions of the country of origin of the patients. Chronic low intakes of protein and vitamin D may prominently influence the magnitude of osteopenia and osteomalacia associated with any given degree of osteitis fibrosa.

The skeletal hallmark of parathyroid overactivity is osteitis fibrosa (fibroosteoclasia).[97] It is now well accepted that the histologic changes in cases of early renal failure are predominantly those of osteitis fibrosa.[69] The latter have been shown to correlate directly with the levels of PTH and parathyroid gland mass.[69, 70, 97] These changes of early renal disease are present long before any clinical or radiologic changes are present in the skeleton. As renal failure progresses, the histologic picture becomes a mixture of varying degrees of osteitis fibrosa and osteomalacia. The latter is represented by numerous broad nonmineralized osteoid seams and is the hallmark of the histologic representation of a deficient or defective action of vitamin D on the skeleton. However, with respect to the interpretation of excess osteoid, we feel it is important to quote the recent critical and perceptive reservations of Ritz and his associates.[97]

Resistance to physiological doses of vitamin D: This leads to *defective mineralization* of osteoid in the skeleton. The appearance of numerous broad osteoid seams points to the presence of *osteomalacia* ("mineralization block"). In contrast to reports in literature, *ricketic* changes in the growth apparatus with accumulation of excessive cartilage are *not typical* for renal osteodystrophy in older growing children. The amount of osteoid has been equated by many authors with the severity of the mineralization block. This misinterpretation certainly does not become more correct by repetition. The amount of osteoid present at any given moment depends on the birth rate of new osteoid seams (increased in high-turnover hyperparathyroidism!) as well as on the lifespan of the individual osteoid seam (prolonged in osteomalacia). The amount of osteoid also depends on the duration of the disease, even more osteoid accumulating during renal insufficiency. A good indication of impaired mineralization is given by the fraction of osteoid seams failing to be stained by *in vivo* double-labelling with tetracycline (active primary mineralization).

The clinician should be familiar with these basic histological facts in order to be able to evaluate bone biopsy findings correctly. Iliac crest cancellous bone is most suitable for biopsy since, due to its rapid turnover, it reflects metabolically induced lesions best.

It is a common feature of both fibro-osteoclastic and osteomalacic lesions to accumulate with increasing duration of disease, causing progressive transformation of the premorbid skeleton into mechanically inferior woven bone or osteoid. This points to the necessity of preventing this process by *early* institution of appropriate therapy.

Excess osteoid and defective mineralization may be seen in patients with early renal failure. However, it usually occurs with significant destruction of renal mass and GFR lower than 30 ml/minute.[106] Whereas in early renal disease the picture is that of parathyroid overactivity (osteitis fibrosa), with advanced renal failure true osteomalacia may become the dominant and, at times, seemingly the only lesion. However, it must be stressed that both may be present in large and florid amounts in the same skeleton, often not recognized because of the limitations of a single bone biopsy representing the entire skeleton.

Hemodialysis Bone Disease

Reports of bone histology in patients on maintenance hemodialysis show considerable variability.[98] As we said before, the histologic picture is that of osteitis fibrosa and osteomalacia. Usually one picture predominates, but the factors that determine which picture will predominate are unknown. Ritz *et al.* found no correlation between plasma $25(OH)D_3$ levels and the degree of mineralization.[99] Other reports indicated a correlation between PTH levels and the type of bone disease.[96, 97] In general, bone histology does not differ qualitatively in hemodialysis patients. Although hemodialysis prolongs life, it also exposes the patient to pathophysiologic factors, e.g., phosphorus retention and depletion, secondary hyperparathyroidism, vitamin D resistance and deficiency, Mg^{2+} excess and even protein depletion. In the past ten years, several factors have been considered important in the prevention and management of hemodialysis bone disease.

HYPERPHOSPHATEMIA. — Reduction of serum phosphorus levels toward normal by means of restricting dietary phosphorus intake to 700 – 1,000 mg/day and the use of phosphate binders has been shown to cause a small increment in the amount of ionized calcium and a fall in the PTH level.[43] However, it has also been proved that despite control of hyperphosphatemia, the secondary hyperparathyroidism progresses in a substantial number of patients.[42, 43]

DIALYSATE CALCIUM. — It has been shown that using a low-dialysate calcium, 2.5 – 2.6 mEq/L, will aggravate secondary hyperparathyroidism, and increasing the dialysate calcium concentration of 3.0 mEq/L will clearly reduce the incidence of overt skeletal disease.[15] However, studies of the use of higher-dialysate calcium have shown that there is no decrease in secondary hyperparathyroidism and bone disease.

DIALYSATE MAGNESIUM. — Hypermagnesemia is the rule in patients with end-stage renal disease. Therefore, the use of a Mg^{2+} level of 0.5 mEq/L is generally recommended, and there are some suggestions that chemical bone composition becomes better with hypomagnesemia.[22] Other factors such as heparin, trace metals and aluminum toxicity have been mentioned as a cause of bone disease in hemodialysis patients, but these have not been studied extensively and the data available today are not sufficient to allow us any conclusions.

PHOSPHATE DEPLETION. — Recently, a very unique syndrome of hypophosphatemia in hemodialysis has been reported, and we feel that, although the data available today are scarce, it is possible that there is a group of hemodialysis patients who are hypophosphatemic and relatively phosphate depleted. Hypophosphatemia in hemodialysis patients was reported to be due to excessive use of phosphate binders. Recently, Ahmed *et al.* reported on hemodialysis patients with hypophosphatemia without the use of phosphate binders.[1] The authors felt that the hypophosphatemia was the result of low dietary intake of phosphate, intestinal malabsorption of phosphate and phosphate loss via dialysis. Furthermore, the bone lesions of these patients were compatible with those of phosphate depletion osteomalacia, while $25(OH)D_3$ was normal in these patients. Moreover, recently it has been shown that a group of hemodialysis patients who were treated with active vitamin D metabolites were resistant to treatment.[2] These patients had bone histology compatible with osteomalacia, and they were hypophosphatemic. It is our feeling that, although hypophosphatemia has not been reported frequently in hemodialysis patients, there are patients fitting this category.

Renal Osteodystrophy and Calcitonin

Three hormones predominate in calcium homeostasis — PTH, vitamin D and calcitonin (TCT). The evidence now suggests that PTH and vitamin D are important in the development of renal osteodystrophy. Naturally, it is tempting to speculate that if two of the hormones are involved in renal osteodystrophy, then obviously the third should be somehow also involved. The primary action of TCT appears to be inhibition of osteoclastic bone resorption antagonizing the action of PTH on the skeleton. Although the role of calcitonin in regulation of calcium and bone metabolism in the day-to-day physiology is probably not major, the histologic picture in renal osteodystrophy of increased osteoclastic activity suggests the possibility that deficiency of calcitonin may be responsible, in part, for this picture. In cases of chronic renal failure, increased concentrations of inorganic (i) TCT may arise from increased secretion of the hormone or delay in degradation. Kanis *et al.* found that bilateral nephrectomy caused acute rises in the level of iTCT and a decrease in bone turnover rates.[59] Ardaillou *et al.* have demonstrated a reduction in clearance rates of iTCT in humans with renal failure.[6] Recently, Kanis *et al.* studied patients with chronic renal failure who were on maintenance hemodialysis.[58] They found a correlation between the levels of iTCT and the severity of bone disease (expressed as bone alkaline phosphatase activity and PTH levels). They suggested that in patients with high levels of TCT, alkaline phosphatase activity and bone disease are less severe than in those with lower levels of calcitonin. They proposed that iTCT may protect the bone in renal osteodystrophy, and that in patients with calcitonin deficiency, bone disease will be more severe. This hypothesis seems to be very promising at first glance; however, one must be very cautious in interpreting these data. The reasons for such caution are: (1) Lee *et al.* recently showed that in patients with chronic renal failure and elevated levels of TCT, there is immunochemical heterogeneity of the hormone,[63] and (2) to date, biologic activity of this fraction has not been studied, and therefore we must await further improvements in the available immuno- and bioassay techniques. Further studies will have to evaluate the role of calcitonin in renal osteodystrophy.

Effects of PTH and Vitamin D Deficiency on the Kidney

Secondary hyperparathyroidism is present in patients at all stages of renal failure. The normal response of a kidney to PTH is an increase in phosphate clearance and a decrease in calcium clearance. These tubular effects continue to be seen in cases of chronic renal disease. In contrast to the skeleton, there is no resistance at the renal level to the action of PTH.

Renal Clearance of Phosphate

In earlier studies, Kleeman *et al.* have shown that the sustained rise in the level of PTH causes an increase in renal clearance of phosphorus within the limits imposed by the degree of renal failure.[60] Although the absolute clearance of phosphate is reduced, the fractional excretion is increased. The two main contributing factors to this phenomenon are: (1) secondary hyperparathyroidism and (2) increased filtered load of phosphorus per nephron.

Renal Handling of Calcium

Kleeman *et al.* showed clearly that almost all patients with renal failure have varying degrees of absolute hypocalciuria.[60]

This hypocalciuria is primarily due to direct action of PTH on the renal tubule.[62] It is very interesting to note that in normal patients, simple vitamin D deficiency will cause hypocalciuria.[62] Kleeman *et al.* suggested that the fractional excretion of calcium is greater in patients with pyelonephritis than in those with glomerular diseases, and in both it was correlated with the renal excretion of sodium.[60] It is possible that the greater hypocalciuria seen in glomerular lesions (more cortical destruction) can be correlated with a greater defect in the synthesis of vitamin D metabolites for a given loss of renal mass.

Renal Handling of Magnesium

As renal failure progresses, there is a significant increase in the fractional clearance of Mg^{2+}, rising to 60–70% of the amount of filtered Mg^{2+}.[60] It is apparent that despite marked reduction of renal mass, the absolute magnesium clearance may remain very close to normal, and plasma Mg^{2+} levels will remain near normal. It is only in patients nearing end-stage renal disease that we see modest hypermagnesemia. The roles of dietary intake of magnesium and dialysate solution concentration of magnesium may be critical in causing the hypermagnesemia of end-stage renal disease.

Vitamin D and the Kidney

The classic biochemical findings of vitamin D deficiency in humans and experimental animals include phosphaturia and hypocalciuria—the same biochemical changes seen in renal failure. The mechanism of phosphaturia has been attributed to the secondary hyperparathyroidism seen in patients with vitamin D deficiency. However, the observation that administration of vitamin D to vitamin D-deficient patients corrects the phosphaturia brought up the possibility that vitamin D has a direct action on the renal tubular handling of phosphorus. The interpretation of this observation is complicated by the fact that vitamin D administration may cause both a direct and an indirect effect on PTH secretion, and this, by itself, will change the amount of urinary excretion of phosphorus. The question of the direct role of vitamin D in the renal tubular handling of phosphate has been a subject for many studies. Several reports and conclusions, using different animal modalities, did not answer this question. Puschett *et al.* found that both 25(OH)D$_3$ and 1,25(OH)$_2$-D$_3$ have a direct hypophosphaturic action in the thyroparathyroidectomized (TPTX) dog.[93, 94] Popovtzer *et al.* found that such an effect occurs in the rat only in the presence of PTH.[90] Brautbar *et al.* reported that administration of 1,25(OH)$_2$D$_3$ to TPTX dogs caused hypophosphaturia only in the presence of PTH and suggested that if there is a direct action of vitamin D on the renal tubular handling of phosphate, it is the result of interaction between parathyroid hormone and vitamin D.[18] We feel that this question has not been resolved yet due to difficulties arising from the use of different animal species, the use of pharmacologic amounts of vitamin D and studying a nonphysiologic situation, TPTX, to determine physiologic actions.

The renal handling of calcium and vitamin D therapy also deserve a special discussion. As was stated before, in pure vitamin D deficiency, the classic urinary picture is hypocalciuria. It is interesting that in cases of renal failure where we have secondary hyperparathyroidism and vitamin D deficiency or resistance, there is also marked hypocalciuria. The mechanism, in both pure vitamin D deficiency and renal failure, is probably the same: increased tubular reabsorption of calcium.[60, 62] It is tempting to speculate that in both vitamin D deficiency and renal failure the administration of vitamin D will correct the hypocalciuria.

Reviewing the available data, this is not the case. The original observation of Liu and Chu demonstrated that with administration of vitamin D$_2$ to the vitamin D-deficient subjects, there was an elevation in the level of plasma calcium.[65] This elevation of plasma calcium, which probably caused a decrease in the level of circulating PTH, should have resulted in relatively higher amounts of urinary calcium. On the contrary, Liu and Chu showed that there was a mild decrease in the level of urinary calcium. Furthermore, recent studies by Bordier *et al.* clearly showed that administration of 25(OH)D$_3$ not only did not increase the amount of urinary calcium excretion, but there was a relatively mild decrease.[14] Kanis *et al.* reported the same observations with the administration of 24,25(OH)$_2$D$_3$.[57] However, the striking observation is that of Bordier *et al.* showing that 1,25(OH)$_2$D$_3$ administration caused a significant increase in the level of urinary calcium with no relation to its filtered load.[14]

There could be two interpretations of these studies: (1) Vitamin D and its metabolites, with the exception of $1,25(OH)_2D_3$, are having a direct effect on the renal tubular reabsorption of calcium, and (2) the administration of vitamin D or its metabolites is causing bone to heal and mineralize normally, and bone is "signaling" to the kidney to increase its reabsorption of calcium. This signal could not be PTH because $25(OH)D_3$, $24,25(OH)_2D_3$ and vitamin D_3 cause elevation of the level of plasma calcium and, as a result, a decrease in the amount of circulating PTH. It is possible that some other humoral factor or factors yet unidentified are signaling the kidney to reabsorb calcium avidly for further bone mineralization. In any event, it is clear that $1,25(OH)_2D_3$ is different in this respect. Although it may increase bone mineralization, it may not do this normally, and in most of the cases studied, the level of urinary calcium increases rather than decreases. It is possible that $1,25(OH)_2D_3$ has a different role in bone-calcium regulation than do vitamin D, dihydrotachysterol and the other metabolites.

Therapy

In an earlier review by Kleeman and Better, the basic approach to therapy for disturbed divalent ion metabolism and renal osteodystrophy was preventive and curative.[61] Unfortunately, despite the massive development of new techniques and the discovery of vitamin D metabolites, we still feel that the therapy is basically (1) maintenance of near-normal or normal concentrations of divalent ion concentration in body fluids, (2) prevention of secondary hyperparathyroidism by increasing the amount of dietary calcium and decreasing phosphorus retention and (3) treatment of the secondary hyperparathyroidism by surgery if it is not manageable by conservative measures and if bone disease and metastatic calcification and its consequences become dangerous. As we stated before, we do feel that hypophosphatemia should be avoided and that there is a small group of patients who have severe bone disease due to hypophosphatemia. For these patients, the use of phosphate binders should be avoided, and increasing dietary intake of phosphorus should be the therapy of choice.

The role of vitamin D and its metabolites deserves special discussion here due to the large number of related clinical studies and case reports from different parts of the world. Before 1969, the forms of vitamin D available were D_2 ergocalciferol and D_3 cholecalciferol, which is the naturally occurring form of vitamin D. Treatment with large doses of vitamin D_2 or D_3 has been shown to improve overt skeletal disease in uremic patients.[50, 107] With the development of knowledge of vitamin D bioconversion and the availability of $25(OH)D_3$ and $1,25(OH)_2D_3$, these metabolites were used in small amounts to correct renal osteodystrophy. Attention has been largely directed toward the use of $1,25(OH)_2D_3$ because of the knowledge that the kidney is required for $1,25(OH)_2D_3$ synthesis and because the production of $1,25(OH)_2D_3$ is impaired in renal failure due to renal parenchymal damage. It has been shown that $1,25(OH)_2D_3$ administration improves bone disease in patients with renal failure[20, 49] and reverses the secondary hyperparathyroidism.[20] Coburn *et al.* showed that administration of $1,25(OH)_2D_3$ caused a substantial improvement of excessive bone resorption, and administration of $1,25(OH)_2D_3$ for three to four months corrected the osteomalacia.[29] These first reports and studies caused enthusiasm all over the world, and reports of the use of $1,25(OH)_2D_3$ were almost the rule. However, due to the expense and the difficulty in the synthesis of $1,25(OH)_2D_3$, investigators started to use $25(OH)D_3$.

Several investigators have shown that $25(OH)D_3$ will cause elevation to normal levels of serum calcium, enhance intestinal absorption of calcium and correct the bone disease toward normal.[13, 109] They suggested that $25(OH)D_3$ in doses lower than needed for vitamin D_3 is effective in treatment of patients with chronic renal failure. It was suggested that $25(OH)D_3$ may have direct action on organ systems that $1,25(OH)_2D_3$ does not. One of these observations was in the study by Birge and Haddad, which reported specific action of $25(OH)D_3$ on in vitro muscle metabolism in vitamin D-deficient animals.[12] Recently, Fournier *et al.* evaluated the role of $1\alpha(OH)D_3$ and $25(OH)D_3$ in patients with renal osteodystrophy.[36] They found that $1\alpha(OH)D_3$ was very potent in increasing intestinal absorption of calcium, but was less effective in treating bone mineralization than is $25(OH)D_3$. Since $1\alpha(OH)D_3$ is effective only after hydroxylation to $1,25(OH)_2D_3$, they concluded that the active metabolite that will cure renal osteodystrophy is not $1,25(OH)_2D_3$. The fact that pharmacologic doses of $25(OH)D_3$ were needed to correct the mineralization led them to conclude that the active metabolite missing is a derivative of $25(OH)D_3$, but not $1,25(OH)_2D_3$ itself. These studies suggested the possibility that the active metabolite may be $24,25(OH)_2D_3$. Indeed, Kanis *et al.* reported that small doses of $24,25(OH)_2D_3$ increased intestinal absorption of calcium both in normal patients and in those with chronic renal failure.[57] Furthermore, the authors showed that in anephric patients, small doses of $24,25(OH)_2D_3$ increased intestinal absorption of calcium, and suggested that the active form is $24,25(OH)_2D_3$. Administration of small doses of $24,25(OH)_2D_3$ also decreased alkaline phosphatase activity and increased the calcification front. All these data together question the statement that $1,25(OH)_2D_3$ is the final active metabolite that is missing. Its use in renal osteodystrophy as a drug superior to other vitamin D preparations is also brought into question. Furthermore, studies on vitamin D-deficient nonuremic patients clearly demonstrated that $25(OH)D_3$ administration corrected the biochemical, as well as the bone histologic, changes, whereas $1,25(OH)_2D_3$ did not and did not produce a normal bone mineralization front. The authors concluded that the active metabolite is probably derived from $25(OH)D_3$ but is not $1,25(OH)_2D_3$.

Strong support for this observation came recently from several centers treating patients with renal osteodystrophy and chronic advanced renal failure. It is clear from these studies that we are dealing with two populations of patients: the responders who share a bone histologic picture of osteitis fibrosa, elevated alkaline phosphatase levels and elevated amounts of PTH; and a second group who clearly show a predominant picture of osteomalacia and low to normal PTH levels, do not respond to treatment and actually will develop hypercalcemia.[28, 56, 86, 87] It is suggested by these recent studies that $1,25(OH)_2D_3$ is not the active metabolite missing, but that some other derivative of D_3 or $25(OH)D_3$ is.

Our personal feeling is that if $1,25(OH)_2D_3$ were the ultimate missing hormone, the smallest physiologic amount of $1,25(OH)_2D_3$ needed to correct vitamin D deficiency in patients without renal failure should be totally effective in treating patients with renal failure. This is not the case. We use fairly high doses of $1,25(OH)_2D_3$ to cause hypercalcemia, hyperphosphatemia and hypercalciuria. We believe that the studies of Bordier *et al.*[14] in vitamin D-deficient humans, and those of Kanis *et al.*[57] prove indirectly that a combination of $24,25(OH)_2D_3$ *and* $1,25(OH)_2D_3$ is needed. To our knowledge, no studies have been carried out in renal osteodystrophy to evaluate the combined use of physiologic doses of $24,25(OH)_2D_3$ *and* $1,25(OH)_2D_3$. Future clinical studies, as well as experimental ones, will answer this question. It is our feeling that for practical purposes of treatment, we can use D_3 or D_2, dihydrotachysterol or $25(OH)D_3$ when caution is taken to avoid hypercalcemia.

References

1. Ahmed, K. Y., Varghese, Z., Meinhard, E. A., Baillod, R. A., Skinner, R. W., Wills, M. R., and Moorhead, J. F.: Hypophosphatemia and osteomalacia in hemodialysis patients not taking phosphate binders, Adv. Exp. Med. Biol. 81:581, 1977.
2. Ahmed, K. Y., Wills, M. R., Skinner, R. W., Varghese, Z., Meinhard, E., and Baillod, R. A.: Persistent hypophosphatemia and osteomalacia in dialysis patients not on oral phosphate binders: Response to dihydrotachysterol therapy, Lancet 2:439, 1976.
3. Alfrey, A. C., Miller, N. L., and Butkus, D.: Evaluation of body magnesium stores, J. Lab. Clin. Med. 84:153, 1974.
4. Alfrey, A. C., Solomons, C. C., and Ciricillo, J.: Extraosseous calcification. Evidence for abnormal pyrophosphate metabolism in uremia, J. Clin. Invest. 57:692, 1976.
5. Alfrey, A. C., and Solomons, C. C.: Bone pyrophosphate in uremia and its association with extraosseous calcification, J. Clin. Invest. 57:700, 1976.
6. Ardaillou, R., Sizonenko, P., Meyrier, A., Vallee, G., and Beaugas, C.: Metabolic clearance rate of radioiodinated human calcitonin in man, J. Clin. Invest. 49:234g, 1970.
7. Arnaud, C. D., Tsao, H. S., and Oldham, S. B.: Native human parathyroid hormone: An immunochemical investigation, Proc. Natl. Acad. Sci. USA 67:415, 1970.
8. Arnaud, C. D., Sizemore, G. W., Oldham, S. B., Fischer, J. A., Tsao, H. S., and Littledike, E. T.: Human parathyroid hormone: Glandular and secreted molecular species, Am. J. Med. 50:630, 1971.
9. Bates, R. F. L., Care, A. D., Peacock, M., Mawer, E. B., and Taylor, C. M.: Inhibitory effects of 24-25-dihydroxy vitamin D_3 on parathyroid hormone secretion in the goat, J. Endocrinol. 64:6, 1974.
10. Bell, H., and Bartter, F. C.: Transient reversal of hyperabsorption of calcium and abnormal sensitivity to vitamin D in a patient with sarcoidosis during episode of nephritis, Ann. Intern. Med. 61:702, 1964.
11. Berson, S. A., and Yalow, R. S.: Immunochemical heterogeneity of parathyroid hormone in plasma, J. Clin. Endocrinol. 28:1037, 1968.
12. Birge, S. J., and Haddad, J. G.: 25-hydroxycholecalciferol stimulation of muscle metabolism, J. Clin. Invest. 56:1100, 1975.
13. Bone, M., Stein, P., Borsseau, V. C., Teitelbaum, S., and Avioli, L. V.: The effects of 25-hydroxycholecalciferol in renal osteodystrophy, in *Abstracts of Free Communications*, Sixth International Congress on Nephrology, Florence, June 8–12, 1976, p. 842.
14. Bordier, P., Ryckwaert, A., Marie, P., Miravet, L., Norman, A. W., Rasmussen, H.: Vitamin D metabolites and bone mineralization in man, in Norman, A. W., Schaeker, K., Coburn, J. W., DeLuca, H. F., Fraser, D., Grigolct, H. G., and Her-

rath, D. V. (eds.): *Vitamin D. Biochemical, Chemical and Clinical Aspects Related to Calcium Metabolism* (New York: Walter de Gruyter, 1977), pp. 897–909.

15. Bouillon, R., Verberckmoes, R., and Moor, P. D.: Influence of dialysate calcium concentration and vitamin D on serum parathyroid hormone during repetitive hemodialysis, Kidney Int. 7:422, 1975.

16. Boyle, I. T., Gray, R. W., and DeLuca, H. F.: Regulation by calcium of *in vivo* synthesis of 1,25-dihydroxycholecalciferol and 21,25-dihydroxycholecalciferol, Proc. Natl. Acad. Sci. USA 68:2131, 1971.

17. Brautbar, N., Lee, D. B. N., Coburn, J. W., and Kleeman, C. R.: Phosphate depletion without hypophosphatemia: The gut as a sensor organ, Clin. Res., in press.

18. Brautbar, N., Yaron, M., and Coburn, J. W.: Interactions between parathyroid hormone and $1,25(OH)_2$-vitamin D_3 on the renal handling of phosphate by the dog, Clin. Res. 25:136A, 1977.

19. Bricker, N. S., Slatopolsky, E., Reiss, E., and Avioli, L. V.: Calcium, phosphorus and bone in renal disease and transplantation, Arch. Intern. Med. 123:543, 1969.

20. Brickman, A. S., Sherrard, D. J., Jowsey, J., Singer, F. R., Baylink, D. J., Maloney, N., Massry, S. G., Norman, A. W., and Coburn, J. W.: 1,25 dihydroxycholecalciferol: Effect on skeletal lesions and plasma parathyroid hormone in uremic osteodystrophy, Arch. Intern. Med. 134:883, 1974.

21. Brickman, A. S., Coburn, J. W., Rome, P. H., Massry, S. G., and Norman, A. W.: Impaired calcium absorption in uremic man: Evidence for defective absorption in the proximal small intestine, J. Lab. Clin. Med. 84:791, 1974.

22. Burnell, J. M., and Teubne, E.: Effects of decreasing magnesium in patients with chronic renal failure, Proc. Dial. Transplant Forum 5:131, 1976.

23. Carr, A. D., Pickard, D. W., Peacock, M., Mawer, B., Taylor, C. M., Redel, J., and Norman, A. W.: Reduction of parathyroid hormone secretion by 24-25 dihydroxycholecalciferol (24-25 DHC), in Norman, A. W., Schaefer, K., Coburn, J. W., DeLuca, H. F., Fraser, D., Grigolet, H. G., and Herrath, D. V. (eds.): *Vitamin D. Biochemical, Chemical and Clinical Aspects Related to Calcium Metabolism* (New York: Walter de Gruyter, 1977), pp. 105–7.

24. Coburn, J. W., Hartenbower, D. L., and Brickman, A. S.: Advances in vitamin D metabolism as they pertain to chronic renal disease, Am. J. Clin. Nutr. 29:1283, 1976.

25. Coburn, J. W., Koppel, M. H., Brickman, A. S., and Massry, S. G.: Study of intestinal absorption of calcium in patients with renal failure, Kidney Int. 3:264, 1973.

26. Coburn, J. W., Hartenbower, D. L., Brickman, A. S., Massry, S. G., and Koppel, J. D.: Intestinal absorption of calcium, magnesium and phosphorus in chronic renal insufficiency, in David, D. S. (ed.): *Calcium Metabolism in Renal Failure and Nephrolithiasis* (New York: John Wiley & Sons, 1977), pp. 77–109.

27. Coburn, J. W., Popovtzer, M. M., Massry, S. G., and Kleeman, C. R.: The physiochemical state and renal handling of divalent ions in chronic renal failure, Arch. Intern. Med. 124:302, 1969.

28. Coburn, J. W., Brickman, A. S., Sherrard, D. S., Wong, E. G. C., Singer, F. R., and Norman, A. W.: Defective skeletal mineralization in uremia without relation to vitamin D, serum Ca or P, Proc. Am. Soc. Nephrol. 10:3, 1977.

29. Coburn, J. W., Brickman, A. S., Sherrard, D. J., Singer, F. R., Balink, D. J., Wong, E. G. C., Massry, S. G., and Norman, A. W.: Clinical efficacy of 1,25 dihydroxy-vitamin D_3 in renal osteodystrophy, in Norman, A. W., Schaefer, K., Coburn, J. W., DeLuca, H. F., Fraser, D., Grigolet, H. G., and Herrath, D. V. (eds.): *Vitamin D. Biochemical, Chemical and Clinical Aspects Related to Calcium Metabolism.* (New York: Walter de Gruyter, 1977), pp. 657–64.

30. DeLuca, H. F.: Metabolism of vitamin D: Current status, J. Clin. Nutr. 29:1258, 1976.

31. Dent, C. E., Harper, C. M., and Philpot, G. R.: Treatment of renal-glomerular osteo-dystrophy, Q. J. Med. 30:1, 1961.
32. Eastwood, J. B., Stamp, T. C. B., Harris, E., and de Wardener, H. E.: Vitamin D deficiency in the osteomalacia of chronic renal failure, Lancet 2:1209, 1976.
33. Evanson, J. M.: The response to the infusion of parathyroid extract in hypocalcemic states, Clin. Sci. 31:63, 1966.
34. Fischer, J. A., Bins Wanger, U., Fanconi, A., Illig, R., Baerlocher, K., and Prader, A.: Serum parathyroid hormone concentrations in vitamin D deficiency rickets of infancy: Effects of intravenous calcium and vitamin D, Horm. Metab. Res. 5:381, 1973.
35. Flueck, J. A., Di Bella, F. P., Edis, A. J., Kehrwald, J. M., and Arnaud, C. D.: Immunoheterogeneity of parathyroid hormone in venous effluent serum from hyperfunctioning parathyroid glands, J. Clin. Invest. 60:1367, 1977.
36. Fournier, A., Bordier, P., Geuris, J., Ferriere, E., Chanard, J., Marie, P., Sebert, J. L., Bedrossian, J., DeLuca, H. F., and Amiens, C. H. U.: Comparison of 1α hydroxyvitamin D_3 and 25 hydroxyvitamin D_3 in treatment of renal osteodystrophy, in Norman, A. W., Schaefer, K., Coburn, J. W., DeLuca, H. F., Fraser, D., Grigolet, H. G., and Herrath, D. V. (eds.): *Vitamin D. Biochemical, Chemical and Clinical Aspects Related to Calcium Metabolism* (New York: Walter de Gruyter, 1977), pp. 667–69.
37. Fraser, D. R., and Kodicek, E.: Unique biosynthesis by kidney of a biologically active vitamin D metabolite, Nature 228:764, 1970.
38. Fraser, D. R., and Kodicek, E.: Regulation of 25, hydroxycholecalciferol-1-hydroxylase activity in the kidney by parathyroid hormone, Nature 241:163, 1973.
39. Friis, T., Hahnemann, S., and Weeke, E.: Serum calcium and serum phosphorus in uremia during administration of sodium phytate and aluminum hydroxide, Acta Med. Scand. 183:497, 1968.
40. Garabedian, M., Pavlovitch, H., Fellot, C., and Balsan, S.: Metabolism of 25-hydroxyvitamin D_3 in anephric rats: a new active metabolite, Proc. Natl. Acad. Sci. USA 71:554, 1974.
41. Genuth, S. M., Vertes, V., and Leonards, J. R.: Oral calcium absorption in patients with renal failure treated by chronic hemodialysis, Metabolism 18:124, 1969.
42. Glassford, D. M., Remmers, A. R., Jr., and Sarles, H. E.: Hyperparathyroidism in the maintenance dialysis patient, Surg. Gynecol. Obstet. 142:328, 1976.
43. Goldsmith, R. S., Furszyfer, J., and Johnson, W. J.: Control of secondary hyperparathyroidism during long-term hemodialysis, Am. J. Med. 50:692, 1971.
44. Goldsmith, R. S., Furszyfer, J., and Johnson, W. J.: Etiology of hyperparathyroidism and bone disease during chronic hemodialysis. III. Evaluation of parathyroid suppressibility, J. Clin. Invest. 52:173, 1973.
45. Gordon, H. E., Coburn, J. W., and Passaro, E., Jr.: Surgical management of secondary hyperparathyroidism, Arch. Surg. 104:520, 1972.
46. Gray, R., Boyle, I., and DeLuca, H. F.: Vitamin D metabolism: The role of kidney tissue, Science 172:1232, 1971.
47. Habener, J. F., and Potts, J. T.: Relative effectiveness of magnesium and calcium on the secretion and biosynthesis of parathyroid hormone in vitro, Endocrinology 98: 197, 1976.
47a. Haussler, M. R., and McCain, T. A.: Circulating 1,25 dehydroxy vitamin D in health and disease, Clin. Res. 26:128A, 1978.
48. Heimberg, K. W., Matthews, C., Ritz, E., Augustino, J., and Hasselbach, W.: Active Ca transport of sarcoplasmic reticulum during experimental uremia, Eur. J. Biochem. 61:207, 1976.
49. Henderson, R. G., Russell, R. G. G., Ledingham, J. G. G., Smith, R., Oliver, D. O., Walton, R. J., Small, D. G., Preston, C., Warner, G. T., and Norman, A. W.: Effects

of 1,25-dihydroxycholecalciferol on calcium absorption, muscle weakness, and bone disease in chronic renal failure, Lancet 1:379, 1974.

50. Holick, M. F., and DeLuca, H. F.: Vitamin D metabolism, Annu. Rev. Med. 25:349, 1974.

51. Horsting, M., and DeLuca, H. F.: *In vitro* production of 25-hydroxy-cholecalciferol, Biochem. Biophys. Res. Commun. 36:251, 1969.

52. Hruska, K. A., Dopelman, R., Rutherford, W. E., Klahr, S., and Slatopolsky, E.: Metabolism of immunoreactive parathyroid hormone in the dog. The role of the kidney and the effects of chronic renal disease, J. Clin. Invest. 56:39, 1975.

53. Hughes, M. R., Brumbaugh, P. F., Haussler, M. R., Wergedal, J. E., and Baylink, D. J.: Regulation of serum 1α 25 dihydroxyvitamin D_3 by calcium and phosphate in the rat, Science 190:578, 1975.

54. Hurst, J. H., and Mayer, G. P.: Assessment of the effect of 1,25-dihydroxy-cholecalciferol on parathyroid secretion rates in calves, in Norman, A. W., Schaefer, K., Coburn, J. W., DeLuca, H. F., Fraser, D., Grigolet, H. G., and Herrath, D. V. (eds.): *Vitamin D. Biochemical, Chemical and Clinical Aspects Related to Calcium Metabolism* (New York: Walter de Gruyter, 1977), pp. 139–141.

55. Jowsey, J.: Calcium release from the skeleton of rachitic puppies, J. Clin. Invest. 51:9, 1972.

56. Junor, B. J. R., Catto, G. R. D., and Macleod, M.: The treatment of renal osteodystrophy with 1α hydroxycholecalciferol, Calcif. Tissue Res. 22(Suppl.):112, 1977.

57. Kanis, J. A., Heynen, G., Russell, R. G. G., Smith, R., Walton, R. J., and Warner, G. T.: Biological effects of 24,25 dihydroxycholecalciferol in man, in Norman, A. W., Schaefer, K., Coburn, J. W., DeLuca, H. F., Fraser, D., Grigolet, H. G., and Herrath, D. V. (eds.): *Vitamin D. Biochemical, Chemical and Clinical Aspects Related to Calcium Metabolism* (New York: Walter de Gruyter, 1977), pp. 792–95.

58. Kanis, J. A., Oliver, D., Ledingham, J. G., and Russell, R. G.: Evidence that endogenous calcitonin protects against renal bone disease, Lancet 2:1322, 1976.

59. Kanis, J. A., Earnshaw, M., Heyman, G., Ledingham, J. G., Oliver, D. O., Price, C., Russell, R. G., and Woods, G. G.: Decreased bone turnover after nephrectomy. Possible mediation by endogenous calcitonin, Proc. Eur. Dial. Transplant Assoc. 13:409, 1977.

60. Kleeman, C. R., Better, O. S., Massry, S. G., and Maxwell, M. H.: Divalent ion metabolism and osteodystrophy in chronic renal failure, Yale J. Biol. Med. 40:1, 1967.

61. Kleeman, C. R., and Better, O. S.: Disordered divalent ion metabolism in kidney disease: Comments on pathogenesis and treatment, Kidney Int. 4:73, 1973.

62. Kleeman, C. R., Bernstein, D., Rockney, R., Dowling, J. T., and Maxwell, M. H.: Studies on the renal clearance of diffusable calcium and the role of the parathyroid gland in its regulation, Yale J. Biol. Med. 34:1, 1961.

63. Lee, E. J., Parthemore, J. G., and Deftos, L. J.: Immunochemical heterogeneity of calcitonin in renal failure, J. Clin. Endocrinol. Metab. 45:528, 1977.

64. Lichtwitz, A., and Parlier, R.: Calcium et maladies métaboliques de l'os, in *Tome III Rein et Métabolism du Calcium à l'Etat Pathologique* (Paris: Expansions Scientifique Française, 1965), pp. 199–246.

65. Liu, S. H., and Chu, H. I.: Studies on calcium and phosphorus metabolism with special reference to pathogenesis and effect of dihydrotachysterol (AT 10) and iron, Medicine 22:103, 1943.

66. Llach, F., Massry, S. G., Singer, F. R., Kurokawa, K., Kaye, J. H., and Coburn, J. W.: Skeletal resistance to endogenous parathyroid hormone in patients with early renal failure. A possible cause of secondary hyperparathyroidism, Clin. Endocrinol. Metab. 41:339, 1975.

67. Llach, F., Massry, S. G., Koffler, A., Malluche, H., Singer, F. R., Brickman, A. S., and Kurokawa, K.: Secondary hyperparathyroidism in early renal failure: role of phosphate retention, Proc. Am. Soc. Nephrol. 10:7, 1977.

68. Loreau, N., Cosyns, J. P., Lepreux, C., and Ardaillou, R.: Renal adenylate, calcitonin receptors and phosphate excretion in rats immunized against tubular basement membrane, in Massry, S. G., and Ritz, E. (eds.): *Proceedings of the Second International Workshop on Phosphate Metabolism* (New York: Plenum Press), pp. 71–72.
69. Malluche, H. H., Ritz, E., Lange, H. P., Kutschera, J., Hodgson, M., Seiffert, U., and Schoppe, W.: Bone histology in incipient and advanced renal failure, Kidney Int. 9: 355, 1976.
70. Malluche, H. H., Ritz, E., Kutschera, J., Krause, G., Werner, E., Gati, A., Seiffert, U., and Lange, H. P., in Norman, A. W., Schaefer, K., Grigolet, H. G., Herrath, D., and Ritz, E. (eds.): *Vitamin D and Problems Related to Uremic Bone Disease* (Berlin: Walter de Gruyter, 1975), pp. 513–18.
71. Massry, S. G., Coburn, J. W., Lee, D. B. N., Jowsey, J., and Kleeman, C. R.: Skeletal resistance to parathyroid hormone in renal failure, Ann. Intern. Med. 78:357, 1973.
72. Massry, S. G., Coburn, J. W., Lee, D. B. N., and Kleeman, C. R., in Frame, B., Parfitt, A. M., and Duncan, H. (eds.): *Clinical Aspects of Metabolic Bone Disease* (Amsterdam: Excerpta Medica, 1973), p. 578.
73. Massry, S. G., Stein, R., Arieff, A. I., Coburn, J. W., Norman, A. W., and Friedler, R. M.: Skeletal resistance to the calcemic action of parathyroid hormone in uremia. Role of 1-25 OH_2D_3, Kidney Int. 9:467, 1976.
74. Massry, S. G., Dua, S., Garty, J., and Friedler, R. M.: Role of uremia in the skeletal resistance to the calcemic action of parathyroid hormone (PTH), Proc. Am. Soc. Nephrol. 9:4, 1976.
75. Massry, S. G., and Coburn, J. W.: Comments on the mechanism of disordered divalent ion metabolism in renal failure: A possible role of magnesium depletion, Am. J. Clin. Nutr. 220:4, 1971.
76. Massry, S. G., Coburn, J. W., and Kleeman, C. R.: Evidence for suppression of parathyroid gland activity by hypermagnesemia, J. Clin. Invest. 49:1619, 1970.
77. Massry, S. G., Coburn, J. W., Peacock, M., and Kleeman, C. R.: Turnover of endogenous parathyroid hormone in uremic patients and those undergoing hemodialysis, Am. Soc. Artif. Intern. Organs 18:416, 1972.
78. Melick, R. A., and Martin, T. J.: Parathyroid hormone metabolism in man: Effect of nephrectomy, Clin. Sci. 37:667, 1969.
79. Messenger, R. P., Smith, H. T., Shapiro, F. L., and Gregory, D. H.: The effect of hemodialysis, vitamin D and renal homotransplantation on the calcium absorption in chronic renal failure, J. Lab. Clin. Med. 74:472, 1969.
80. Norman, A. W., Midgett, R. J., Myrtle, J. F., and Nowicki, H. G.: Studies on calciferol metabolism. I. Production of vitamin D metabolite 4B from 25-OH-cholecalciferol by kidney homogenates, Biochem. Biophys. Res. Commun. 42:1082, 1971.
81. Omdahl, J. L., Gray, R. W., Boyle, I. T., Knutson, J., and DeLuca, H. F.: Regulation of metabolism of 25-hydroxycholecalciferol by kidney tissue in vitro by dietary calcium, Nature 237:63, 1972.
82. Papenheimer, A. M., and Willens, S. L.: Enlargement of parathyroid gland in renal disease, Am. J. Pathol. 2:73, 1935.
83. Parfitt, A. M.: The actions of parathyroid hormone on bone: relation to bone remodeling and turnover, calcium homeostasis and metabolic bone disease, Metabolism 25:1157, 1976.
84. Parfitt, A. M.: Relation between parathyroid cell mass and plasma calcium concentration in normal and uremic subjects. A theoretical model with an analysis of the concept of autonomy and speculation on the mechanism of parathyroid hyperplasia, Arch. Intern. Med. 124:269, 1969.
85. Pavlovitch, H., Fontaine, O., and Balsan, S.: Maintenance of a calcemic response to parathyroid hormone in D-deficient rats by the prevention of severe hyperparathyroidism, Calcif. Tissue Res. 23:277, 1977.
86. Pierides, A. M., Ellis, H. A., Ward, M. K., Simpson, W., and Kerr, D. N. S.: 1α-hy-

droxycholecalciferol in renal osteodystrophy, Calcif. Tissue Res. 22(Suppl.):105, 1977.

87. Pierides, A. M., Simpson, N., Ward, M. K., Ellis, H. A., Dewar, J. H., and Err, D. N. S.: Variable response to long term 1α hydroxycholecalciferol in hemodialysis osteodystrophy, Lancet 1:1092, 1976.

88. Ponchon, G., Kennan, A. L., and DeLuca, H. F.: "Activation" of vitamin D by the liver, J. Clin. Invest. 48:2032, 1969.

89. Popovtzer, M. M., Schainuck, L. I., Massry, S. G., and Kleeman, C. R.: Divalent ion excretion in chronic kidney disease. Relation to degree of renal insufficiency, Clin. Sci. 38:297, 1970.

90. Popovtzer, M. M., Robinette, J. B., DeLuca, H. F., and Holick, M. F.: The acute effects of 25-hydroxycholecalciferol on renal handling of phosphorus. Evidence for a parathyroid hormone dependent mechanism, J. Clin. Invest. 53:913, 1974.

91. Posner, A. S., Betts, F., and Blumenthal, N. C.: Role of ATP and Mg in the stabilization of biological and synthetic amorphous calcium phosphates, Calcif. Tissue Res. 22(Suppl.):208, 1977.

92. Potts, J. T., Niall, H. O., Tregrar, G. W., van Rietschosen, J., Habener, J. F., Serge, G. V., and Keutmann, H. T.: Chemical and biological studies on parathyroid hormone: Analysis of hormone biosynthesis and metabolism, Mt. Sinai J. Med. NY. 40: 448, 1973.

93. Puschett, J. B., Moranz, J., and Kurnick, W. S.: Evidence for a direct action of cholecalciferol and 25-hydroxycholecalciferol on the renal transport of phosphate, sodium and calcium, J. Clin. Invest. 51:373, 1972.

94. Puschett, J. B., Fernandez, P. C., Boyle, I. T., Gray, R. W., Omdahl, J. L., and De-Luca, H. F.: The acute renal tubular effects of 1,25 dihydroxycholecalciferol, Proc. Soc. Exp. Biol. Med. 141:379, 1972.

95. Raisz, L. G., and Neimann, I.: Effect of phosphate, calcium and magnesium on bone resorption and hormonal responses in tissue culture, Endocrinology 85:446, 1969.

96. Randall, R. E., Cohen, M. D., and Spray, C. C.: Hypermagnesemia in renal failure. Etiology and toxic manifestations, Ann. Intern. Med. 61:73, 1964.

97. Ritz, E., Malluche, H., Bommer, J., Mehls, O., and Krempien, B.: Metabolic bone disease in patients on maintenance hemodialysis, Nephron 12:393, 1974.

98. Ritz, E., Malluche, H. H., and Krempien, B.: Bone histology in renal insufficiency, in David, D. S. (ed.): *Calcium Metabolism in Renal Failure and Nephrolithiasis* (New York: John Wiley and Sons, 1976), pp. 197–234.

99. Ritz, E., Krempien, B., and Mehls, O.: Skeletal complications of renal insufficiency and maintenance haemodialysis, Nephron 10:195, 1973.

100. Rude, R. K., Oldham, S. B., and Singer, F. R.: Functional hypoparathyroidism and parathyroid hormone end organ resistance in human magnesium deficiency, Clin. Endocrinol. 5:209, 1976.

101. Serge, G. V., Habener, J. F., Powell, D., Treager, G. W., and Potts, J. T.: Parathyroid hormone in human plasma. Immunochemical characterization and biological implications, J. Clin. Invest. 52:524, 1972.

102. Serge, G. V., Niall, H. D., Habener, J. F., and Potts, J. T.: Metabolism of parathyroid hormone: physiologic and clinical significance, Am. J. Med. 56:774, 1974.

103. Slatopolsky, E., Caglar, S., Gradowska, L., Canterbury, J., Reiss, E., and Bricker, N. S.: On the prevention of secondary hyperparathyroidism in experimental chronic renal disease using "proportional reduction" of dietary phosphorus intake, Kidney Int. 2:147, 1972.

104. Slatopolsky, E., Caglar, S., Pennell, J. P., Tagart, D. B., Canterbury, J. M., Reiss, E., and Bricker, N. S.: On the pathogenesis of hyperparathyroidism in chronic experimental renal insufficiency in the dog, J. Clin. Invest. 50:492, 1971.

105. Stanbury, S. W.: Azotemic renal osteodystrophy, Br. Med. Bull. 13:57, 1957.

106. Stanbury, S. W., Mawer, E. B., Lumb, G. A., Hill, L. F., Holman, C. A., Taylor,

C. M., and Torkington, P., in Frame, B., Parfitt, A. M., and Duncan, H. (eds.): *Clinical Aspects of Metabolic Bone Disease* (Amsterdam: Excerpta Medica, 1973), pp. 562–70.

107. Stanbury, S. W., and Lumb, G. A.: Metabolic studies of renal osteodystrophy. I. Calcium, phosphorus and nitrogen metabolism in rickets, osteomalacia and hyperparathyroidism complicating chronic uremia and in the osteomalacia of the adult Fanconi syndrome, Medicine 41:1, 1962.
108. Swenson, R. S., Weisinger, J. R., Ruggeri, J. L., and Reaven, G. M.: Evidence that parathyroid hormone is not required for phosphate homeostasis in renal failure, Metabolism 24:199, 1975.
109. Teitelbaum, S. L., Bone, M., Gilden, J., Stein, P. M., Borsseau, V. C., Bates, M., and Avioli, L. V.: The effects of 25-hydroxyvitamin D therapy on renal osteodystrophy: A morphometric analysis, in *Abstracts of Free Communications*, Sixth International Congress on Nephrology, Florence, June 8–12, 1976, p. 840.
110. Tomlinson, S., Barling, P. M., Albano, J. D. M., Brown, B. L., and O'Riordan, J. L. H.: The effects of exogenous parathyroid hormone on plasma and urine adenosine 3-5 cyclic monophosphate in man, Clin. Sci. 47:481, 1974.

Part III

DIALYSIS AND TRANSPLANTATION

11

Early Renal Failure after Cadaver Kidney Transplantation

H. KREIS, M.D., T. W. FINCH, M.D.,
J. F. MOREAU, M.D., L. H. NOËL, M.D.,
M. LACOMBE, M.D., AND J. CROSNIER, M.D.

Hôpital Necker, Paris, France

Episodes of renal failure frequently follow kidney transplantation. In general they are thought to be of immunologic origin, whether they occur early or later on, and are referred to as hyperacute rejection or acute rejection, according to their time sequence and course. In fact, in many cases renal failure is the consequence of traumatic injury of the transplant during harvesting, or of surgical complication. The diverse types of postoperative damage make diagnosis difficult. The failure of immunologic follow-up tests to forecast a rejection episode or even to definitely recognize the presence of one probably stems from this diversity.[17]

These implications are serious, since renal failure can compromise the viability of the transplant short or long term if appropriate medical or surgical therapy is not started immediately. Nevertheless, an early diagnosis of posttransplant renal failure is probably the key for better long-term survival, since the failure can be totally or partially reversed with adequate treatment. Therefore, we have attempted to analyze renal failure that occurred within the first month following cadaver kidney transplantation.

0084-5957/79/080209-24$3.75

Materials and Methods

We studied 172 patients who received cadaver kidney transplants at Necker Hospital between January 1, 1970, and July 1, 1975. Female recipients (65) accounted for 37.8% of the total population.

DRUG PROTOCOL

Azathioprine was given to all recipients according to the same protocol: 5 mg/kg body weight per day for three days, and 3 mg/kg/day thereafter. This dosage was reduced only in cases of bone marrow intolerance.

Prednisone was started at 5 mg/kg body weight per day for five days and then tapered off gradually to 0.25 mg/kg/day 10 weeks later. In 58 patients, this protocol was started in the immediate posttransplant period, whereas in the remaining 114, it was begun only when an episode of renal failure occurred.

In addition, 81 patients were given an intravenous pulse of 500 mg furosemide during surgery.

Thus, there were three different therapeutic protocols.

Protocol I: Twenty-three patients treated with furosemide during surgery and then azathioprine, but without steroids, until the first evidence of acute renal failure. Protocol II: Fifty-eight patients treated with furosemide during the operation and with azathioprine and steroids immediately after transplantation. Protocol III: Ninety-one patients given azathioprine without furosemide; steroids were given only if renal failure occurred.

SOURCE OF KIDNEYS

In 167 cases, kidneys were harvested from ventilated donors with intact heartbeat. Warm ischemia time was less than 10 minutes. In the five remaining cases, kidneys were removed from donors after cardiac arrest had occurred, and the warm ischemia time was between 20 and 50 minutes. Compatibility for HL-A A and B antigens was checked routinely in all 172 donor–recipient combinations. A compatibility coefficient was calculated according to the method of Hors *et al.*[10] A crossmatch reaction was always performed on the donor's cells in the laboratory of Professor Dausset. In only one case was a transplantation done despite a positive reaction.

Factors that could indicate possible HL-A presensitization were always sought: previous blood transfusions and previous pregnancies were recorded whenever possible. Sera from all recipients were tested every two months for cytotoxic anti-HL-A antibodies using the microcytotoxicity technique proposed by Terasaki.[18]

Follow-up Parameters

Serum and urinary sodium and creatinine levels were determined daily, as was proteinuria in all recipients. Special attention was paid to the creatinine U/P ratio, the urinary sodium concentration and variation of proteinuria during the three days preceding and the three days following the occurrence of renal failure. Within the same period of time a rise in temperature to or above 38 C, a diastolic blood pressure of or exceeding 100 mm Hg and/or a urinary output of less than 300 ml/24 hours was recorded.

Microscopic examinations of the transplanted kidneys were performed in 52 cases (36 open biopsies and 16 nephrectomies). All sections were evaluated by light microscopy using Masson's trichrome, hematoxylin and eosin and Weigert staining. All sections were pooled and examined "blind" at random. Five types of changes were categorized: severe vascular changes (24 cases); tubular necrosis (7 cases); interstitial edema and cellular infiltration (9 cases); normal kidney (10 cases); and miscellaneous (2 cases).

Arteriography of the transplanted kidney was performed in 79 patients via a catheter inserted into the femoral artery, according to a technique published elsewhere.[14]

Arteriographic findings were classified into five different types.

Type I: Acute vascular syndrome: 14 cases, distinguished by (1) delayed contrast medium transit time, (2) a faint vascular nephrogram, (3) multiple narrowing of renal artery branches and lack of arteriolar filling, and (4) infarcts of different size and number, or cortical necrosis.

Type II: Syndrome reported by Hollemberg et al.:[9] 22 cases, consisting of markedly delayed transit time of the contrast medium with a faint vascular nephrogram and no defined cortico-medullary junction. Although the intraparenchymatous vessels may be distorted or crowded, their total distribution is normal.

Type III: The "low renal blood flow" syndrome: 13 cases, with only mild decrease in contrast medium transit time. The vascular nephrogram is less dense than in normal arteriography, but the corticomedullary junction is well defined.

Type IV: Normal arteriogram: 19 cases.

Type V: Miscellaneous: 11 cases.

CRITERIA FOR DEFINITION OF RENAL FAILURE

The patients considered to have episodes of renal failure were those in which there was no decrease in the pretransplant serum creatinine level 24 hours after surgery; the serum creatinine level, after initial improvement, stabilized at an abnormal level or increased more than 0.3 mg/100 ml for at least two consecutive days. In case of immediate renal failure, the day of operation was considered the first day. For secondary renal failure episodes, the first day was that on which the first rise in the serum creatinine clearance occurred. The end of the episode was considered to be the first day of a spontaneous decrease in the serum creatinine clearance, provided it lasted at least 48 hours.

Results

A total of 215 renal failure episodes were observed in 156 patients during the first 30 posttransplantation days. They may be distributed as shown on Table 11–1: 16 patients (9.3%) had no episodes of renal failure (group O); 65 episodes of renal failure

TABLE 11–1.—DISTRIBUTION OF RENAL
FAILURE EPISODES ACCORDING TO
TREATMENT PROTOCOLS

PROTOCOL*	GROUP O†	GROUP A	GROUP B	GROUP C
I	1/23	6/23	10/11	. . .
II	11/58	14/58	42/53	. . .
III	4/91	45/91	39/43	. . .
Total	16/172	65/172	91/107	59/52

*See text for description of the drugs used in each patient.
†See text for clinical descriptions of each group.

TABLE 11-2.—TOTAL ISCHEMIA TIME OF THE GRAFT

PROTOCOL	GROUP O	GROUP A	GROUP B
I	17 hr 30 min	16 hr 57 min	15 hr 33 min
	—	(± 2 hr 57 min)	(± 63 min)
II	15 hr 37 min	17 hr 40 min	16 hr 57 min
	(±43 min)	(± 1 hr 12 min)	(± 42 min)
III	6 hr 52 min	9 hr 49 min	8 hr 35 min
	(± 3 hr 17 min)	(± 59 min)	(± 49 min)

were observed immediately following surgery (group A); 91 episodes of renal failure occurred later in patients who had not had immediate episodes (group B); and 59 recurrent episodes of renal failure occurred in 52 patients (group C).

Group O

As seen on Table 11-1, group O includes 12 of the 81 (14.8%) patients treated either by furosemide (1 of 23) or prednisone (11 of 58), but only four patients of 91 (4.4%) who received azathioprine only.

The mean total ischemia time (TIT) of the 16 group O grafts was 13 hours, 33 ± 80 minutes. But the TIT was shorter (6 hours, 52 ± 197 minutes) in the four cases of group O III than in the 11 cases of group O II (15 hours, 37 ± 43 minutes) (Table 11-2).

There were relatively more women (62.5%) in group O than in the overall population (37.8%) ($p < .05$). Moreover, 40% of patients had a previous history of pregnancy (6 of 15), whereas only 12.5% had been pregnant in all 152 patients who developed renal failure (19 of 152) ($p < .005$). Percentages of previously transfused recipients (92.9%), recipients with detectable preformed anti-HL-A cytotoxic antibodies (42.9%) and HL-A-compatible donor-recipient combinations (66.7%) were similar to those observed in the overall population.

Group A

INFLUENCE OF FUROSEMIDE AND/OR STEROIDS.—Among the 91 recipients treated by protocol III (azathioprine alone), 45 (49.4%) had immediate renal failure (IRF), (group A III). On the contrary, of 58 protocol II patients receiving both steroids and furo-

TABLE 11–3.–FACTORS THAT MIGHT PLAY A ROLE IN IMMUNOLOGIC REJECTION PHENOMENON FREQUENCY (%) IN GROUPS A I & II AND A III

GROUPS	WOMEN	PREVIOUS HISTORY OF PREGNANCY	NONTRANSFUSED	ANTI-HL-A CYTOTOXIC ANTIBODIES	WELL MATCHED
A I+II	25 (20)*	10 (20)	12.5 (16) ⎱ $p < .02$	50 (16)	62.5 (16)
A III	42.2 (45)	9.3 (43)	0 (43) ⎰	33.3 (42)	45.2 (42)
Total	36.9 (65)	9.5 (63)	3.4 (59)	37.9 (58)	50 (58)
Total population	37.8 (172)	15.9 (157)	9.6 (146)	39.7 (156)	56.7 (157)

*Total number of patients studied.

semide, and of 23 protocol I patients receiving furosemide alone, 24.1% (group A II), ($p < 0.005$) and 26.1% (group A I), (not significant), respectively, had IRF. Thus 24.7% of 81 group A I + II patients had IRF ($p < .001$).

INFLUENCE OF TOTAL ISCHEMIA TIME (TIT) (Table 11–2).–It can been seen in Table 11–2 that TIT was not different between patients with IRF (group A) and patients with no IRF (groups O and B). Moreover, in group A III, where the percentage of IRF was the highest, the TIT was the shortest.

HL-A COMPATIBILITY AND PRESENSITIZATION FACTORS (Table 11–3).– When comparing groups A I + II, A III and the overall population, no differences could be demonstrated in the sex ratio, the proportion of recipients with a previous history of pregnancy, those with preformed cytotoxic HL-A antibodies or the percent of HL-A-compatible donor–recipient pairs. The 45 group A III patients, on the contrary, had all received at least a single blood unit before transplantation, but 12.5% of the 16 group A I + II patients and 9.6% of the overall population had never received blood transfusions.

COMPLICATIONS AND FACTORS CONTRIBUTING TO IMMEDIATE RENAL FAILURE.–It was possible in 27 of 65 group A patients (41.5%) to discover one or more factors that could have caused or contributed to the occurrence of renal failure, such as those reported in Table 11–4. They were present with a similar frequency in groups A I (33.3%), A II (35.7%) and A III (44.4%). Nevertheless, it is worthwhile to note that a warm ischemia period of more than 20 minutes and technical problems during harvesting were present in 17 of the 65 group A patients, and in only 16 of 107 patients without IRF.

TABLE 11–4.–MAJOR FACTORS RESPONSIBLE
FOR OR CONTRIBUTING TO THE OCCURRENCE
OF IMMEDIATE RENAL FAILURE EPISODES

Infarcts	4
Frozen kidney	1
Rupture	3
Technical accident	14
Urinary tract fistula	3
Warm ischemia time (10–50 min)	5
Perirenal collection	1
Cortical necrosis	3
Miscellaneous	2

CLINICAL ASPECTS AND BIOCHEMICAL PARAMETERS. — As there were no significant differences between group A I and A II patients in clinical or laboratory data (Table 11–5), results of both groups were pooled and compared with the data from the patients treated with azathioprine only (group A III). Fever was significantly less frequent in group A I + II patients who received steroids than in group A III patients ($p < .02$). The creatinine U/P ratio was lower than 10 in 50% of group A I + II patients (mean value, 10.8 ± 1.5) and in 53.1% of group A III patients (mean value, 9.2 ± 0.8). Urinary sodium concentrations were higher than 30 mEq/L in 73.7% of the 19 patients of groups A I and II in whom the urines could be collected (mean value, 45.2 ± 5.2 mEq/L) and in 85% of 40 group A III patients (mean value, 58.2 ± 4.7 mEq/L).

Figure 11–1 shows that there was no correlation between the creatinine U/P ratio, which was always relatively low because of high serum levels, and urinary sodium concentration.

PATHOLOGY. — Pathologic examination was obtained in 11

TABLE 11–5.–FREQUENCY (%) OF MAJOR CLINICAL AND
BIOCHEMICAL FEATURES AT THE ONSET OF IMMEDIATE
RENAL FAILURE

GROUPS	TEMPERATURE ≥ 38 C	HYPERTENSION	ANURIA	CREATININE U/P <10	URINE Na ≥ 30 mEq/L
A I	66.6 (6)*	0 (6)	100 (6)	50 (4)	66.6 (6)
A II	35.7 (14)	14.3 (14)	64.3 (14)	50 (8)	76.9 (13)
A I+II	45 (20) $\Big\}\, p < .02$	10 (20)	75 (20)	50 (12)	73.7 (19)
A III	71.1 (45)	29.5 (44)	86.6 (45)	53.1 (32)	85 (40)

*Total number of patients studied.

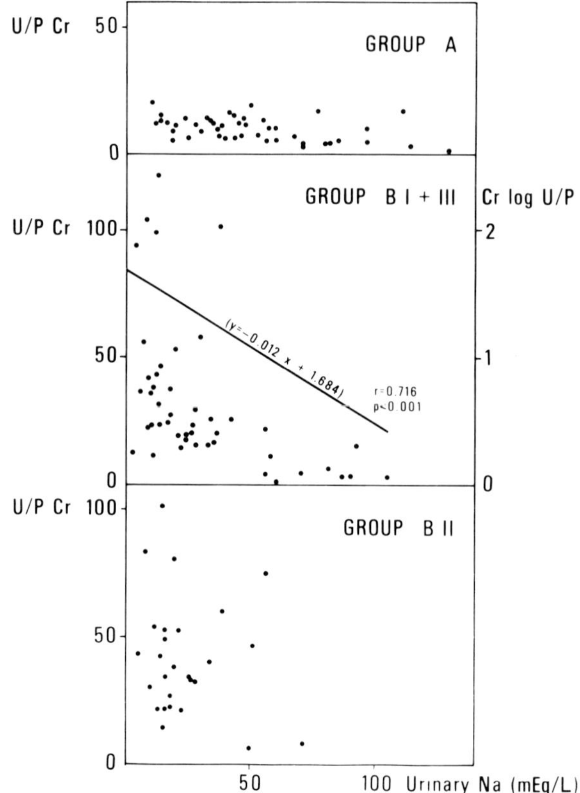

Fig. 11−1.−Relationship between the creatinine U/P ratio and urinary sodium concentration during episodes of immediate renal failure (group A) and delayed renal failure (group B I + III and group B II).

cases (three biopsies and eight nephrectomies), and 10 of these could be interpreted. Results are given on Table 11−6. In spite of the small number of cases, it should be noted that in the group with severe vascular lesions, five of six patients had no other treatment than azathioprine (group A III); only one patient received a compatible kidney and he was the only one to develop reversible kidney failure; and in all six cases, the creatinine U/P ratio was lower than 10 and the urinary sodium concentration was higher than 30 mEq/L.

ARTERIOGRAPHY.−Arteriography was performed in 28 cases. In the 25 interpretable arteriographies, the observed aspects

TABLE 11-6.—PATHOLOGIC CHANGES IN TEN
IMMEDIATE RENAL FAILURE EPISODES (GROUP A)

	A I+II	A III	CREATININE U/P <10	URINARY NA ≥30 mEq/L	NONREVERSIBLE COURSE	WELL-MATCHED PATIENTS
Severe vascular lesions (6)	1	5	100%	100%	5	1
Acute tubular necrosis (2)	1	1	100%	100%	1 (Torsion of the artery)	2
No changes (2)	1	1	. . .	. . .	1 (Pulmonary embolism)	1

were: (1) Acute vascular syndrome: three cases were confirmed by pathologic examination. In these three cases, evolution was irreversible. (2) Syndrome described by Hollemberg: 12 cases. For 12 patients, the average time of renal failure was 15.5 days. (3) Low renal blood flow syndrome: five cases. Average time of renal failure was 16 days. (4) Normal arteriography: five cases. Average time of renal failure was 10.2 days.

COURSE.—Irreversible renal failure was observed immediately after transplantation in eight patients of the 65 in group A

Fig. 11-2.—Duration of immediate renal failure episodes: comparison of group A I + II and group A III.

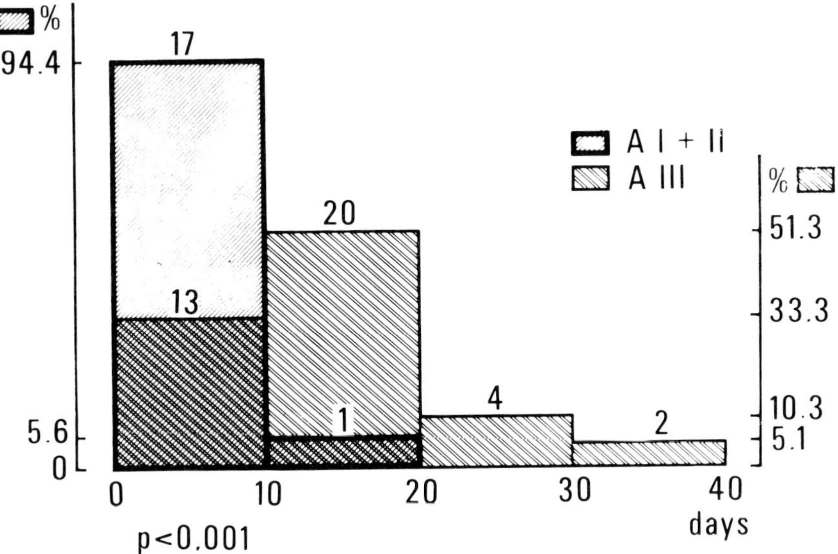

(12.3%). In three cases it was associated with death of the patients, and in five cases it was due to major vascular lesions. Of the 18 reversible renal failure episodes in group A I + II patients, 94.4% lasted less than 10 days, although only 33.3% of the 39 similar episodes observed in group A III patients lasted less than 10 days ($p<.001$) (Fig. 11–2).

In group A III patients, who had received neither furosemide nor initial steroid treatment, 40% of the transplants (2 of 5) were functional less than five days after treatment was started, provided that steroids were given before the third day of renal failure; this was the case for only 17.6% of patients (6 of 34) when treatment was started later. Although the number of cases in both groups was too small for the difference to be significant, steroids may act favorably when they are given early enough.

GROUP B

A delayed renal failure episode was observed in 91 of 107 patients (85%) whose kidney transplants had originally functioned well. Forty-two were already on steroid therapy when renal failure occurred (prescribed routinely at transplantation in 33 cases or for diverse reasons in nine cases), and were thus recorded as group B II (53 patients). The 49 patients who were not treated by steroids were recorded as group B I + III (54 cases).

Table 11–1 indicates that there is no significant difference in the frequencies of renal failure between group B II and group B I + III patients.

DATE OF ONSET. — In 87.8% (43 of 49) of patients not pretreated with steroids (group B I + III), the onset of renal failure took place one to five days after transplantation, whereas it started after day 5 in 95.2% (40 of 42) of patients already receiving steroid therapy ($p < .001$) (Fig. 11–3). In two group B II patients, renal failure started before day 5, but there was a warm ischemia period of 36 minutes in one, and surgical shock occurred in the other.

INFLUENCE OF TOTAL ISCHEMIA TIME. — The mean TIT of group B transplants was 13 hours, 17 ± 38 minutes, which is similar to the mean TIT of group O transplants (13 hours, 33 ± 80 minutes). As shown on Table 11–2, the mean TIT of group B I + III

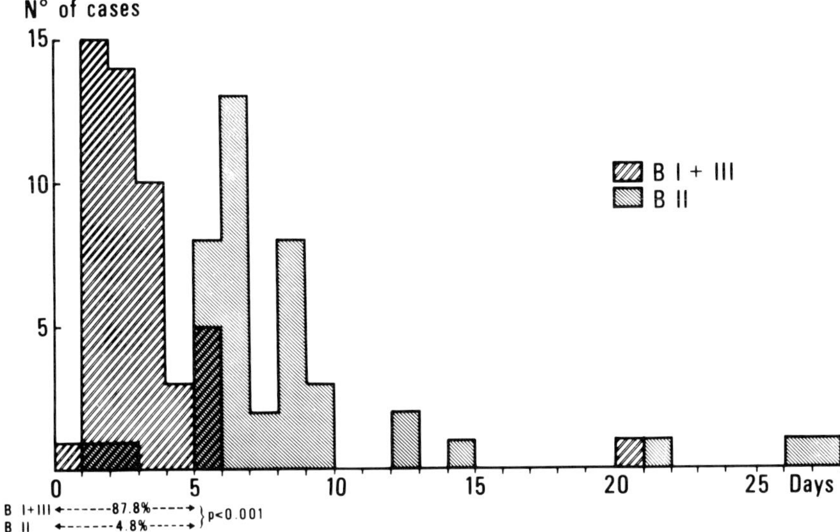

Fig. 11–3. — Date of onset of renal failure episodes in group B.

patients was significantly shorter than that of group B II subjects.

HL-A COMPATIBILITY AND PRESENSITIZATION FACTORS. — Table 11–7 indicates that there were no differences between group B II, group B I + III and the overall population with regard to the proportion of female patients, the percent of recipients with a previous history of pregnancy or with preformed cytotoxic HL-A antibodies, or the percent of HL-A-compatible donor-recipient pairs.

TABLE 11–7. — FACTORS THAT MIGHT PLAY A ROLE IN IMMUNOLOGIC REJECTION PHENOMENON FREQUENCY (%) IN GROUP B AND IN GROUPS B I+III AND B II

GROUPS	WOMEN	PREVIOUS HISTORY OF PREGNANCY	NONTRANSFUSED	ANTI-HL-A CYTOTOXIC ANTIBODIES	WELL-MATCHED PATIENTS
B I+III	32.6 (49)*	18.7 (48)	9.3 (43) ⎱ p = .05	34.1 (44)	58.7 (46)
B II	38.1 (42)	9.7 (41)	26.7 (30) ⎰	48.7 (39)	60.5 (38)
Total	35.2 (91)	14.6 (89)	16.4 (73)	41 (83)	59.5 (84)
Total population	37.8 (172)	15.9 (157)	9.6 (146)	39.7 (156)	56.7 (157)

*Total number of patients studied.

TABLE 11-8.—MAJOR FACTORS
RESPONSIBLE FOR OR
CONTRIBUTING TO THE OCCURRENCE
OF GROUP B RENAL FAILURES;
FREQUENCY (%) OF RENAL
FAILURE EPISODES ASSOCIATED
WITH SUCH FACTORS

Groups	B I+III	B II
Technical accident	5	3
Infections		
Urinary	2	1
Wound	2	7
Lung ⎫ Blood ⎭	1	3
Rupture	2	2
Infarcts	1	1
Ureter fistula	5	4
Miscellaneous	2	2
No. of patients with a complication	18	23
Total no. of patients	49	42
Percent	36.7	54.8

On the other hand, 26.7% of group B II recipients had never received any blood transfusion before transplantation, versus only 9.3% of group B I + III recipients ($p < .05$).

COMPLICATIONS AND FACTORS CONTRIBUTING TO RENAL FAILURE.—In 41 of the 91 group B patients (45%), a factor responsible for, or at least contributing to, the occurrence of renal failure was found (Table 11-8). This was the case in 36.7% of group B I + III patients and in 54.8% in group B II patients (not significant). The difference between these two groups is the consequence of a higher percentage of infectious complications in group B II patients (22.4%) than in group B I + III patients (10.2%), ($p < .05$).

CLINICAL SIGNS.—The only significant differences in the clinical presentation between group B II (steroids) and group B I + III (no steroids) patients was the higher incidence of fever in the latter (97.9%) (Table 11-9) than in the former (41.5%) group ($p < .01$).

BIOCHEMICAL DATA.—The creatinine U/P ratio was higher than 10, with a mean value of 41.4 ± 4.5, in 92.6% of group B II patients. In group B I + III patients, the creatinine U/P ratio was higher than 10 in 86.9% of cases, with a mean value of

TABLE 11-9.—FREQUENCY (%) OF MAJOR CLINICAL
FEATURES AT THE ONSET OF DELAYED RENAL FAILURE
(GROUP B)

GROUPS	FEVER	HYPERTENSION	ANURIA	PROTEINURIA
B II	41.5 (41)*	30.9 (42)	38.1 (42)	51.2 (41)
B I+II	97.9 (49) } $p < .001$	38.8 (49)	51 (49)	41.9 (43)

*Total number of patients studied.

31.6 ± 4.3. Urinary sodium concentrations also differ between
the two groups, being less than 30 mEq/L in 80.5% of group B II
patients, but in only 63.8% of group B I + III patients (Fig.
11-4). An inverse correlation was found between the creatinine
U/P ratio and the urinary sodium concentration (r = .716,

Fig. 11-4.—Respective values of urinary sodium concentration (mEq/L) and of the
creatinine U/P ratio during episodes of delayed renal failure (group B).

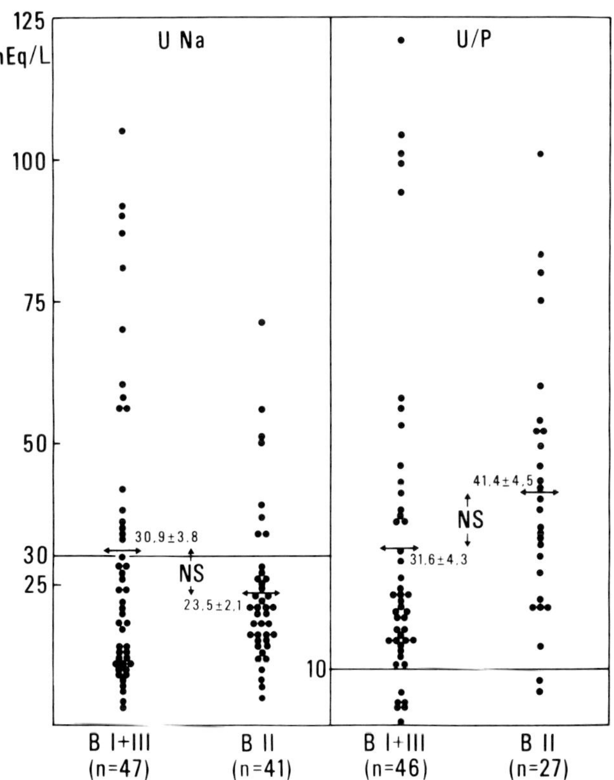

TABLE 11–10.—PATHOLOGIC CHANGES IN 24 CASES OF GROUP B RENAL FAILURE EPISODES

	B II	B I$^+$III	CREATININE U/P < 10	URINARY NA ≥30 mEq/L	IRREVERSIBLE COURSE	AVERAGE LENGTH (DAYS)	WELL-MATCHED RECIPIENTS
Severe vascular changes (12)	9	3	22.2%	18.2%	66.7%	…	6
Acute tubular necrosis (3)	2	1	…	100%	33.3%	15.5	1
Interstitial edema and cellular infiltration (2)	1	1	…	0	0	9.5	1
No changes (5)	5	0	…	—	0	9.2	4
Miscellaneous	1	1	…	—	100%	—	1

$p < .001$) in group B I + III patients, but not in group B II patients (see Fig. 11–1).

PATHOLOGY. — The pathologic data of group B recipients are summarized in Table 11–10. Contrary to group A data, the creatinine U/P ratio was higher than 10 and the urinary sodium concentration was less than 30 mEq/L in many group B patients with severe vascular lesions of the transplant. On the other hand, recovery was observed in four Group B II patients despite the presence of vascular lesions. In three of them the graft was well matched with the recipient, whereas 62.5% of irreversible renal failures supervened in mismatched donor-recipient combinations.

RADIOLOGY. — Thirty-four arteriograms were available (Table 11–11) and the following changes were seen: (1) an acute vascular syndrome in five cases, in full agreement with pathologic data — the outcome was always unfavorable; (2) the "Hollemberg syndrome" in ten cases — the mean duration of renal failure was 9.2 days; (3) low renal blood flow syndrome in five cases — the average length of renal failure was 16 days; (4) normal arteriograms in nine cases — the average length of renal failure was 9.5 days; and (5) five cases were unclassifiable.

COURSE. — According to our plan of stratification, seven patients were classified as having irreversible renal failure. In four cases, severe vascular damage in the transplanted kidneys necessitated their removal. The remaining three patients died of extrarenal causes. Since their kidneys showed only tubulointerstitial lesions, the renal failure might have been reversible had they not died. In 84 patients a favorable course was observed, and renal function started to improve in less than six days in 58.3% of patients. Recovery took more than ten days in only

TABLE 11–11. — RENAL ARTERIOGRAMS IN 34 EPISODES
OF DELAYED RENAL FAILURE (GROUP B)

	B II	B I+III	CREATININE U/P < 10	URINARY Na ≥30 mEq/L
Vascular changes	3	2	40%	40%
Hollemberg syndrome	3	7	33% (9)*	66 % (9)*
Low renal blood flow	4	1	25% (4)*	60%
No changes	1	8	0 (7)*	22.2%
Nondescript	—	—	—	—

*Number of patients with available urinary samples.

17.8% of cases. Courses were similar in patients from both groups B I + III and B II.

When considering only those group B I + III patients having a reversible course and in whom no known factors contributing to renal failure were present, there was a shorter course (3.15 days) when the urinary sodium level was less than 30 mEq/L (10 patients) than when the urinary sodium level was equal to or greater than 30 mEq/L (20 patients = 8.9 days), ($p < .01$).

Group C

Fifty-two patients with a previous history of either IRF (21 cases) or delayed renal failure (31 cases) had second (52 cases) or even third (7 cases) episodes of renal failure. In this group, nine patients died, but only six had severe injury of the transplant vessels.

The number of episodes of renal failure was not related to the long-term outcome of the graft, as a 65.4% success rate was observed in the 52 group C patients as compared with 63.3% in 120 patients with no or only one episode.

No conclusions could be drawn from the 17 renal biopsies and 17 arteriograms available, due to the wide disparity between episodes of renal failure in this group.

Irreversible Renal Failure

In 24 of 215 cases (11.2%) the renal failure was irreversible and led to transplant removal. In five cases, this was associated with the recipient's death, although there was only a mild decrease in renal function. In four cases, the transplant had to be removed as the consequence of a urinary tract fistula (three cases) or torsion of the renal artery (one case). In the remaining 15 patients irreversible renal failure was associated with severe renal parenchymatous damage. This was the case in six of 52 group C patients (11.5%), five of 65 group A patients (7.7%) and four of 91 group B patients (4.4%), (not significant).

Discussion

More than 90% of all kidneys transplanted by our group have a cadaver origin. Our study was therefore restricted to cadaver kidney transplantation.

It is common practice to consider most renal failure episodes occurring after kidney transplantation to be rejection phenomena, although many of them are not the consequence of an immunologic process. In fact, they can be related to various causes,[13] and are encountered more frequently in cadaver kidney transplantation than in transplantation of a kidney from a living related donor. Among these nonimmunologic factors, some are the consequence of immunosuppressive therapy, especially corticosteroids; others are the consequence of surgical mishaps during harvesting or transplantation; and still others can arise from a prolonged agonal phase or faulty preservation methods.

Posttransplant renal failure episodes are frequent. Ninety percent of our patients had at least one and nearly one third of the recipients had two or more episodes. It has not been possible, due to the lack of reliable immunologic criteria, to accurately diagnose a rejection episode. It is, therefore, easy to understand how contradictory the results of correlation may be between follow-up immunologic tests and clinical episodes. For these reasons, and because of the important therapeutic implications, a reappraisal of early posttransplant renal failure was necessary.

First, we differentiated the renal failure episodes by their date of onset after transplantation. It is known that renal failure that occurs immediately prior to transplant function is most probably of nonimmunologic origin. The term *"hyperacute rejection"* has been used to describe irreversible renal failure occurring immediately after revascularization of the graft.[19] This rejection might be due to anti-HL-A cytotoxic antibodies in the recipient that are directed against the donor and, thus, are injurious to the vascular endothelium.[1, 18] Such an interpretation is weakened, however, when the donor-recipient crossmatch is negative, as is the general rule.

There were only five episodes in our study of this type of hyperacute rejection. Pathologic examination showed severe vascular lesions in all five cases. Three of the four arteriograms performed during these episodes revealed a typical appearance of vascular rejection. It is impossible to be certain, however, that these so-called hyperacute rejection episodes were actually responsible for the inception of renal failure. In fact, they could have occurred secondarily in patients who already had acute tubular necrosis. This hypothesis is supported by creatinine U/P ratios and urinary sodium concentrations in the first 24 hours following transplantation when the patient was not totally anuric. In our five patients, the creatinine U/P ratios were less than 10 and the urinary sodium concentrations were greater than 30 mEq/L, which is characteristic of acute tubular necrosis. Otherwise, it would be hard to understand how a rejection phenomenon could occur so quickly in immunodepressed patients who have not as yet developed antibodies against the donor. There is the possibility that routinely used crossmatch techniques are not sensitive enough to detect low titers of antibodies or even presensitization that is no longer detectable in the serum. An argument in favor of this hypothesis is that in our patients the percentage of recipients with circulating antibodies directed against the panel was significantly higher in those subjects who had had hyperacute rejection episodes.

Delayed hyperacute rejection or acute irreversible rejection has already been described as irreversible renal failure that occurs after the transplanted kidney has functioned for several days.[13] The frequency of these delayed irreversible renal failure episodes was the same as that of the immediate irreversible episodes. Three occurred before the 10th day after transplantion, and the fourth was observed on the 22d day. The fact that steroids had not been given previously did not seem to affect the frequency of these episodes. In each case the transplanted kidney was the site of severe vascular lesions (Class I), which resulted in necrosis of the graft. The arteriograms of three patients made diagnosis possible by showing characteristic aspects of vascular rejection.

It is less surprising to have these episodes occur ten days after transplantation than immediately. These episodes are often correlated with the appearance in recipient serum of cytotoxic HL-A antibodies specifically directed against the donor, which were not present prior to transplantation.[3] In most cases, although the pathologic and radiologic alterations were identical with those seen in cases of immediate hyperacute rejection, the creatinine U/P ratio was greater than 10 and the urinary sodium concentration was less than 30 mEq/L. Thus, we think that irreversible renal failure episodes are almost always the result of severe vascular lesions, of which the clinical or biologic manifestations are delayed. Diagnosis of these episodes is particularly difficult when the patient already has acute tubular necrosis.

More than one third of the patients studied had *reversible renal failure immediately after the transplantation*. It is tempting to relate this phenomenon to the total ischemia time of the graft. But the frequency was much lower in the patients of group A I + II who had received kidneys with a much longer ischemia time than in the group A III patients. We have demonstrated elsewhere that total ischemia time had no influence on the recovery of graft function as long as it was less than 30 hours.[11] Furosemide given to the recipient during surgery was probably responsible for a significant decrease in the frequency of immediate renal failure in patients in groups A I and II.

It should be observed that the cause of renal failure could not be explained in more than 50% of our cases, and in the other 50% it was not always possible to assume that the findings were not in fact the consequence of a rejection. Such could be the case for rupture of the kidney or necrosis of the ureter secondary to rejection.

No differences, however, were found between clinical or biologic manifestations of explicable or inexplicable immediate renal failure episodes, whether or not patients were receiving steroids and/or furosemide. Fever was the only factor that was significantly more frequent in group A I and III patients than in group A II patients who had received high doses of steroids. The high urinary sodium concentration and the low creatinine U/P ratio found in patients with immediate renal failure indicated acute tubular necrosis. All these signs were more clear-cut in group A III patients, in whom anuria and hypertension were more frequent. All immediate renal failure episodes should therefore be regarded as the consequence of injury to the kidney that may induce posttransplantation acute tubular necrosis.

Furosemide has an unquestionable influence, not only in preventing the occurrence of immediate renal failure episodes but also in shortening their course. Steroids, on the other hand, did not influence the duration of these immediate renal failure episodes. The presence of a possible immunologic mechanism is therefore debatable. Biopsies of the transplanted kidney at this stage would have been useful. Unfortunately, sections of only three kidneys were available in our study: lesions of acute tubular necrosis were observed in one, vascular changes similar to those usually described in cases of hyperacute rejection were seen in another and the last was normal.[2]

The delayed acute renal failure episodes are usually considered as secondary to an acute rejection phenomenon. In fact, this is a misuse of the word "rejection," since in approximately half of our cases of group B renal failures, it was possible to demonstrate either a renal lesion secondary to surgery (such as urinary tract fistula, rupture or infarcts of the transplant) or a nonrenal complication (such as infection) that is possibly responsible for the renal failure. It is noteworthy that cases in which such complications were found were more frequent in patients treated with steroids.

The overall frequency of delayed reversible renal failures is much higher in patients having cadaver rather than related living kidney transplantation.[4] However, this is not proof of immunologic origin since nonimmunologic complications are also much more frequent in cadaver kidney transplantation. It is tempting to think that the institution of high doses of steroids immediately after surgery would have prevented most of those delayed renal failure episodes. As a matter of fact, as early as 1963, Dormont[6] and Goodwin et al.[7] showed the efficacy of prednisone treatment in reversing the kind of episode that has been called "transplant crises" since 1959. Despite this, delayed renal failure episodes were still observed in pretreated patients (group B II), and their frequency was only slightly less than that in non-pretreated patients (group B I+III). But if renal failure secondary to infectious complications (18%) and directly related to corticosteroids is excluded from group B II, the frequency of the remaining renal failure episodes becomes significantly lower than that observed in group B I + III patients ($p < .005$).

The occurrence of renal failure in patients receiving high doses of steroids could be attributed to two factors. (1) The percentage of nontransfused patients was higher in this group. The influence of pretransplantation blood transfusions on the outcome of the graft is well known today,[15, 16] but the similarity in the course of delayed renal failure in the two groups makes this explanation unlikely. (2) The mean total ischemia time undergone by the graft was greater for group B II patients than for the nontreated patients. However, it is difficult to understand how the duration of the storage period could be responsible for late renal failure episodes, since it has been shown that it had no influence on the occurrence of immediate renal failures.

Finally, even when renal failure possibly related to complication is excluded in both groups, we are still faced with a large number of episodes of renal failure for which an immunologic origin cannot be easily proved. In patients receiving steroids from the first day following transplantation, the frequency of this kind of renal failure is lower (45%) than that observed in nontreated patients (63%). Such a difference can probably be explained by the presence of two different types of renal failure. One type would be sensitive to steroids and is consequently not found in pretreated patients; it agrees with the classical description of transplant crisis. The other type would be independent of steroid treatment. Although the latter type has been considered probable for many years, it has never been proven.

Significant differences between the clinical and biologic data are in favor of this hypothesis. In nontreated patients (group B), renal failure episodes almost always occur within the first five days, whereas they are observed only after the fifth posttransplantation day in treated recipients. More important is the fact, demonstrated by Figure 11−1, that two different types of biologic data are found in nontreated patients: (1) a high creatinine U/P ratio with a low urinary sodium concentration, and (2) a low creatinine U/P ratio with a high urinary sodium concentration. The latter type is also observed in patients with immediate renal failure but not in those with delayed renal failure occurring in pretreated patients. We therefore feel that there are two varieties of delayed renal failure. One, with a high urinary sodium output, can respond to steroids and will be prevented by the institution of high doses of steroids immediately after transplantation. The other, with a low urinary sodium output, does not respond to steroids, occurs a few days later and has a spontaneously favorable course.

Sensitivity to steroids cannot be considered an argument in favor of an immunologic origin of a renal failure episode. Although interstitial edema and cellular infiltration of the transplant, considered characteristic of transplant crisis, are not always the result of an immunologic episode,[12] they could easily be responsible for renal failure that responds to anti-inflammatory drugs such as steroids.[13] On the other hand, hyperacute rejection of the vascular type, related to the presence in the recipient of specific antidonor cytotoxic antibodies, is never influenced by steroids, even when very high doses are used. Finally, the biologic aspect of steroid-independent delayed renal failure is similar to that described in patients with ischemic kidneys. On the contrary, in patients with steroid-sensitive delayed renal failure, as well as in those with immediate renal failure, the biologic features are similar to what is usually observed in cases of acute tubular necrosis.

The general characteristics as well as the frequency of renal failure episodes supervening in a transplant recipient are closely related to the type of treatment used. Thus, it would be excessive and maybe even dangerous to consider all posttransplantation renal failure episodes as rejections, because this misconception could result in inappropriate therapy in some cases that could have a spontaneously favorable outcome.

Summary and Conclusion

A total of 215 episodes of renal failure occurring within the first month following a cadaver kidney transplantation were analyzed in 172 patients.

Only 16 patients had no episodes of renal failure. Among them, the percentage of women as well as the percentage of patients with previous pregnancies were significantly higher than those in the 156 patients who developed renal failure.

First-month posttransplant renal failure episodes, as observed in 156 patients, were of various types according to their clinical and biologic aspects.

IRREVERSIBLE RENAL FAILURE. — Irreversible renal failure due to severe vascular lesions of the graft did not occur immediately after transplantation, were distinguishable by a low urinary sodium concentration, preceded by acute tubular necrosis that modified the biologic data, and were completely unresponsive to treatment.

IMMEDIATE OR DELAYED REVERSIBLE RENAL FAILURES. — *Immediate renal failures.* — In most cases (80%) they originated from acute tubular necrosis, with a high urinary sodium output. A specific cause was found in nearly half of the cases. This type of renal failure was prevented, and its course shortened, by systematic preoperative use of furosemide.

Delayed renal failures. — They were sometimes related to a specific but not always obvious cause, but most of the time they were idiopathic. Two varieties of idiopathic renal failure were distinguished. (1) A steroid-sensitive type, occurring within the first five days following transplantation. A low creatinine U/P ratio associated with a high urinary sodium concentration was a salient feature. This type was prevented by the institution of high doses of steroids immediately after transplantation. (2) A steroid-nonresponsive type, occurring during the second week following transplantation and having a spontaneously reversible course. The creatinine U/P ratio was high and the sodium urinary concentration low.

The pathologic changes, the time of occurrence and the sensitivity to steroids cannot be considered as valid arguments for an immunologic mechanism of these renal failure episodes. Therefore, the systematic use of the terms "hyperacute rejection," "delayed hyperacute rejection" or "acute rejection" to describe a renal failure episode occurring after transplantation should be avoided in order to prevent unnecessary treatment of a case that could reverse spontaneously.

References

1. Boehmig, H. J., Giles, G. R., Amemiya, H., Wilson, C. B., Coburg, A. J., Genton, E., Bunch, D. L., Dixon, F. J., and Starzl, T. E.: Hyperacute rejection of renal homografts: with particular reference to coagulation changes, humoral antibodies and formed blood elements, Transplant. Proc. 3:1105, 1971.
2. Busch, G. J., Reynolds, E. S., Galvanek, E. G., Braun, W. E., and Dammin, G. J.: Human renal allografts. The role of vascular injury in early graft failure, Medicine 50:29, 1971.
3. Descamps, B., Gagnon, R., Barbanel, C., Debray-Sachs, M., and Crosnier, J.: Complement dependent and lymphocyte dependent antibodies in human allograft recipients, Transplant. Proc. 7:1, 1975.
4. Descamps, B., Hinglais, N., and Crosnier, J.: Renal transplantation between 33 HLA identical siblings, Transplant. Proc. 5:231, 1973.
5. Descamps, B., and Kreis, H.: Recipient presensitization: a critical survey, in Hamburger, J., Crosnier, J., and Maxwell, M. H. (eds.): *Advances in Nephrology* (Chicago: Year Book Medical Publishers, Inc., 1975), Vol. 6, pp. 443–461.
6. Dormont, J.: Perspectives actuelles de la transplantation rénale chez l'homme, *Actual. Nephrol. Hôpital Necker* (Paris: Flammarion, 1963), pp. 267–92.
7. Goodwin, W. E., Kaufman, J. J., Mins, M. M., Turner, R. D., Glassock, R., Goldman, R., and Maxwell, M. H.: Human renal transplantation: clinical experiences with 6 cases of renal homotransplantation, J. Urol. 89:13, 1963.
8. Hamburger, J., Vaysse, J., Crosnier, J., Tubiana, M., Lalanne, M., Antoine, B., Auvert, J., Soulier, J. P., Dormont, J., Salmon, J., Maisonnet, C., and Amiel, J. L.: Transplantation d'un rein entre jumeaux non-monozygotes après irradiation du receveur. Bon fonctionnement au 4ème mois, Nouv. Presse Med. 67:1771, 1959.
9. Hollemberg, N. K., Adams, D. F., Merrill, J. P., and Abrams, H. L.: Renal angiography in oliguria, in Abrams, H. L. (ed.): *Angiography* (New York; Little, Brown and Co., 1971), vol. 2, p. 887.
10. Hors, J., Feingold, N., Fradelizi, D., and Dausset, J.: Critical evaluation of histocompatibility in 179 renal transplants, Lancet 1:609, 1971.
11. Kreis, H., Noel, L. H., Moreau, J. F., Barbanel, C., and Crosnier, J.: Biologic, pathologic and radiologic studies of cadaver kidneys preserved in Collins' solution, Transplant. Proc. 9:1611, 1977.

12. Lund, B.: *Renal Transplantation in Rabbits* (Copenhagen: Munksgaard, 1973), p. 748.
13. Maher, J. F.: A logical approach to the diagnosis of renal transplant rejection. Immunologic, ischemia and inflammatory impairment of renal function, Am. J. Med. 56: 275, 1974.
14. Moreau, J. F., Kleinknecht, D., Grunfeld, J. P., Reboul, F., Sabto, J., and Michel, J. R.: Arteriographic patterns of renal cortical necrosis, J. Radiol. Electrol. Med. Nucl. 55:1, 1974.
15. Opelz, G., Sengar, D. P. S., Mickey, M. R., and Terasaki, P. I.: Effect of blood transfusions on subsequent kidney transplants, Transplant. Proc. 5:253, 1973.
16. Persijn, G. G., Van Hooff, J. P., Kalff, M. W., et al.: Effect of blood transfusions and HLA matching on renal transplantation in the Netherlands, Transplant. Proc. 9: 503, 1977.
17. Stiller, C. R., Sinclair, N. R., Abrahams, S., McGirr, D., Harinderjit, S., Howson, W. T., and Ulan, R. A.: Anti-donor immune responses in prediction of transplant rejection, N. Engl. J. Med. 294:978, 1976.
18. Terasaki, P. I., Kreisler, M., and Mickey, R. M.: Presensitization and kidney transplant failures, Postgrad. Med. J. 47:89, 1971.
19. Williams, G. M.: Clinical aspects of allograft rejection, Transplant. Proc. 6:71, 1974.

12

Amino Acid Metabolism in Patients with Advanced Uremia and in Patients Undergoing Chronic Dialysis

JOEL D. KOPPLE, M.D., AND
MICHAEL R. JONES, PH.D.

Medical and Research Services, Veterans Administration, Wadsworth Medical Center and Schools of Medicine and Public Health, UCLA, Los Angeles, California

The metabolism of several amino acids is abnormal in patients with renal failure. Although the clinical significance of these alterations is uncertain, they may contribute to uremic toxicity, the high prevalance of malnutrition and wasting[79] and the disability and feeling of unwellness that are common in even well-dialyzed patients. This chapter reviews current knowledge of abnormal amino acid metabolism in patients with uremia and the relationship of these alterations to the accumulation of metabolic products, malnutrition and wasting and the uremic syndrome in general.

Plasma and Muscle Amino Acid Concentrations

PLASMA AMINO ACIDS

The most obvious evidence for altered amino acid metabolism in patients with uremia are the changes in fasting plasma lev-

233

0084-5957/79/080233-36$3.75

TABLE 12-1.—ALTERED PLASMA AMINO ACID CONCENTRATIONS
IN CHRONIC RENAL FAILURE

ESSENTIAL	CONCENTRATION	NONESSENTIAL	CONCENTRATION
Histidine	Normal-low	Alanine	Normal-low-high
Isoleucine	Normal-low	Arginine	Normal
Leucine	Normal-low	Aspartic acid	Normal-high
Lysine	Normal-low	Glutamic acid	Normal-high
Methionine	Normal	Asparagine	Normal-low
Phenylalanine	Normal	Glutamine	Normal
Tryptophan	Low	Glycine	Normal-high
Valine	Low	Proline	Normal-high
Total essential	Low	Serine	Normal-low
Cystine*	High	Ornithine	Normal-high
Tyrosine*	Low	*Total nonessential*	Normal
RATIOS		Citrulline	High
Essential-nonessential	Low	1-Methylhistidine	High
Valine-glycine	Low	3-Methylhistidine	High
Serine-glycine	Low	Hydroxyproline	Normal-high
Tyrosine-phenylalanine	Low	Taurine	Normal-high

*Semi-essential amino acids.

els. Table 12-1 lists typical alterations in the amino acid pattern in uremic patients. It is noteworthy that there are many discrepancies in reports of plasma amino acid levels in cases of uremia. These differences are probably due to variations in techniques of specimen preparation and analysis, in the clinical condition and particularly in the nutritional status of the patients. The pattern in plasma is not markedly affected by maintenance hemodialysis unless the nutritional status of the patient changes. Indeed, in nonuremic patients, protein intake and malnutrition have a major effect on plasma amino acid levels.[124, 141]

Kopple and Swendseid evaluated the effects of protein intake on plasma amino acid levels in cases of renal failure.[81] A series of 53 studies were conducted in 11 normal subjects and 18 chronically uremic patients ingesting 20-, 40- or 60-gm protein diets, and in seven patients undergoing maintenance hemodialysis with varying protein intakes. Energy intake was high and diets were rigidly controlled. In 79% of the studies, subjects lived in a metabolic research ward for 25 ± 12 (SD) days.

These studies suggested the following conclusions: Certain plasma amino acids are altered primarily by renal failure.

These include elevated levels of citrulline, cystine, and 1- and 3-methylhistidine* and low concentrations of tryptophan and ratios of tyrosine-phenylalanine and serine-glycine. Low protein intakes cause other alterations in plasma amino acid levels. These include low levels of histidine, isoleucine, leucine and lysine, decreased ratios of essential-nonessential amino acids and high levels of glycine. Both uremia and low protein intake contribute to decreased valine and tyrosine levels and to the low valine-glycine ratio. In uremic patients severe malnutrition will lead to altered plasma concentrations of many other amino acids. Indeed, the plasma amino acid pattern in chronically uremic patients who are ingesting low-protein diets or who are malnourished is similar in many respects to the pattern in nonuremic subjects eating decreased quantities of protein or suffering from protein-calorie malnutrition.[124, 141] For certain amino acids there was a direct or inverse correlation between protein intake and plasma levels, and this relationship often differed in chronically uremic or hemodialysis patients as compared with normal subjects. Hence, the response to protein restriction is also abnormal in uremic patients.

MUSCLE AMINO ACIDS

Much less is known about intracellular amino acid levels in uremia and their response to nutritional factors. Muscle contains the largest pool of free amino acids and hence is of particular interest for understanding amino acid metabolism. Bergström *et al.* measured intracellular concentrations of amino acids in muscle tissue of chronically uremic patients and patients undergoing regular peritoneal dialysis.[14] They found in both groups of patients low concentrations of threonine, valine, tyrosine and carnosine, and increased levels of 1- and 3-methylhistidine. In addition, the nondialyzed patients had low levels of intracellular lysine and histidine, and increased amounts of phenylalanine and aspartic acid. The dialysis patients also manifested increased concentrations of lysine, isoleucine and leucine, as well as the nonessential amino acids, glutamine, glutamic

---

*The IUPAC-IUB Commission on Biochemical Nomenclature has recommended the use of N^τ-methylhistidine in lieu of 3-methylhistidine and N^π-methylhistidine for 1-methylhistidine.[61] Since the older terms are more commonly recognized by nephrologists, they will continue to be used in this chapter.

acid, alanine, citrulline, ornithine, arginine and taurine. Normally, intracellular concentrations of many amino acids are maintained against a gradient, and Bergström and co-workers found that the intracellular-extracellular ratio was increased for asparagine and leucine in chronically uremic patients. In the peritoneal dialysis patients, the ratio was increased for several amino acids. The authors point out that the amino acid values in their patients may have been affected by malnutrition, particularly in those undergoing peritoneal dialysis. Serum albumin levels in these latter patients were low, and they were prescribed only 60 gm protein per day.

Altered Metabolism of Specific Amino Acids

The foregoing comments concerning plasma and muscle amino acid concentrations are descriptive; unfortunately the causes of disordered amino acid metabolism in patients with renal failure are usually not well defined. It is perhaps fortunate that abnormal plasma amino acid concentrations in chronically uremic rats and dogs resemble those in humans with renal failure.[40, 138] These animals have served as experimental models for investigating amino acid metabolism.

PHENYLALANINE AND TYROSINE

Plasma tyrosine levels are usually low, and the concentrations of phenylalanine, the precursor of tyrosine, are normal in uremic patients.[66, 71, 83] In our experience, chronically uremic and hemodialysis patients ingesting very low-protein diets (e.g., 20 – 26 gm/day) have the lowest tyrosine levels.[83] Most striking is the low ratio of tyrosine-phenylalanine in the plasma and muscle of chronically uremic dialysis patients.[14, 66, 83, 98] The tyrosine-phenylalanine ratio is directly correlated with the glomerular filtration rate in normal, chronically uremic and dialysis patients and in the latter two groups alone.[83] In patients with chronic uremia, it is the conversion of phenylalanine to tyrosine that is impaired,[66, 85, 98] and the rate of degradation of tyrosine appears normal.[83]

Wang *et al.* assayed the in vitro activities of the enzymes phenylalanine hydroxylase, which catalyzes the hydroxylation of phenylalanine to tyrosine, and tyrosine aminotransferase, the enzyme catalyzing the first step along the major catabolic pathway for tyrosine.[139] They found that activities of these enzymes in liver homogenates were normal in chronically uremic rats as compared with pair-fed controls. Phenylalanine hydroxylase activity in the kidneys of uremic rats was reduced. However, the activity of this enzyme in the kidney is small and probably insignificant relative to that in the liver.[7, 93] Young and Parsons report that sera from uremic patients inhibited hepatic phenylalanine hydroxylase activity in normal rats by an average of 15%.[149] Whether this effect is sufficient to account for the impaired conversion of phenylalanine to tyrosine is uncertain.

It has been suggested that impaired conversion of phenylalanine to tyrosine in uremic patients might lead to a metabolic shunt, with increased synthesis of potentially toxic metabolites of phenylalanine, such as occurs in phenylketonuria. Jones, Kopple and Swendseid measured 13 acidic metabolites of phenylalanine and tyrosine in normal subjects, chronically uremic patients and patients undergoing maintenance hemodialysis.[66] Studies were conducted during fasting and after an oral phenylalanine load, 100 mg/kg body weight. In the normal subjects and dialysis patients, L-[^{14}C(U)]-phenylalanine was given with the load. During fasting, the levels of plasma phenyllactic acid, p-hydroxyphenylacetic acid and p-hydroxybenzoic acid were elevated, the last compound markedly so, in both uremic and dialysis patients. Plasma phenylpyruvic and mandelic acid were detected only in dialysis patients (Fig. 12–1). After the load, in both the uremic and dialysis patients, the level of plasma phenylalanine rose higher and fell more gradually and the amount of tyrosine rose more slowly. These results are consistent with the findings of Pickford, McGale and Aber.[98] Quantitatively, the major change in plasma phenylalanine and tyrosine metabolites after the load was the increase in the level of conjugated phenylacetic acid in some uremic subjects and dialysis patients (Fig. 12–1). Urinary excretion of phenylacetic acid was decreased in chronically uremic patients compared with normal subjects. In the dialysis patients, levels of urinary benzoic acid and conjugated p-hydroxybenzoic acid were decreased and phenylpyruvic acid was sometimes increased. Expiration of $^{14}CO_2$ during the 24-hour period after the load was decreased in the dialysis patients.

These findings suggest that the hydroxylation of phenylalanine to form tyrosine is only mildly impaired in uremic patients

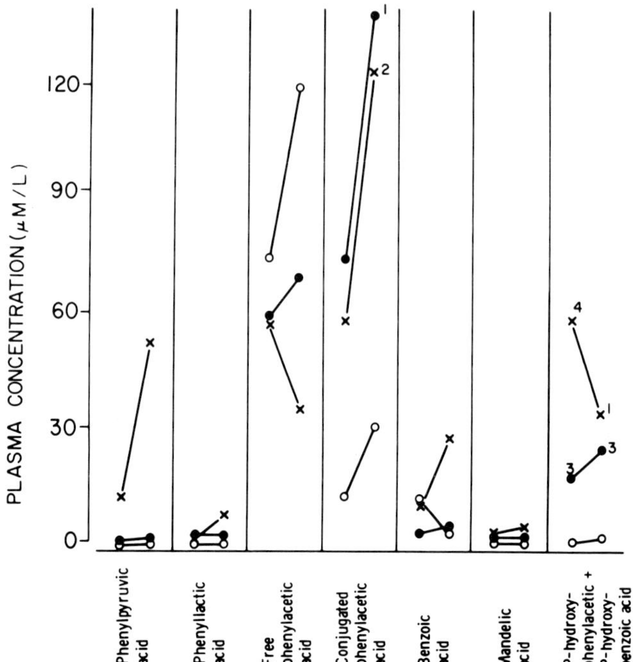

Fig. 12–1.—Plasma concentrations of metabolites of phenylalanine and tyrosine in the fasting state and the maximum values or minimum levels (if plasma concentrations fell) attained two to four hours after ingestion of an oral phenylalanine load, 100 mg/kg. Open circles indicate normal subjects; closed circles, nondialyzed chronically uremic patients; and crossed lines, patients undergoing maintenance hemodialysis. *1*—differs from fasting levels in the same subjects, $p < 0.05$. *2*—differs from values in normal subjects obtained after the load, $p < 0.05$. *3*—differs from values in normal subjects, $p < 0.05$. *4*—differs from values in chronically uremic patients, $p < 0.05$.

and does not result in marked increases in the levels of metabolites of phenylalanine in plasma. Since the amount of phenylpyruvic acid was increased in both plasma and urine of some dialysis patients, production of this compound was probably increased. In support of this finding, Giordano *et al.* reported increased levels of urinary phenylpyruvic acid in uremic patients both before and after a phenylalanine load.[49] Although these data and those of others indicate that the amount of plasma tyrosine is low and that some plasma metabolites of phenylalanine and tyrosine are increased in cases of renal failure,[71] it is not known whether these alterations have adverse clinical effects.[71]

TRYPTOPHAN

Plasma tryptophan levels are decreased in patients with uremia and do not normalize with hemodialysis. Tryptophan differs from other amino acids in plasma in that a substantial fraction is bound to protein.[34] In cases of renal failure, low tryptophan levels are due primarily to decreased binding to albumin, and unbound concentrations may actually be increased.[55] This decreased binding appears to be due to competition by other substances for binding sites on the albumin molecule.[34]

The clinical significance of altered tryptophan binding is unclear. Tryptophan has an important role in the induction of polysomal aggregation, an initial step in protein synthesis.[92] Also, tryptophan is converted in brain to serotonin (5-hydroxytryptamine) and then to 5-hydroxyindoleacetic acid. These reactions may be controlled by the tryptophan content in the brain.[69] Moreover, tryptophan transport into the brain is determined by the ratio of plasma total or free tryptophan to the five other amino acids that compete for the blood-brain transport system — valine, leucine, isoleucine, phenylalanine and tyrosine.[39, 69]

Recently, Siassi and co-workers investigated the relation between plasma tryptophan and brain serotonin metabolism in chronically uremic rats.[115] These animals also manifested low total and increased free tryptophan concentrations in plasma. The results indicated that with a diet relatively high in casein (18%), the ratio in plasma of total tryptophan to the five competing amino acids was decreased in the uremic rats, and this was associated with low levels of brain tryptophan and serotonin. With a lower (11%) casein diet, brain tryptophan and serotonin levels were normal and the amount of 5-hydroxyindoleacetic acid was increased in uremic rats, suggesting increased serotonin turnover. Moreover, in a separate study, Siassi and associates gave pargyline, a monoamine oxidase inhibitor, to chronically uremic and sham-operated pair-fed control rats to assess brain serotonin turnover.[114] They corroborated the increased turnover of this compound in the brains of the uremic rats.

In platelets of uremic patients, Tam and co-workers found that the level of serotonin is reduced and the activity of monoamine oxidase, which catabolizes serotonin, is increased.[125] Monoamine oxidase activity is also increased in plasma and heart, reduced in kidney and skeletal muscle and unchanged in liver and cerebrum of chronically uremic rats.[137] The clinical significance of these changes is unclear. Low serotonin content may contribute to abnormal platelet function in uremic subjects. Also, it is possible that altered brain serotonin metabolism might contribute to isomnia, hypothermia and impaired mentation in uremic patients.

BRANCHED-CHAIN AMINO ACIDS—
VALINE, LEUCINE, ISOLEUCINE

Valine levels are consistently low in plasma and are also decreased in muscle in cases of renal failure.[14, 65, 71] Leucine and isoleucine levels are frequently reduced in plasma.[71] However, Bergström *et al.* found muscle levels of leucine and isoleucine to be normal in chronically uremic patients and increased in subjects undergoing peritoneal dialysis.[14] These altered concentrations may be clinically important for the following reasons: (1) The branched-chain amino acids and their ketoacid analogues appear to have anabolic effects. In fasting obese subjects, the ketoacid analogues of the branched-chain amino acids reduce urea excretion and improve nitrogen balance.[108] These effects persist beyond the infusion of these compounds. Also, in in vitro studies, leucine enhances protein synthesis in the rat diaphragm.[42] These observations have been interpreted as indicating a specific pharmacologic stimulation of protein synthesis by one or more branched-chain amino acids or ketoacids. However, Waterlow, Garlick and Millward suggested that the concentrations of branched-chain amino acids may be limiting for protein synthesis, and supplemental doses may promote anabolism simply by making them more available.[140] (2) The branched-chain amino acids are all essential. (3) Unlike other amino acids, they are degraded primarily in muscle.[150] (4) Chronically uremic patients often suffer from muscle wasting,[72, 79] and this could be related to altered metabolism of the branched-chain amino acids.

In a series of metabolic diet studies in normal subjects described earlier, we observed that plasma valine levels correlated with protein intake.[81] However, in chronically uremic and hemodialysis patients, the amount of plasma valine was low and did not vary with dietary protein unless patients were clearly malnourished. Hence, it appears that factors in addition to dietary intake affect plasma valine levels in uremic patients. Plasma leucine and isoleucine levels were slightly but not significantly less than normal in our uremic and dialysis patients.

We conducted kinetic studies of valine metabolism in five normal subjects, three chronically uremic patients and eight patients undergoing maintenance hemodialysis.[65] After an overnight fast, patients received an intravenous injection of L-valine labeled with ^{14}C in the carboxyl carbon, and the fall in plasma specific activity and the expiration of $^{14}CO_2$ were monitored for 120 minutes. The chronically uremic patients were ingesting 53 ± 13 gm protein per day and normal subjects were fed 40 ± 1 gm protein diets. Many of the subjects were fed these diets in a metabolic research unit for a mean of 16 ± 8 days.

From the data, two rapidly exchangeable pools were identified; a smaller pool roughly corresponding to plasma free valine and a larger pool containing intracellular and probably most of the extracellular free valine (Fig. 12–2). The amounts in both valine pools were decreased in the chronically uremic patients and normal in the subjects undergoing maintenance hemodialysis. Fractional and absolute rates of valine oxidation, calculated from the $^{14}CO_2$ expiration and pool sizes, were decreased in the chronically uremic patients and normal in the dialysis patients. These observations were puzzling because we had hypothesized that the low valine pools were caused by an enhanced rate of oxidation. It is not likely that poor nutrition could account for

Fig. 12–2.—A two-pool kinetic model for valine metabolism in normal subjects and chronically uremic patients. Pool 1 represents primarily plasma free valine. Pool 2 includes intracellular free valine and probably most extracellular valine.

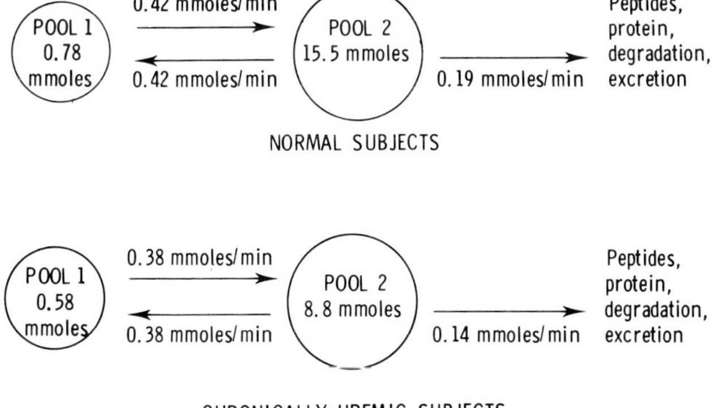

the low pools, since protein intake in the chronically uremic patients was at least as great as that in the normal subjects. Urinary valine excretion was not sufficient in the uremic patients to account for the low valine pools. The normal pool sizes and rates of oxidation in the dialysis patients may reflect improvement in uremic toxicity by hemodialysis or the fact that these patients, by coincidence, were particularly well-nourished and robust.

The possibility was considered that enhanced oxidation of valine led to decreased valine pools which, in turn, reduced the rate of oxidation. Three chronically uremic patients were therefore restudied after receiving their same diets supplemented with 1.25–1.5 gm L-valine per day in divided doses, which increased valine intake by 65%. Surprisingly, neither the two valine pools nor valine oxidation increased. Also, the level of urinary valine could not account for the failure of valine pool levels to rise. These kinetic studies were conducted during fasting conditions, and it is possible that valine oxidation is enhanced in cases of uremia only postprandially.

HISTIDINE

Interest in histidine metabolism was stimulated by observations that the level of plasma histidine is sometimes low in uremic patients,[49, 71] and by the findings of Bergström et al. that addition of histidine to histidine-free diets improved the nitrogen balance.[11] Giordano and co-workers found increased incorporation of ^{14}C-leucine into globin in the blood of two chronically uremic patients when histidine was added to histidine-free diets.[52]

Kopple and Swendseid evaluated the essentiality of histidine in both chronically uremic and normal men.[80] In these studies, three chronically uremic men and four normal men were fed, in chronological order, a 40-gm protein diet, a semisynthetic amino acid diet almost completely devoid of histidine (60 mg/day) and a histidine-repletion diet (1,200 mg/day) that was usually similar to the second diet. Diets were fed for approximately one month each and were essentially isocaloric and isonitrogenous, providing 39.3 ± 4.9 kcal/kg/body weight per day and 6.6 ± 0.2 gm nitrogen per day. With the 40-gm protein diet, nitrogen balance during equilibration was neutral or positive in all subjects (Fig. 12–3). After ingestion of the histidine-free diet,

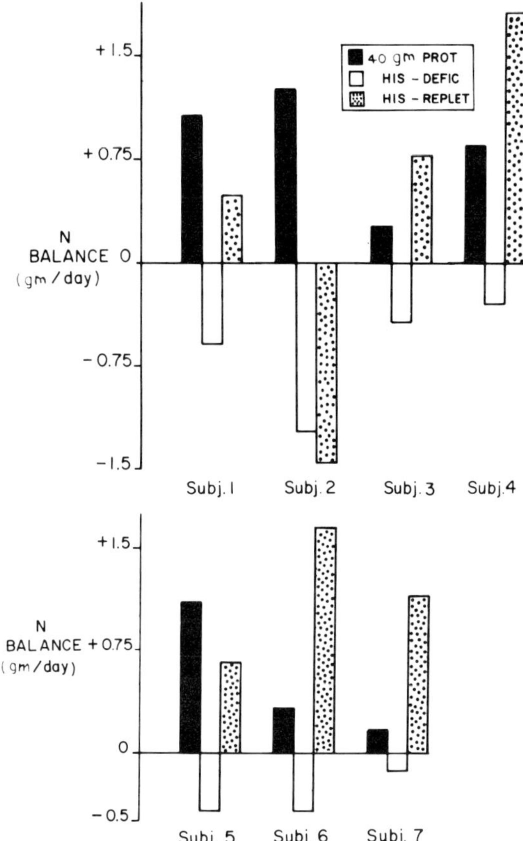

Fig. 12–3.—Nitrogen balance in four normal (subjects 1–4) and three chronically uremic subjects (subjects 5–7) after stabilization on 40-gm protein, histidine-deficient and histidine-repletion diets. Balances are adjusted for changes in body urea content but not for unmeasured losses. [From: *Defined Formula Diets for Medical Purposes* (Chicago: American Medical Assoc., 1977), p. 113. Used by permission.]

balance gradually became negative in each individual, and serum albumin levels decreased in six subjects. With administration of the histidine-repletion diet, balance became positive in all uremic patients and in three of the four normal subjects. Serum albumin amounts rose in five subjects and were unchanged in two after beginning this last diet.

Postabsorptive plasma histidine levels fell slightly but not significantly with the 40-gm protein diet (Fig. 12–4). However,

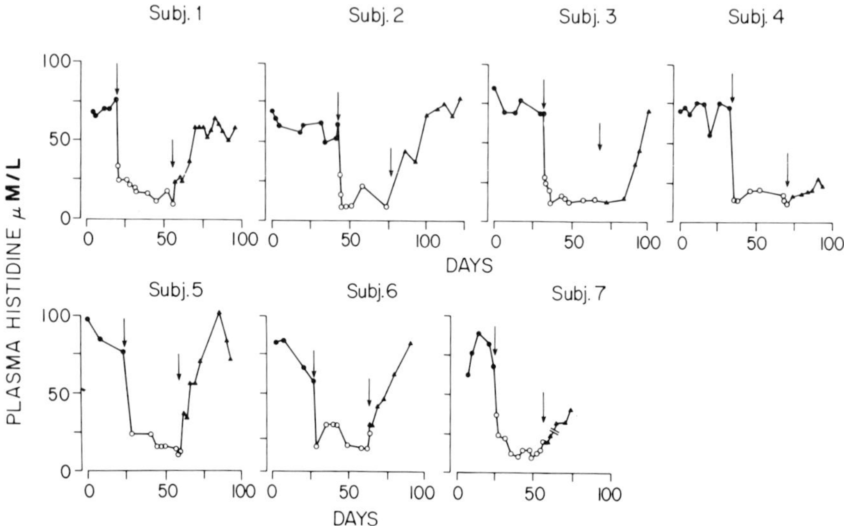

Fig. 12–4. – Plasma histidine levels in four normal men and three chronically uremic patients during ingestion of 40-gm protein *(closed circles)*, histidine-deficient *(open circles)*, and histidine-repletion *(closed triangles)* diets. For each subject, the first arrow indicates the time of onset of the histidine-deficient diet, and the second arrow, the beginning of the histidine-repletion diet. The break in the data in Subject 7 indicates a period of three days during which he did not participate in the study. (From Kopple, J. D., and Swendseid, M. E.: Evidence that histidine is an essential amino acid in normal and chronically uremic man, J. Clin. Invest. 55:881, 1975. Used by permission.)

within the first day after ingestion of the histidine-deficient diet, the plasma histidine level fell by more than 50%. Plasma histidine values continued to decrease, and by the end of the study with each diet, mean levels had fallen to $17 \pm 2\%$ of the concentrations present at the termination of the 40-gm protein diet. With the histidine-repletion diet, plasma levels rose in each subject.

Histidine concentrations in the gastrocnemius muscle, measured at the end of the study with each diet, are shown in Figure 12–5. Muscle histidine levels decreased markedly with the histidine-deficient diet to $38 \pm 19\%$ of the levels present with the 40-gm protein diet. With histidine repletion, muscle histidine increased to control levels.

Serial hematocrit readings, reticulocyte counts and serum iron levels during the course of study are shown in Figure 12–6. With the 40-gm protein diet, the hematocrit value fell slightly in both uremic and normal subjects, and this probably reflects

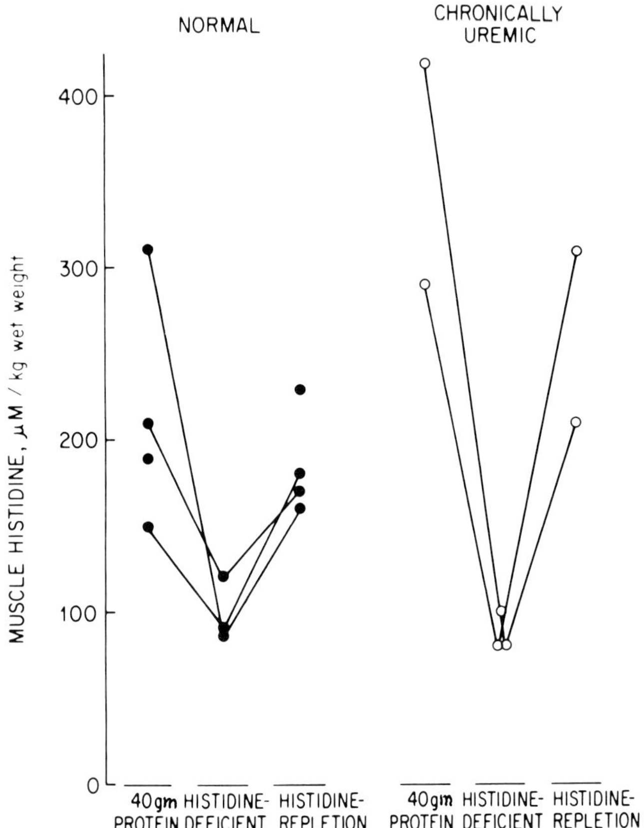

Fig. 12–5.—Histidine concentrations in the gastrocnemius muscles of four normal and three chronically uremic subjects after ingestion of 40-gm protein, histidine-deficient and histidine-repletion diets. Lines connect data from the same subject. [From: *Defined Formula Diets for Medical Purposes* (Chicago: American Medical Assoc., 1977), p. 113. Used by permission.]

the magnitude of blood drawing. During ingestion of the histidine-deficient diet, the hematocrit reading fell progressively. Coincidentally, the level of serum iron rose and the reticulocyte count remained low. With administration of the histidine-repletion diet, the serum iron level fell abruptly. This was followed by a rise in the reticulocyte count, and the hematocrit value then began to rise.

During ingestion of the histidine-depletion diet, a clinical syndrome gradually developed which was characterized by mal-

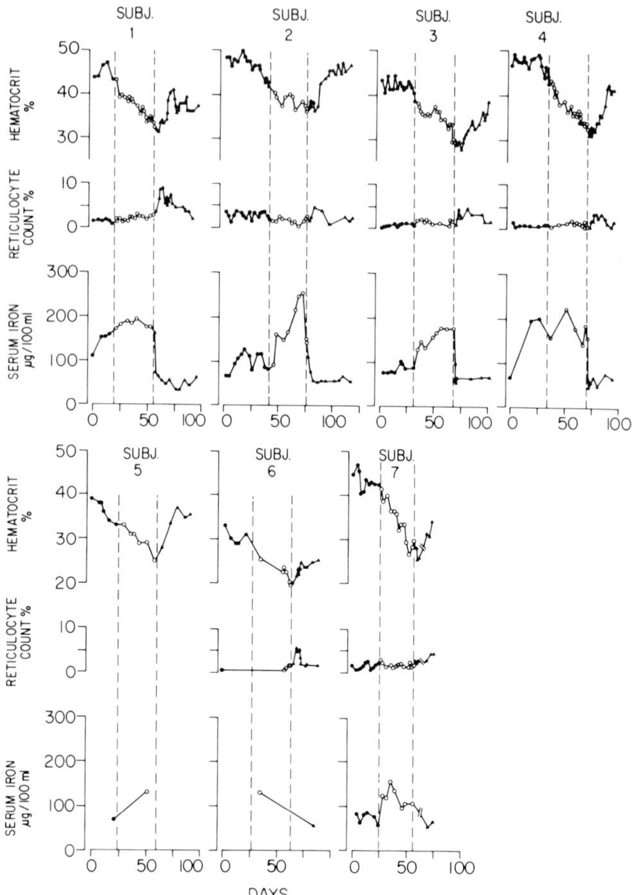

Fig. 12–6.—Serial hematocrit readings, reticulocyte counts and serum iron levels in four normal men and three chronically uremic patients during ingestion of 40-gm protein, histidine-deficient and histidine-repletion diets. For each case, the first and second broken vertical lines indicate the times of onset of the histidine-depletion and histidine-repletion diets, respectively. Other symbols are defined in the legend of Figure 12–4. (From Kopple, J. D., and Swendseid, M. E.: Evidence that histidine is an essential amino acid in normal and chronically uremic man, J. Clin. Invest. 55:881, 1975. Used by permission.)

aise, anorexia, nausea, agitation, memory loss, confusion and a skin eruption resembling asteatosis. With histidine repletion, the syndrome reversed over many days.

Thus, histidine appears to be an essential amino acid in both normal and chronically uremic men. The absence of dietary histidine leads to decreased erythropoiesis.

There is now other evidence for the essentiality of histidine in healthy adults. Anderson *et al.* found that nitrogen balance tended to be more positive and urea excretion decreased when histidine or histidine and arginine were added to isonitrogenous diets devoid of these amino acids.[2, 3] Cho, Krause and Anderson also found that fasting and postprandial plasma histidine concentrations fell and fasting serum urea levels rose when amino acid diets lacking in histidine or histidine and arginine were fed.[24] Similarly, we found in our three uremic patients that serum urea nitrogen levels rose with the histidine-depletion diet and fell during histidine repletion.[80] Wixom and co-workers found low plasma histidine levels in one subject receiving parenteral nutrition for 27 days with amino acid solutions devoid of histidine, although nitrogen balance was not negative.[146]

There is some evidence that histidine metabolism may be abnormal in uremic patients. Fürst gave ^{15}N-ammonium chloride or ^{15}N-urea to one normal subject, one catabolic patient and two uremic patients.[43] He found the ^{15}N-label in histidine from plasma or muscle protein in the normal subject and the catabolic patient but not in the uremic patients. The inference was that synthesis of imidazolepyruvic acid and/or transamination of this precursor to form histidine does not occur in uremic patients. However, Giordano and co-workers gave ^{15}N-urea and found the ^{15}N-label in histidine from plasma albumin of both normal and uremic subjects.[48] Interestingly, Sheng and co-workers fed ^{15}N-ammonium chloride to one normal man deprived of histidine.[111] They reported the ^{15}N-label in both the α-amino nitrogen and the imidazole ring from histidine and 3-methylhistidine isolated from globin or urine. These findings suggest that some histidine may be synthesized in normal humans at least during histidine deficiency. It is not clear whether such synthesis occurs in intestinal bacteria.

In patients with renal failure, loss of renal biochemical activity might also affect histidine metabolism. Histidine is reported to be released from the kidney in dogs, pregnant sheep and rats, although this has not been confirmed in all studies.[9, 40, 122] In dogs with uranyl nitrate-induced chronic renal failure, Fukuda and Kopple found that less histidine was released into renal venous plasma than in normal dogs.[41] The amount of peripheral venous histidine was also decreased in the uremic dogs. The finding that the kidney is a net contributor of histidine is puzzling in view of the evidence that histidine is essential. It is possible that histidine can be synthesized but in insufficient amounts for daily needs. Also, the kidney contains carnosinase,[84] and may release histidine by hydrolyzing carnosine (β-alanylhistidine). Indeed, Fukuda and Kopple infused carnosine into the renal artery of dogs and observed a marked increase in histidine concentrations in renal venous plasma.[41] The relevance of these findings to humans will not be clear until it is established whether or not histidine is released by the human kidney.

Schmid *et al.* also found evidence for altered histidine metabolism in chronically uremic rats.[110] These animals had normal plasma histidine, decreased muscle histidine, and increased brain levels of both histidine and its decarboxylation product, histamine, in comparison with sham-operated pair-fed controls.

In studies evaluating the dietary requirements for histidine and the metabolism of histidine using tracer ^{14}C-histidine, Kopple and co-workers observed no differences in the metabolism of histidine in normal and in chronically uremic patients.[74, 77, 82] In our experience, in normal and chronically uremic patients fed 20-, 40- or 60-gm protein diets, postabsorptive plasma histidine levels were similar at each level of protein intake.[81] We found a direct correlation between fasting morning plasma histidine levels and 24-hour urinary histidine excretion in normal and chronically uremic subjects.[76] But for each level of plasma histidine, the amount of urinary excretion was lower in the uremic patients. Whitehouse *et al.* report that urinary clearance of histidine is directly correlated with the inulin clearance.[143] However, the percent of tubular reabsorption of histidine falls, and thus fractional excretion rises as the glomerular filtration rate decreases.[143] Hence, the fall in histidine clearance is proportionally less than the decrease in inulin clearance. Other investigators also report increased fractional excretion of histidine in cases of advanced renal failure.[15, 54, 94]

There is controversy concerning the therapeutic benefits of supplemental histidine in uremic patients. Giordano and co-workers fed L-histidine monohydrochloride, usually 1 gm/day, to patients undergoing maintenance hemodialysis.[51] They reported a rise in the levels of plasma histidine and iron, serum transferrin, and in the hematocrit reading, and a fall in the reticulocyte count. However, Blumenkrantz and co-workers were unable to confirm these benefits in a double-blind controlled study in chronically uremic patients and patients undergoing maintenance dialysis prescribed L-histidine, 4 gm/day, or placebo.[17] There were no differences in hematologic parameters in the chronically uremic or dialysis patients fed histidine supplements as compared with those given the placebo. Other studies support these results.[67, 91, 101] These findings suggest that histidine may act analogously to folic acid or vitamin B_{12}. A deficiency causes failure in erythropoiesis. However, in subjects already receiving sufficient amounts, additional intake provides no benefits.

Histidine binds divalent cations, and in iron-depleted rats, oral histidine intake enhances gastrointestinal absorption of iron.[129] Jontofsohn *et al.* report that in chronically uremic patients fed supplements of iron, 300 mg/day, and L-histidine, 1.5 gm/day, hemoglobin, serum transferrin and serum histidine levels rose.[67] In similar patients receiving oral iron alone, the amount of hemoglobin rose more slowly and serum transferrin levels also increased. In patients administered histidine alone or given no therapy, there were no significant changes in hemoglobin and transferrin levels.

1- AND 3-METHYLHISTIDINE

Levels of plasma 1-methylhistidine and 3-methylhistidine are elevated in uremic patients.[14, 49, 71] Bergström *et al.* report elevated levels of these compounds intracellularly in muscle.[14] Normally 1- and 3-methylhistidine are excreted in the urine, and increased levels reflect impaired excretion. 3-Methylhistidine has elicited much interest because it is an indicator of muscle protein breakdown. It is present in actin and myosin of skeletal muscle and in actin of cardiac muscle.[4, 62, 126] Histidine is methylated in the 3-position only after it has been incorporated into protein.[32, 151] Once released from muscle protein, 3-methylhistidine is apparently not reutilized and is excreted in the urine.[86, 151] Whitehouse *et al.* report a direct relation between clearances of 3-methylhistidine and inulin and a hyperbolic relation between serum 3-methylhistidine and inulin clearance.[143] The tubular reabsorption of 3-methylhistidine was $48 \pm 12\%$ in patients with varying degrees of renal failure and did not vary with renal function. They suggest that serum 3-methylhistidine may be a sensitive indicator of renal failure.

Urinary excretion of 3-methylhistidine is decreased in clinically stable chronically uremic patients (Kopple and Swendseid, unpublished observations). We have observed this phenomenon even when comparisons were made between normal and uremic subjects ingesting amino acid diets containing no meat, which is a source of 3-methylhistidine. These observations suggest that in patients with renal failure, either muscle protein turnover is decreased or the formation or metabolism of 3-methylhistidine is altered. It is possible that because of the elevated plasma levels in uremic patients, 3-methylhistidine may be either degraded or incorporated into larger molecules.

HYDROXYPROLINE AND PROLINE

Plasma levels of total, free and peptide-bound hydroxyproline are elevated in cases of renal failure.[16, 35, 46, 70, 130] Hydroxyproline in the body is present primarily in collagen.[68, 100] In conditions with increased bone turnover, such as primary hyperparathyroidism, Paget's disease and chronic renal failure, hydroxyproline is released from bone, and free and peptide hydroxyproline levels may be elevated in both plasma and urine.[68, 70] A correlation has been demonstrated between the severity of renal osteodystrophy and the degree of elevation of plasma free and peptide hydroxyproline levels.[16, 35, 70, 130] However, Avioli, Sharp and Birge have suggested that a major cause of increased free hydroxyproline levels in uremic patients is decreased degradation of this amino acid due to impaired activity of hepatic hydroxyproline oxidase.[5] Renal osteodystrophy has also been implicated as a cause of elevated plasma proline levels.[16, 130]

GLYCINE, SERINE AND THE SERINE-GLYCINE AND VALINE-GLYCINE RATIOS

The kidney synthesizes serine from glycine and may be a major source of free serine in the body.[99] In dogs with renal failure, release of serine from the kidney decreases.[40] Hence, low plasma serine levels[71] and decreased plasma and muscle serine-glycine ratios[14, 71] in patients with renal failure probably reflect decreased synthesis of serine. The plasma glycine level often remains normal or is increased in malnourished patients.[124, 141]

Thus, elevated plasma glycine levels in uremic patients may reflect both poor nutritional intake and decreased conversion to serine. Since nutritional intake affects both valine (discussed above) and glycine, it is not surprising that the plasma valine-glycine ratio varies directly with protein intake. However, the plasma valine-glycine ratio is lower in chronically uremic patients compared with normal subjects ingesting the same levels of protein, and this probably reflects the non-nutritional causes for low valine and high glycine levels in such patients.

ALANINE

Alanine is of particular interest because it is the principal precursor of hepatic gluconeogenesis. Reports concerning plasma alanine in patients with renal failure are conflicting and describe alanine levels as normal, low or increased.[71] Variations in protein intake may account for the discrepancies among different studies since the plasma alanine level tends to rise when protein intake is decreased. Bergström *et al.* report that the amount of muscle intracellular alanine is normal in chronically uremic patients and increased in patients undergoing maintenance peritoneal dialysis.[14]

Harter and co-workers studied the release of alanine from isolated rat epitrochlearis muscle.[56] They found increased release of alanine but not of glutamine or glutamic acid in uremic as compared with control rats pair-fed either 20% or 40% casein diets. Insulin decreased alanine release from the muscles of uremic rats fed either diet but not from controls. Garber found increased release of alanine and total amino acids from epitrochlearis muscle of uremic rats as compared with control rats.[44] Parathyroid hormone administration increased the release of alanine, glutamine and glutamic acid from the muscles of control rats but enhanced the release of only glutamic acid in uremic rats. These observations suggest that there is increased proteolysis in muscle of uremic rats and that hormonal control of this process may be altered in cases of uremia. In addition, the increased release of alanine from muscle is consistent with the observations of Garber that alanine turnover is enhanced in uremic patients.[45] He also reported that a greater fraction of alanine is converted to glucose in uremia.

CYSTINE

Cystine is consistently observed to be elevated in the plasma of uremic patients. Recently, Cohen *et al.* reported elevated plasma and urinary levels of homocysteine, a metabolic intermediate between methionine and cystine.[29] The causes of these alterations are unclear.

UREA CYCLE AMINO ACIDS—ORNITHINE, CITRULLINE, ARGININE

These amino acids give rise to urea and other potentially toxic products. In patients with renal failure, plasma levels of citrulline are virtually always increased.[71] Chan *et al.* report increased levels of citrulline in plasma, liver and muscle of chronically uremic rats as compared with pair-fed, sham-operated controls.[23] Most reports indicate that arginine concentrations are normal, and ornithine is either normal or increased.[71] In muscle, Bergström and co-workers report that intracellular concentrations of all three urea cycle amino acids are normal in chronically uremic patients and increased in those undergoing maintenance peritoneal dialysis.[14]

Several investigators have analyzed in vitro activities of enzymes that catalyze the synthesis or degradation of these amino acids (Fig. 12–7). Brown *et al.* investigated the activity of the arginine synthetase system, which converts citrulline to arginine.[20] They found increased enzyme activity in the livers of chronically uremic rats as compared with control animals who were offered the same diets. However, animals were not pair-fed, and the differences between animals may have reflected variations in dietary intake. Chan and co-workers evaluated enzyme activities in chronically uremic and pair-fed, sham-operated control rats.[23] They found in uremic rats increased activity of ornithine transcarbamoylase in liver and decreased activity of arginine synthetase in kidney, whether calculated per milligram of protein or per total kidney mass. Liver arginase activity was decreased or increased in uremic animals, depending on the protein intake. In rats, the kidney is considered to take up citrulline and to be the main source of free arginine for extrahepatic protein synthesis.[37] Hence, impaired kidney arginine synthetase activity could lead to reduced citrulline utilization, a fall

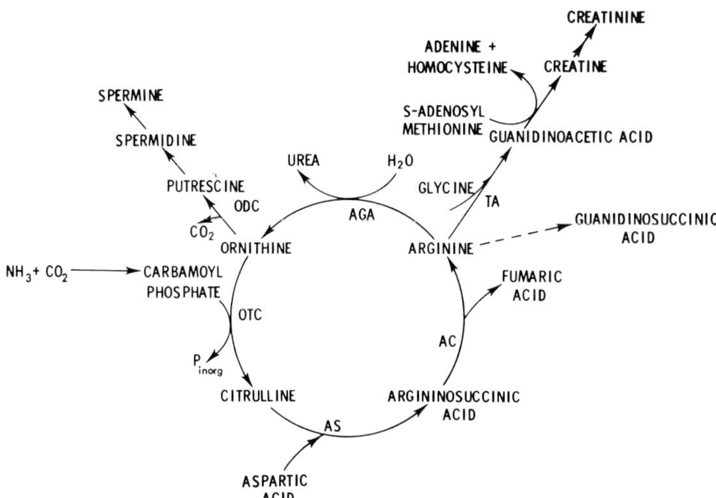

Fig. 12–7.—The urea cycle and adjoining metabolic pathways. Enzymes catalyzing the various reactions are as follows: OTC = ornithine transcarbamoylase; AS = argininosuccinate synthetase; AC = argininosuccinase; AGA = arginase; ODC = ornithine decarboxylase; TA = transamidinase.

in arginine production and increased plasma citrulline levels.[23] However, in human studies, data regarding the uptake of citrulline and release of arginine by the normal kidney are inconclusive.[38, 96]

Arginine is essential for normal growth in rats. Since the rat kidney is thought to be a major source of arginine for extrahepatic protein synthesis, it is possible that uremic rats might have a special need for dietary arginine. Wang *et al.* fed chronically uremic and pair-fed, sham-operated control rats amino acid diets that either contained arginine or were devoid of this amino acid.[135] The uremic rats fed the arginine-containing diet had a reduced weight gain relative to control rats. However, there was no further decrease in weight gain when the uremic rats were fed the arginine-free diet. In the control rats pair-fed this latter diet, weight gain fell to the level of the chronically uremic rats. In the uremic rats ingesting the arginine-free diet as compared with pair-fed controls, free arginine levels were similar in plasma, muscle and kidney and were increased in the brain; moreover, in uremic rats ingesting the arginine-free diet as compared with pair-fed controls, incorporation of ^{14}C-arginine into protein in muscle, kidney and brain was decreased. These findings suggest that uremic rats, as compared with pair-fed, sham-operated controls, responded somewhat differently to arginine deficiency; but the evidence does not demonstrate a greater need for dietary arginine.

Some investigators have added arginine to the essential amino acid preparations for uremic patients.[1] However, Bergström and co-workers[10] and Giordano *et al.*[52] could not demonstrate that arginine was essential for chronically uremic patients when it was added to essential amino acid diets. However, in several of our studies, there was a tendency for plasma arginine levels to fall when arginine-free diets were fed to chronically uremic patients.[78]

Urea, guanidines and polyamines are products formed from the urea cycle amino acids (Fig. 12−7). Each of these substances is potentially toxic, and investigators have questioned whether their biosynthesis is altered in patients with renal failure.[71] There are reports that urea production in the perfused liver is increased in acutely or chronically uremic rats.[97] However, in these studies animals were not pair fed. Also, data from acutely uremic rats may not be applicable to chronically uremic animals because the former are often hypercatabolic.

Arginine contains a guanidino moiety ($-NH-\overset{\displaystyle NH}{\overset{\|}{C}}-NH_2$) and probably participates in the formation of many guanidines. In chronically uremic patients, the levels of guanidinoacetic acid and creatinine are increased in plasma and reduced in urine.[28, 30, 53, 109] The creatine level is increased in plasma and normal in urine.[28, 109] Guanidinosuccinic acid and methylguanidine amounts are increased in serum and urine in patients with renal failure, suggesting increased synthesis or, less likely, reduced degradation of these compounds.[28, 30, 75, 109, 123] Disordered synthesis or metabolism of these compounds in uremic patients has been previously reviewed.[71, 75] Dimethylguanidine and 1,3-diphenylguanidine levels are also reported to be increased in uremic sera.[71]

The urea cycle amino acids also give rise to the polyamines — putrescine, spermidine and spermine (Fig. 12−7). Campbell *et al.* report increased levels of serum free polyamines in uremic patients which fall with dialysis therapy.[22] Swendseid and colleagues observed increased spermidine levels in the red cells of chronically uremic patients and patients undergoing maintenance hemodialysis. Wang *et al.* observed that in chronically uremic rats, the amount of ornithine decarboxylase, which converts ornithine to putrescine, is slightly decreased in liver and markedly decreased in kidney.[136] Thus, synthesis of polyamines may be decreased in uremia, and elevated blood levels may reflect impaired excretion or other factors. Polyamine levels are increased in rapidly proliferating tissues,[18, 106] in blood of pregnant and lactating rats[87] and in urine in patients with many types of cancer.[104, 127] There is evidence that the formation and accumulation of polyamines may affect RNA and DNA synthesis and cellular growth.[36, 105] The clinical significance of elevated polyamine levels in uremic patients should be a fruitful area for further research.

Contribution of the Kidney and Gastrointestinal Tract

KIDNEY FUNCTION

The kidney participates in net utilization and production of several amino acids.[38, 40] Also, it catabolizes a large number of peptides, small proteins and other compounds[72] and by this process may also release amino acids into renal venous plasma. Thus, under normal conditions, the kidney may help to control the pool sizes of certain amino acids, such as serine, as discussed earlier.[38] In patients with renal failure, loss of these activities may alter the metabolism of a number of amino acids. Also, the kidney has a major role in the degradation of many peptide hormones, including insulin, glucagon and parathyroid hormone.[72] In cases of renal failure, impaired catabolism of these hormones may contribute to elevated circulating levels and altered amino acid and protein metabolism.[112, 113] Sherwin *et al.* reported that the hyperglycemic effects of glucagon are increased in chronically uremic patients and fall after institution of maintenance dialysis therapy.[112] Failure of the diseased kidney to synthesize 1,25-dihydroxycholecalciferol and erythropoietin may lead, respectively, to altered bone and muscle metabolism and impaired red blood cell production.[19, 72, 89]

In patients with renal failure, the percent of tubular reabsorption of most amino acids is decreased; thus fractional excretion is increased, often markedly so.[15, 54, 94] The absolute quantity excreted may be normal, decreased or increased.[15, 54, 94] Elevated parathyroid hormone levels may be a cause of the increased fractional excretion of amino acids.[113] Investigators have questioned whether enhanced urinary losses of amino acids might affect pool sizes or metabolism.[15, 54] However, the urinary excretion of amino acids in both normal subjects and patients with renal failure is so low relative to the dietary intake that this is unlikely.

GASTROINTESTINAL FUNCTION

Gulyassy, Peters and Schoenfeld found decreased plasma levels of ^{14}C-cycloleucine after an oral load in hemodialysis patients,[55] suggesting that gastrointestinal absorption of this nonmetabolized amino acid is decreased. Also, Williams and Dick found increased amounts of nonprotein nitrogen in the liquid portion of diarrheal stools of patients with renal failure.[144] Wilson *et al.* found increased total nitrogen in fecal dialysates obtained in vivo from uremic patients.[145] However, in 11 chronically uremic men and 7 healthy men who were ingesting 40-gm protein diets in a metabolic unit, we found similar quantities of fecal nitrogen excretion in both groups, 1.32 ± 0.29 gm/day versus 1.37 ± 0.39 gm/day.[71] As in normal subjects,[121] fecal nitrogen amounts can be reduced in uremic patients by feeding low-fiber (e.g., amino acid) diets.[78]

There appear to be increased numbers of bacteria in the intestinal tract of uremic patients,[118, 131] and bacteria can be identified in areas as high as the duodenum. Such altered bacterial flora might have adverse effects, particularly in the presence of elevated circulating levels of many nitrogenous and non-nitrogenous compounds that may diffuse into the gut and be metabolized.

Many compounds are synthesized or catabolized in the intestinal tract. Among them, ammonia, dimethylamine and trimethylamine are produced,[88, 116-118, 147] and urea, uric acid, creatinine, choline, certain indoles, and probably guanidinosuccinic acid, amino acids, peptides and proteins are degraded or incorporated into other compounds.[33, 60, 63, 90, 119, 120, 131, 147]

Clinical Implications

ASSESSMENT OF NUTRITIONAL STATUS

Fasting levels of many plasma amino acids may be used to indicate nutritional status. The ratios of essential-nonessential amino acids and valine-glycine correlate directly with protein intake.[79] In malnourished uremic patients, these ratios may be markedly decreased, and in addition, the plasma levels of each individual essential amino acid and the sum of all essential amino acids are often very low. Elevated free and bound hydroxyproline levels may indicate renal osteodystrophy.

The use of plasma amino acids to assess nutritional status may be limited by the rapidity with which plasma levels may change. When dietary protein intake changes in nonuremic subjects, postabsorptive plasma amino acid levels may respond rapidly, often within two or three days, and long before serum proteins and anthropometric measurements become normal.[142] Also, discrepancies between amino acids that are altered in plasma and those that are abnormal intracellularly in muscle indicate that caution must be exercised in using plasma levels to indicate the pool sizes of amino acids.[14]

KETOACIDS AND HYDROXYACIDS

α-Ketoacid and α-hydroxyacid analogues of essential amino acids have been used to treat such nitrogen storage diseases as renal and liver failure and inborn errors of the urea cycle.[8, 50, 132] Since these ketoacids and hydroxyacids lack the α-amino nitrogen, administering them is almost tantamount to giving amino acids without increasing the nitrogen load. From studies in various tissues as well as in normal and chronically uremic humans, it appears that most or all of the ketoacid and hydroxyacid analogues, except lysine and threonine, can be readily converted to the corresponding essential amino acids.[6, 21, 50, 102, 103, 107, 134]

It is currently believed that amino groups are taken up by ketoacids and hydroxyacids prior to their incorporation into urea, although some amino groups may be derived from the hydrolysis of urea.[133] Studies of nitrogen balance in humans and of growth in rats indicate that the ketoacids and hydroxyacids are not used as efficiently as equimolar quantities of the essential amino acids.[25-27, 103] The efficiency of utilization appears to increase when nitrogen intake is reduced.[26, 27]

THERAPY WITH AMINO ACIDS, α-KETOACIDS OR α-HYDROXYACIDS

Amino acid and ketoacid or hydroxyacid diets generally contain low quantities (e.g., 16–30 gm/day) of mixed-quality protein supplemented with the nine essential amino acids or a mixture of calcium or sodium salts of ketoacid or hydroxyacid analogues of five essential amino acids (valine, leucine, isoleucine, phenylalanine and methionine) and small quantities of the other essential amino acids.[12, 59, 73, 78, 95, 132-134, 148] Diets virtually devoid of protein but that provide essential amino acids or mixtures of essential and nonessential amino acids have also been used.[47, 73, 78]

The potential benefits of these diets relate to their capability for improving nutritional status, correcting disorders in amino acid metabolism and reducing uremic toxicity. These diets appear to be utilized more efficiently for maintaining nitrogen balance and reducing urea appearance than diets providing similar quantities of protein. Such effects may be related to the greater proportion of protein given as essential amino acids or their ketoacid or hydroxyacid precursors, the lower amounts of nonamino acid nitrogen, possibly to the increased quantities of branched-chain amino acids or ketoacids, and the greater gastrointestinal absorption of amino acids or their precursors as compared with higher-fiber diets. These diets also offer the possibility of normalizing the amino acid patterns in plasma and tissue by modifying the dietary composition of amino acids and ketoacids.[13, 73, 148] In patients with very low glomerular filtration rates (e.g., less than 4.0–5.0 ml/minute) who are not undergoing regular dialysis therapy, these amino acid and ketoacid diets appear preferable to low protein intakes.

Walser *et al.* report that low-protein diets supplemented with ketoacids are utilized more efficiently than similar diets supplemented with amino acids.[132, 134] As previously indicated, they reported a nitrogen-sparing effect of ketoacids which persisted beyond the period of their administration,[107, 132] and they suggest that this may be due to the branched-chain ketoacids.[108] These investigators also report improvement in renal function with ketoacid diets,[132] although this has not been generally confirmed. It may be worth noting that, with the exception of metabolites containing the α-amino nitrogen, these compounds should give rise to the same potentially toxic metabolites as would equimolar quantities of their corresponding amino acids.

Despite reports concerning the benefits of amino acid or ketoacid diets in treating patients with chronic renal failure, it is still unclear whether these diets maintain nutrition and minimize uremic toxicity as well as maintenance dialysis therapy with more liberal protein diets. These semisynthetic diets contain only marginal quantities of amino acids or ketoacids and may not be as nutritious as higher protein intakes. Since regular dialysis therapy is readily available in most Western nations and uremic patients are often wasted,[72, 79] this is a question of considerable importance. An objective evaluation of the benefits of these diets would probably require a large-scale cooperative study of their effects on nutritional status, clinical signs and symptoms, and uremic toxicity as compared with maintenance dialysis therapy.

Supplemental essential amino acids or essential amino acids and ketoacids have also been used with varying success in patients undergoing maintenance hemodialysis. Heidland and Kult infused 17 gm of the essential amino acids during the last 90 minutes of each dialysis treatment to patients undergoing maintenance hemodialysis who were prescribed 1 gm protein/kg body weight per day.[58] Serum levels of many proteins and hemoglobin were low initially and increased during therapy. When infusions were discontinued for 16 weeks, some serum protein levels fell. Reinstitution of therapy was associated with a rise in the amount of serum proteins. However, several studies did not confirm these benefits in children or adults undergoing maintenance hemodialysis who received essential amino acids or the ketoacids orally or intravenously.[31, 57, 128] In these latter studies patients were prescribed liberal food intakes; and it is possible that essential amino acid or ketoacid supplements may improve nutrition only in patients ingesting marginal or submarginal protein intakes.

MODIFYING INTAKE OF SPECIFIC AMINO ACIDS

The finding that histidine is an essential amino acid indicates that it should be included in all nutritional preparations of essential amino acids. Current evidence suggests that both chronically uremic patients and normal adults require between 8 and 12 mg L-histidine per kilogram body weight per day.[74] However, the observation that in uremic patients L-histidine given as a single amino acid supplement does not improve anemia[17, 91, 101] suggests that there is no value to administering it in this manner. The value of dietary histidine to enhance intestinal absorption of iron must still be clarified.[67]

Some investigators have questioned whether impaired conversion of phenylalanine to tyrosine has created a dietary requirement for tyrosine in uremic patients. Similarly, the increased plasma phenylalanine level following a phenylalanine load has raised questions regarding whether the phenylalanine content of diets should be reduced. Currently, there are no definitive data concerning these questions. However, recent findings that the defect in conversion of phenylalanine to tyrosine is mild suggests that there is probably no requirement for tyrosine.[66]

The observation that brain metabolism of tryptophan and serotonin is abnormal in chronically uremic rats[114, 115] may indicate a role for dietary treatment of neurologic disorders in uremic patients. It is tempting to speculate whether modifying the relative proportions of tryptophan and the five competing amino acids (valine, leucine, isoleucine, phenylalanine and tyrosine) in the diet might alter the transport of tryptophan into the brain and normalize the metabolism of tryptophan and serotonin in this organ.

Conclusions

There are many alterations in amino acid metabolism in patients with renal failure. Currently the causes and clinical consequences of these abnormalities are not well defined, but many alterations do not appear to be improved by dialysis therapy. Abnormal amino acid metabolism may contribute to the malnutrition and wasting that commonly occur in chronically uremic patients and patients undergoing chronic dialysis. The use of amino acids and ketoacids or hydroxyacids may be beneficial as dietary therapy for conservative management of chronically uremic patients. Further studies are necessary to determine whether these compounds may be used to treat specific disorders of amino acid metabolism.

Acknowledgments

This work was supported by NIH Contract AM 3-2210 and PHS Grant AM 15197. It is VA Project Number 5016-01.

References

1. Abitbol, C. L., and Holliday, M. A.: Total parenteral nutrition in anuric children, Clin. Nephrol. 5:153, 1976.
2. Anderson, H. L., Cho, E. S., Hanson, K. C., and Krause, G. F.: Effects of low histidine intake on nitrogen utilization of men, Fed. Proc. 34:879, 1975 (Abstract).
3. Anderson, H. L., Cho, E. S., Krause, P. A., Hanson, K. C., Krause, G. F., and Wixom, R. L.: Effects of dietary histidine and arginine on nitrogen retention of men, J. Nutr. 107:2067, 1977.
4. Asatoor, A. M., and Armstrong, M. D.: 3-Methylhistidine, a component of actin, Biochem. Biophy. Res. Commun. 26:168, 1967.
5. Avioli, L. V., Scharp, C., and Birge, S. J.: Catabolism of free hydroxyproline in chronic uremia, Am. J. Physiol. 217:536, 1969.
6. Awapara, J., and Seale, B.: Distribution of transaminases in rat organs, J. Biol. Chem. 194:497, 1952.
7. Ayling, J. E., Helfand, G. D., and Pirson, W. D.: Phenylalanine hydroxylase from human kidney, Enzyme 20:6, 1975.
8. Batshaw, M., Brusilow, S., and Walser, M.: Treatment of carbamyl phosphate synthetase deficiency with keto analogues of essential amino acids, N. Engl. J. Med. 292:1085, 1975.
9. Bergman, E. N., Kaufman, C. F., Wolff, J. E., and Williams, H. H.: Renal metabolism of amino acids and ammonia in fed and fasted pregnant sheep, Am. J. Physiol. 226:833, 1974.
10. Bergström, J., Fürst, P., Josephson, B., and Norée, L. O.: Factors affecting the nitrogen balance in chronic uremic patients receiving essential amino acids intravenously or by mouth, in Kluthe, R., Berlyne, G., and Burton, B. (eds.): *Uremia. An International Conference on Pathogenesis, Diagnosis and Therapy* (Stuttgart: Georg Thieme Verlag, 1972), pp. 264–70.
11. Bergström, J., Fürst, P., Josephson, B., and Norée, L. O.: Improvement of nitrogen balance in a uremic patient by the addition of histidine to essential amino acid solutions given intravenously, Life Sci. 9:787, 1970.
12. Bergström, J., Fürst, P., and Norée, L. O.: Treatment of chronic uremic patients with protein-poor diet and oral supply of essential amino acids. I. Nitrogen balance studies, Clin. Nephrol. 3:187, 1975.
13. Bergström, J., Fürst, P., Norée, L. O., and Vinnars, E.: Intracellular free amino acids in uremic patients as influenced by amino acid supply, Kidney Int. 7:S345, 1975.
14. Bergström, J., Fürst, P., Norée, L. O., and Vinnars, E.: Intracellular free amino acids in muscle tissue of patients with chronic uraemia: effect of peritoneal dialysis and infusion of essential amino acids, Clin. Sci. Mol. Med. 54:51, 1978.

15. Betts, P. R., and Green, A.: Plasma and urine amino acid concentrations in children with chronic renal insufficiency, Nephron 18:132, 1977.
16. Bishop, M. C., Smith, R., Ledingham, J. G. G., and Oliver, D.: Biochemical markers in renal bone disease, Proc. Eur. Dial. Transplant Assoc. 8:122, 1971.
17. Blumenkrantz, M. J., Shapiro, D. J., Swendseid, M. E., and Kopple, J. D.: Histidine supplementation for treatment of anaemia of uraemia, Br. Med. J. 2:530, 1975.
18. Brandt, J. T., Pierce, D. A., and Fausto, N.: Ornithine decarboxylase activity and polyamine synthesis during kidney hypertrophy, Biochim. Biophys. Acta 279:184, 1972.
19. Brickman, A. S., Sherrard, D. J., Coburn, J. W., Poelns, L. S., Baylink, D. J., Friedman, G. S., Massry, S. G., and Norman, A. W.: Management of renal osteodystrophy with $1,25(OH)_2$ and $1\alpha(OH)$-Vitamin D_3: Experience with 36 patients, Kidney Int. 8:407, 1975 (Abstract).
20. Brown, C. L., Houghton, B. J., Souhami, R. L., and Richards, P.: The effects of low-protein diet and uraemia upon urea-cycle enzymes and transaminases in rats, Clin. Sci. Mol. Med. 43:371, 1972.
21. Cammarata, P. S., and Cohen, P. P.: The scope of the transamination reaction in animal tissues, J. Biol. Chem. 187:439, 1950.
22. Campbell, R. A., Bartos, D., Bartos, F., Grettie, D. P., Talwalkar, Y. B., and Musgrave, J. E.: Serum free polyamines (SFPs) in human renal disease by radioimmunoassay (RIA), Clin. Res. 24:199A, 1976 (Abstract).
23. Chan, W., Wang, M., Kopple, J. D., and Swendseid, M. E.: Citrulline levels and urea cycle enzymes in uremic rats, J. Nutr. 104:678, 1974.
24. Cho, E. S., Krause, G. F., and Anderson, H. L.: Effects of dietary histidine and arginine on plasma amino acid and urea concentrations of men fed a low nitrogen diet, J. Nutr. 107:2078, 1977.
25. Chow, K. W., and Walser, M.: Substitution of five essential amino acids by their alpha-keto analogues in the diet of rats, J. Nutr. 104:1208, 1974.
26. Chow, K. W., and Walser, M.: Effect of nitrogen restriction on the utilization of α-ketoisovalerate for growth in the weanling rat, J. Nutr. 105:119, 1975.
27. Chow, K. W., and Walser, M.: Effects of substitution of methionine, leucine, phenylalanine, or valine by their α-hydroxy analogs in the diet of rats, J. Nutr. 105:372, 1975.
28. Cohen, B. D.: Guanidinosuccinic acid in uremia, Arch. Intern. Med. 126:846, 1970.
29. Cohen, B. D., Patel, H., and Kornhauser, R. S.: Proteins in atherogenesis, Abstracts of First International Congress of Nutrition in Renal Disease, Würzburg, Federal Republic of Germany, May 23, 1977.
30. Cohen, B. D., Stein, I. M., and Bonas, J. E.: Guanidinosuccinic aciduria in uremia: A possible alternate pathway for urea synthesis, Am. J. Med. 45:63, 1968.
31. Counahan, R., El-Bishti, M., and Chantler, C.: Oral essential amino acids in children on regular hemodialysis, Clin. Nephrol. 9:11, 1978.
32. Cowgill, R. W., and Freeburg, B.: The metabolism of methylhistidine compounds in animals, Arch. Biochem. Biophys. 71:466, 1957.
33. De La Huerga, J., and Popper, H. J.: Urinary excretion of choline metabolites following choline administration in normals and patients with hepatobiliary diseases, J. Clin. Invest. 30:463, 1951.
34. De Torrente, A., Glazer, G. B., and Gulyassy, P.: Reduced in vitro binding of tryptophan by plasma in uremia, Kidney Int. 6:222, 1974.
35. Dubovský, J., Dubovská, E., Pacovský, V., and Hrba, J.: Free and peptide hydroxyproline in chronic uremia, Clin. Chim. Acta 19:387, 1968.
36. Dykstra, W. G., Jr., and Herbst, E. J.: Spermidine in regenerating liver: Relation to rapid synthesis of ribonucleic acid, Science 149:428, 1965.
37. Featherston, W. R., Rogers, Q. R., and Freedland, R. A.: Relative importance of kidney and liver in synthesis of arginine by the rat, Am. J. Physiol. 224:127, 1973.

38. Felig, P., Owen, O. E., Warren, J., and Cahill, G. F., Jr.: Amino acid metabolism during prolonged starvation, J. Clin. Invest. 48:584, 1969.

39. Fernstrom, J. D., and Wurtman, R. J.: Brain serotonin content: physiological regulation by plasma neutral amino acids, Science 178:414, 1972.

40. Fukuda, S., and Kopple, J. D.: Renal production and degradation of amino acids in normal and uremic dogs, Kidney Int. 12:525, 1977 (abstract).

41. Fukuda, S., and Kopple, J. D.: Carnosine increases release of histidine by the dog kidney, Fed. Proc. 37:281, 1978 (Abstract).

42. Fulks, R. M., Li, J. B., and Goldberg, A. L.: Effects of insulin, glucose and amino acids on protein turnover in rat diaphragm, J. Biol. Chem. 250:290, 1975.

43. Fürst, P.: ^{15}N-studies in severe renal failure. II. Evidence for the essentiality of histidine, Scand. J. Clin. Lab. Invest. 30:307, 1972.

44. Garber, A. J.: Abnormalities of carbohydrate metabolism in chronic uremia, Ninth Annual Contractors' Conference, Artificial Kidney – Chronic Uremia Program, 5, 1976 (Abstract).

45. Garber, A. J.: Abnormalities of carbohydrate metabolism in chronic uremia, Eleventh Annual Contractors' Conference, Artificial Kidney – Chronic Uremia Program, 47, 1978 (abstract).

46. Giordano, C.: Diet and amino acids in uraemia, Proc. Eur. Dial. Transplant Assoc. 9:419, 1972.

47. Giordano, C.: Use of exogenous and endogenous urea for protein synthesis in normal and uremic subjects, J. Lab. Clin. Med. 62:231, 1963.

48. Giordano, C., De Pascale, C., Balestrieri, C., Cittadini, D., and Crescenzi, A.: Incorporation of urea ^{15}N in amino acids of patients with chronic renal failure on low nitrogen diet, Am. J. Clin. Nutr. 21:394, 1968.

49. Giordano, C., De Pascale, C., De Cristofaro, D., Capodicasa, G., Balestrieri, C., and Baczyk, K.: Protein malnutrition in the treatment of chronic uremia, in Berlyne, G. M. (ed.): *Nutrition in Renal Disease* (Baltimore: Williams & Wilkins Co., 1968), pp. 23–34.

50. Giordano, C., De Pascale, C., Phillips, M. E., De Santo, N. G., Fürst, P., Brown, C. L., Houghton, B. J., and Richards, P.: Utilisation of ketoacid analogues of valine and phenylalanine in health and uraemia, Lancet 1:178, 1972.

51. Giordano, C., De Santo, N. G., Rinaldi, S., Acone, D., Esposito, R., and Gallo, B.: Histidine for treatment of uraemic anaemia, Br. Med. J. 4:714, 1973.

52. Giordano, C., De Santo, N. G., Rinaldi, S., De Pascale, C., and Pluvio, M.: Histidine and glycine essential amino acids in uremia, in Kluthe, R., Berlyne, G., and Burton, B. (eds.): *Uremia: An International Conference on Pathogenesis, Diagnosis and Therapy* (Stuttgart: Georg Thieme Verlag, 1972), pp. 138–143.

53. Goldman, R.: Creatinine excretion in renal failure, Proc. Soc. Exp. Biol. Med. 35:446, 1954.

54. Gulyassy, P. F., Aviram, A., and Peters, J. H.: Evaluation of amino acid and protein requirements in chronic uremia, Arch. Intern. Med. 126:855, 1970.

55. Gulyassy, P. F., Peters, J. H., and Schoenfeld, P.: Transport and protein binding of tryptophan in uremia, in Kluthe, R., Berlyne, G., and Burton, B. (eds.): *Uremia: An International Conference on Pathogenesis, Diagnosis and Therapy* (Stuttgart: Georg Thieme Verlag, 1972), pp. 163–170.

56. Harter, H., Karl, I., Klahr, S., and Kipnis, D.: Demonstration of increased proteolysis in isolated uremic muscle, Clin. Res. 24:402A, 1976 (Abstract).

57. Hecking, E., Port, F. K., Brehm, H., Zobel, R., Brandl, M., Prellwitz, W., and Opferkuch, I.: A controlled study of the value of oral supplementation with essential amino acids (EAA) and α-ketoanalogs (αKA) in chronic hemodialysis, Kidney Int. 12:482, 1977 (Abstract).

58. Heidland, A., and Kult, J.: Long-term effects of essential amino acids supplementation in patients on regular dialysis treatment, Clin. Nephrol. 3:234, 1975.

59. Heidland, A., Kult, J., Röckel, A., and Heidbreder, E.: Evaluation of essential amino acids and keto acids in uremic patients on low protein diet, Am. J. Clin. Nutr. 31:1784, 1978.

60. Houssay, B. A.: Phenolemia and indoxylemia. Their origin, significance, and regulation, Am. J. Med. Sci. 192:615, 1936.

61. IUPAC-IUB Commission on Biochemical Nomenclature: Symbols for amino-acid derivatives and peptides, recommendations (1971), J. Biol. Chem. 247:977, 1972.

62. Johnson, P., and Perry, S. V.: Biological activity and the 3-methylhistidine content of actin and myosin, Biochem. J. 119:293, 1970.

63. Jones, J. D., and Burnett, P. C.: Creatinine metabolism in humans with decreased renal function: creatinine deficit, Clin. Chem. 20:1204, 1974.

64. Jones, J. D., and Burnett, P. C.: Implication of creatinine and gut flora in the uremic syndrome: induction of "creatininase" in colon contents of the rat by dietary creatinine, Clin. Chem. 18:280, 1972.

65. Jones, M. R., and Kopple, J. D.: Valine metabolism in normal and chronically uremic man, Am. J. Clin. Nutr. 31:1660, 1978.

66. Jones, M. R., Kopple, J. D., and Swendseid, M. E.: Phenylalanine metabolism in uremic and normal man, Kidney Int. 14:169, 1978.

67. Jontofsohn, R., Heinze, V., Katz, N., Stuber, U., Wilke, H., and Kluthe, R.: Histidine and iron supplementation in dialysis and pre-dialysis patients, Proc. Eur. Dial. Transplant Assoc. 2:391, 1975.

68. Kivirikko, K. I.: Urinary excretion of hydroxyproline in health and disease, Int. Rev. Connect. Tissue Res. 5:93, 1970.

69. Knott, P. J., and Curzon, G.: Free tryptophan in plasma and brain tryptophan metabolism, Nature 239:452, 1972.

70. Koevoet, A. L.: Plasma hydroxyproline in primary hyperparathyroidism and in chronic uremia, Clin. Chim. Acta 12:230, 1965.

71. Kopple, J. D.: Nitrogen metabolism, in Massry, S. G., and Sellers, A. L. (eds.): *Clinical Aspects of Uremia and Dialysis* (Springfield, Ill.: Charles C Thomas, Publisher, 1976), pp. 241–73.

72. Kopple, J. D.: Abnormal amino acid and protein metabolism in uremia, Kidney Int. 14:340, 1978.

73. Kopple, J. D.: Treatment with low protein and amino acid diets in chronic renal failure, *Proc. Eighth International Congress on Nephrology, Montreal* (Berlin: S. Karger, 1978), pp. 497–507.

74. Kopple, J. D., Figueroa, W. G., and Swendseid, M. E.: The dietary histidine requirement in normal and uremic man, Fed. Proc. 36:1092, 1977 (Abstract).

75. Kopple, J. D., Gordon, S. I., Wang, M., and Swendseid, M. E.: Factors affecting serum and urinary guanidinosuccinic acid levels in normal and uremic subjects, J. Lab. Clin. Med. 90:303, 1977.

76. Kopple, J. D., Jones, M. R., Fukuda, S., and Swendseid, M. E.: Amino acid and protein metabolism in renal failure, Am. J. Clin. Nutr. 31:1532, 1978.

77. Kopple, J. D., Paniagua, M., and Swendseid, M. E.: Histidine and 3-methylhistidine in plasma and urine and nitrogen balance in subjects receiving diets varying in histidine content, Fed. Proc. 34:931, 1975 (Abstract).

78. Kopple, J. D., and Swendseid, M. E.: Nitrogen balance and plasma amino acid levels in uremic patients fed an essential amino acid diet, Am. J. Clin. Nutr. 27:806, 1974.

79. Kopple, J. D., and Swendseid, M. E.: Protein and amino acid metabolism in uremic patients undergoing maintenance hemodialysis, Kidney Int. 8:S64, 1975.

80. Kopple, J. D., and Swendseid, M. E.: Evidence that histidine is an essential amino acid in normal and chronically uremic man, J. Clin. Invest. 55:881, 1975.

81. Kopple, J. D., and Swendseid, M. E.: Effect of protein intake and uremia on plasma amino acid levels, Kidney Int. 10:560, 1976 (Abstract).

82. Kopple, J. D., Swendseid, M. E., Paniagua, M., and Wang, M.: Effects of histidine deficient diets on histidine levels and oxidation rates in uremic and normal man, Fed. Proc. 32:916, 1973 (Abstract).

83. Kopple, J. D., Wang, M., Vyhmeister, I., Baker, N., and Swendseid, M. E.: Tyrosine metabolism in uremia, in Kluthe, R., Berlyne, G., and Burton, B. (eds.): *Uremia: An International Conference on Pathogenesis, Diagnosis and Therapy* (Stuttgart: Georg Thieme Verlag, 1972), pp. 150–163.

84. Lenney, J. F.: Specificity and distribution of mammalian carnosinase, Biochim. Biophys. Acta 429:214, 1976.

85. Letteri, J. M., and Scipione, R. A.: Phenylalanine metabolism in chronic renal failure, Nephron 13:365, 1974.

86. Long, C. L., Haverberg, L. N., Young, V. R., Kinney, J. M., Munro, H. N., and Geiger, J. W.: Metabolism of 3-methylhistidine in man, Metabolism 24:929, 1975.

87. Lundgren, D. W., and Oka, T.: Marked increase in free spermidine concentration in blood during pregnancy and lactation in rats, Fed. Proc. 36:1128, 1977 (Abstract).

88. McDermott, W. V., Jr., Adams, R. D., and Riddell, A. G.: Ammonia metabolism in man, Ann. Surg. 140:539, 1954.

89. Matthews, C., Heimberg, K. W., Ritz, E., Agostini, B., Fritzsche, J., and Hasselbach, W.: Effect of 1,25-dihydroxycholecalciferol on impaired calcium transport by the sarcoplasmic reticulum in experimental uremia, Kidney Int. 11:227, 1977.

90. Milstien, S., and Goldman, P.: Role of intestinal microflora in the metabolism of guanidinosuccinic acid, J. Bacteriol. 114:641, 1973.

91. Mirahmadi, K. S., Imparato, B., Gorman, J. T., and Rosen, S. M.: Histidine supplementation in management of anemia in dialysis patients, Kidney Int. 6:77A, 1974 (Abstract).

92. Munro, H. N.: Role of amino acid supply in regulating ribosome function, Fed. Proc. 27:1231, 1968.

93. Murthy, L. I., and Berry, H. K.: Phenylalanine hydroxylase activity in liver from humans and subhuman primates: its probable absence in kidney, Biochem. Med. 12:392, 1975.

94. Nádvorníková, H., Schück, O., Malý, J., Pechar, J., Dobersky, P., and Tomková, D.: Renal clearance of amino acids in patients with severe chronic renal failure, Nephron 20:83, 1978.

95. Norée, L. O., and Bergström, J.: Treatment of chronic uremic patients with protein-poor diet and oral supply of essential amino acids. II. Clinical results of long-term treatment, Clin. Nephrol. 3:195, 1975.

96. Owen, E. E., and Robinson, R. R.: Amino acid extraction and ammonia metabolism by the human kidney during the prolonged administration of ammonium chloride, J. Clin. Invest. 42:263, 1963.

97. Perez, G. O., and Schiff, E. R.: Kinetics of urea synthesis by perfused rat liver in uremia, Kidney Int. 12:533, 1977 (Abstract).

98. Pickford, J. C., McGale, E. H. F., and Aber, G. M.: Studies on the metabolism of phenylalanine and tyrosine in patients with renal disease, Clin. Chim. Acta 48:77, 1973.

99. Pitts, R. F., and MacLeod, M. B.: Synthesis of serine by the dog kidney in vivo, Am. J. Physiol. 222:394, 1972.

100. Prockop, D. J., and Kivirikko, K. I.: Relationship of hydroxyproline excretion in urine to collagen metabolism, Ann. Intern. Med. 66:1243, 1967.

101. Reeves, R. D., Barbour, G. L., Robertson, C. S., and Crumb, C. S.: Failure of histidine supplementation to improve anemia in chronic dialysis patients, Am. J. Clin. Nutr. 30:579, 1977.

102. Richards, P., Ell, S., and Halliday, D.: Direct evidence for synthesis of valine in man, Lancet 1:112, 1977.

103. Rudman, D.: Capacity of human subjects to utilize keto analogues of valine and phenylalanine, J. Clin. Invest. 50:90, 1971.
104. Russell, D. H.: Clinical relevance of polyamines as biochemical markers of tumor kinetics, Clin. Chem. 23:22, 1977.
105. Russell, D. H., Levy, C. C., and Taylor, R. L.: Increased DNA associated with rat liver nucleoli when isolated with spermidine, Biochem. Biophys. Res. Commun. 47: 212, 1972.
106. Russell, D. H., and McVicker, T. A.: Polyamine biogenesis in the rat mammary gland during pregnancy and lactation, Biochem. J. 130:71, 1972.
107. Sapir, D. G., Owen, O. E., Pozefsky, T., and Walser, M.: Nitrogen sparing induced by a mixture of essential amino acids given chiefly as their keto-analogues during prolonged starvation in obese subjects, J. Clin. Invest. 54:974, 1974.
108. Sapir, D. G., and Walser, M.: Nitrogen sparing induced early in starvation by infusion of branched-chain ketoacids, Metabolism 26:301, 1977.
109. Sasaki, M., Takahara, K., and Natelson, S.: Urinary guanidinoacetate/guanidinosuccinate ratio: An indicator of kidney dysfunction, Clin. Chem. 19:315, 1973.
110. Schmid, G., Przuntek, H., Fricke, L., Heidland, A., and Hempel, K.: Increased histidine and histamine content in the brain of chronic uremic rats. Cause of enhanced cerebral cAMP in uremia? Am. J. Clin. Nutr. 31:1665, 1978.
111. Sheng, Y. B., Badger, T. M., Asplund, J. M., and Wixom, R. L.: Incorporation of $^{15}NH_4Cl$ into histidine in adult man, J. Nutr. 107:621, 1977.
112. Sherwin, R. S., Bastl, C., Finkelstein, F. O., Fisher, M., Black, H., Hendler, R., and Felig, P.: Influence of uremia and hemodialysis on the turnover and metabolic effects of glucagon, J. Clin. Invest. 57:722, 1976.
113. Short, E. M., Elsas, L. J., and Rosenberg, L. E.: Effect of parathyroid hormone on renal tubular reabsorption of amino acids, Metabolism 23:715, 1974.
114. Siassi, F., Wang, M., Kopple, J. D., and Swendseid, M. E.: Brain serotonin turnover in chronically uremic rats, Am. J. Physiol. 1:E526, 1977.
115. Siassi, F., Wang, M., Kopple, J. D., and Swendseid, M. E.: Plasma tryptophan levels and brain serotonin metabolism in chronically uremic rats, J. Nutr. 107:840, 1977.
116. Simenhoff, M. L., Burke, J. F., Saukkonen, J. J., Wesson, L. G., and Schaedler, R. W.: Amine metabolism and the small bowel in uraemia, Lancet 2:818, 1976.
117. Simenhoff, M., and Saukkonen, J.: Amine metabolism in uremia, Clin. Res. 21:707, 1973 (Abstract).
118. Simenhoff, M. L., Wesson, L. G., Schaedler, R., Saukkonen, J., Gordon S., Lasker, N., Burke, J., Dunn, S., and Spainhour, J.: Amine metabolism in uremia, Seventh Annual Contractors' Conference, Artificial Kidney — Chronic Uremia Program, 7, 1974 (Abstract).
119. Sorensen, L. B.: Degradation of uric acid in man, Metabolism 8:687, 1959.
120. Sorensen, L. B., and Levinson, D. J.: Origin and extrarenal elimination of uric acid in man, Nephron 14:7, 1975.
121. Southgate, D. A. T., and Durnin, J. V. G. A.: Calorie conversion factors. An experimental reassessment of the factors used in the calculation of the energy value of human diets, Br. J. Nutr. 24:517, 1970.
122. Squires, E. J., Hall, D. F., and Brosnan, J. T.: Arteriovenous differences for amino acids and lactate across kidneys of normal and acidotic rats, Biochem. J. 160:125, 1976.
123. Stein, I. M., Perez, G., Johnson, R., and Cummings, N. B.: Serum levels and urinary excretion of methylguanidine in chronic renal failure, J. Lab. Clin. Med. 77:1020, 1971.
124. Swendseid, M. E., Yamada, C., Vinyard, E., and Figueroa, W. G.: Plasma amino acid levels in young subjects receiving diets containing 14 or 3.5 g nitrogen per day, Am. J. Clin. Nutr. 21:1381, 1968.

125. Tam, C. F., Kopple, J. D., Wang, M., and Swendseid, M. E.: Alterations of mono-amine oxidase activity in uremia, Kidney Int. 7:S328, 1975.
126. Trayer, I. P., Harris, C. I., and Perry, S. V.: 3-Methyl histidine and adult and foetal forms of skeletal muscle myosin, Nature 217:452, 1968.
127. Tsuji, M., Nakajima, T., and Sano, I.: Putrescine, spermidine, N-acetylspermidine and spermine in the urine of patients with leukaemias and tumors, Clin. Chim. Acta 59:161, 1975.
128. Ulm, A., Neuhäuser, M., and Leber, H. W.: Influence of essential amino acids and ketoacids on protein metabolism and anemia of patients on intermittent hemodialysis, Am. J. Clin. Nutr. 31:1827, 1978.
129. Van Campen, D.: Effect of histidine and ascorbic acid on the absorption and retention of ^{59}Fe by iron-depleted rats, J. Nutr. 102:165, 1972.
130. Varghese, Z., Moorhead, J. F., Tatler, G. L., Baillod, R. A., and Wills, M. R.: Plasma hydroxyproline in renal osteodystrophy, Proc. Eur. Dial. Transplant Assoc. 10:187, 1973.
131. Vince, A., Down, P. F., Murison, J., Twigg, F. J., and Wrong, O. M.: Generation of ammonia from non-urea sources in a faecal incubation system, Clin. Sci. Mol. Med. 51:313, 1976.
132. Walser, M.: Ketoacids in the treatment of uremia, Clin. Nephrol. 3:180, 1975.
133. Walser, M.: Treatment of renal failure with keto acids, Hosp. Pract. 1:59, 1975.
134. Walser, M., Coulter, A. W., Dighe, S., and Crantz, F. R.: The effect of keto-analogues of essential amino acids in severe chronic uremia, J. Clin. Invest. 52:678, 1973.
135. Wang, M., Kopple, J. D., and Swendseid, M. E.: Effects of arginine-devoid diets in chronically uremic rats, J. Nutr. 107:495, 1977.
136. Wang, M., Kopple, J. D., and Swendseid, M. E.: Metabolism of 1,4-^{14}C-putrescine in chronically uremic rats, Fed. Proc. 37:536, 1978 (Abstract).
137. Wang, M., Tam, C. F., Swendseid, M. E., and Kopple, J. D.: Monoamine and diamine oxidase activities in uremic rats, Life Sci. 17:653, 1975.
138. Wang, M., Vyhmeister, I., Kopple, J. D., and Swendseid, M. E.: Effect of protein intake on weight gain and plasma amino acid levels in uremic rats, Am. J. Physiol. 230:1455, 1976.
139. Wang, M., Vyhmeister, I., Swendseid, M. E., and Kopple, J. D.: Phenylalanine hydroxylase and tyrosine aminotransferase activities in chronically uremic rats, J. Nutr. 105:122, 1975.
140. Waterlow, J. C., Garlick, P. J., and Millward, D. J.: Amino acid supply and protein turnover, in Greene, H. L., Holliday, M. A., and Munro, H. N. (eds.): *Clinical Nutrition Update: Amino Acids* (Chicago: American Medical Association, 1977), pp. 1–9.
141. Whitehead, R. G., and Dean, R. F. A.: Serum amino acids in kwashiorkor. I. Relationship to clinical condition, Am. J. Clin. Nutr. 14:313, 1964.
142. Whitehead, R. G., and Dean, R. F. A.: Serum amino acids in kwashiorkor. II. An abbreviated method of estimation and its application, Am. J. Clin. Nutr. 14:320, 1964.
143. Whitehouse, S., Katz, N., Schaeffer, G., and Kluthe, R.: Histidines and renal function, Clin. Nephrol. 3:24, 1975.
144. Williams, J. L., and Dick, G. F.: The excretion of nonprotein nitrogen substances by the intestine, J.A.M.A. 100:484, 1933.
145. Wilson, D. R., Ing, T. S., Metcalfe-Gibson, A., and Wrong, O. M.: The chemical composition of faeces in uraemia, as revealed by in vivo faecal dialysis, Clin. Sci. 35:197, 1968.
146. Wixom, R. L., Anderson, H. L., Terry, B. E., and Sheng, Y. B.: Total parenteral nutrition with selective histidine depletion in man. I. Responses in nitrogen metabolism and related areas, Am. J. Clin. Nutr. 30:887, 1977.

147. Wrong, O., Houghton, B. J., Richards, P., and Wilson, D. R.: The fate of intestinal urea in normal subjects and patients with uremia, in Schmidt-Nielsen, B. (ed.): *Urea and the Kidney* (Amsterdam: Excerpta Medica, 1970), pp. 461–70.
148. Young, G. A., Oli, H. I., Davison, A. M., and Parsons, F. M.: The effects of calorie and essential amino acid supplementation on plasma proteins in patients with chronic renal failure, Am. J. Clin. Nutr. 31:1802, 1978.
149. Young, G. A., and Parsons, F. M.: Impairment of phenylalanine hydroxylation in chronic renal insufficiency, Clin. Sci. Mol. Med. 45:89, 1973.
150. Young, V. R.: The role of skeletal and cardiac muscle in the regulation of protein metabolism, in Munro, H. N. (ed.): *Mammalian Protein Metabolism,* Vol. 4 (New York: Academic Press, 1970), pp. 585–674.
151. Young, V. R., Alexis, S. D., Baliga, B. S., and Munro, H. N.: Metabolism of administered 3-methylhistidine, lack of muscle transfer ribonucleic acid charging and quantitative excretion as 3-methylhistidine and its N-acetyl derivative, J. Biol. Chem. 247:3592, 1972.

13

Liver Disease in Patients Undergoing Hemodialysis and Kidney Transplantation

C. TOUSSAINT, M.D., E. DUPONT, M.D.,
J. L. VANHERWEGHEM, M.D., R. CAPPEL, M.D.,
G. DE ROY, M.D., P. VEREERSTRAETEN, M.D.,
P. KINNAERT, M.D., L. THIRY, M.D.,
AND J. VAN GEERTRUYDEN, M.D.

*Departments of Nephrology, Surgery and Pathology, Brugmann University Hospital,
and Department of Virology, Pasteur Institute, Brussels, Belgium*

Patients admitted to a dialysis-transplantation program are prone to develop liver dysfunction (LD) of uncertain etiology.[9, 10, 23, 35, 43, 52, 55, 67, 80] Hepatitus B virus (HBV) has been incriminated as the cause in most cases,[4, 28, 38, 39, 47, 66, 68] but other viruses must also be considered, such as cytomegalovirus (CMV),[2, 3, 7, 15, 25, 32, 36, 42, 43, 45, 77, 80] hepatitus A virus (HAV), hepatitis C virus (HCV),[17, 18, 24, 33, 53, 79] Epstein-Barr virus (EBV)[3, 14] and possibly other, still unidentified viruses.[46] In addition, due its hepatotoxicity in dogs,[30, 65] azathioprine, which is administered to practically all graft recipients, has traditionally been incriminated.[43, 64, 83]

During the past few years, several reports presented contradictory data on the role of HBV in the prognosis of the kidney recipient as well as in the survival of the graft itself.[10, 11, 26, 39, 50, 52, 55, 60, 66] It was therefore justified to reexamine, with some recent virologic data, the incidence of LD in 267 patients admitted to a dialysis-transplantation program between 1969 and 1976. In this eight-year period, the prevalence of HBV decreased markedly in our unit, without affecting the overall morbidity and mortality of hepatic origin.

Patients and Methods

PATIENTS. — From January 1, 1969, to December 31, 1976, 267 patients were admitted to a dialysis-transplantation program; 185 of those patients received 211 kidney transplants after dialysis periods of variable duration.

HEMODIALYSES. — All hemodialyses were conducted using arteriovenous fistulas,[37] with a schedule of two or three weekly dialyses. The artificial kidneys used were the coil or sandwich type, connected to a central dialysate delivery system. Until 1974 the artificial kidneys were contained in re-used cannisters, which were subsequently replaced by disposable material. Since that time, the patients have been using, in the ward as well as in the dialysis unit, disposable bed sheets, cups, plates, forks and spoons, and strict adherence to the use of disposable garments and gloves has been enforced among the professional staff.

KIDNEY TRANSPLANTATIONS. — Of the 211 transplantations, 13 were performed from related living donors, and brain-death cadaver donors were used in 94% of the cases. A total of 185 patients received one, and 25 received two successive transplants, while a third graft was used in one case. Most of the kidneys were rinsed with and stored in Collins solution prior to transplantation,[13] only a few having been harvested on a pump device, with human serum albumin as a perfusate.[12] Immunosuppressive therapy consisted of the administration of azathioprine and prednisolone.[75] From January 1969 to December 1975, most patients were also treated with antilymphocyte globulins for 2 to 12 weeks following the operation. Rejection crises were managed by increasing corticosteroid doses and by local irradiation.

The following symbols are used to designate the successive periods of therapy of each patient: D1 = first dialysis period, T1 = period with a functioning first transplant, D2 = second dialysis period following the failure of the first transplant, T2 = period with a functioning second transplant, D3 = third dialysis period following the failure of the second transplant, and T3 = period with a functioning third transplant.

DEFINITION OF LIVER DYSFUNCTION. — Liver function was assessed at more or less regular intervals by measurement of bilirubin, lactic dehydrogenase, transaminase and alkaline phosphatase serum levels. In a few patients, bromsulphalein (BSP) clearance and liver scanning were also performed. Using clinical and biochemical criteria, three forms of LD could be delineated: (1) *acute hepatitis*: in which the duration of LD, with or without symptoms, did not exceed three months; (2) *intermittent hepatitis*, in which signs of LD recurred intermittently, usually without symptoms; and (3) *chronic hepatitis*, in which LD persisted usually beyond 12 months and often led to portal hypertension, jaundice with bleeding tendencies or cirrhosis of the liver.

VIROLOGIC STUDIES. — The following virologic studies were performed monthly on the patients' sera.

Hepatitis B. — Hepatitis B surface antigen (HBsAg) was detected by complement fixation,[58] which was replaced after July 1976 by radioimmunoassay (AUS RIA Kit, Abbott). Anti-HBs was detected by radioimmunoassay (AUS AB Kit, Abbott).

Cytomegalovirus. — Complement fixation was used for anti-CMV titer determinations.[58] The CMV antigen used was prepared from the AD 169 strain (Microbiological Associates). Seroconversion was considered present when a fourfold increase in anti-CMV titer was observed.

HISTOPATHOLOGIC STUDIES. — Liver biopsies were not performed, but liver specimens were obtained at autopsy from 16 HBsAg-positive and 9 HBsAg-negative patients.

Results

Of the 267 patients admitted to the dialysis-transplantation program, 88 (33%) showed evidence of LD at some time. Due to the major role attributed to HBV in the pathogenesis of hepatitis occurring in patients with kidney transplants, we also reviewed the records of 66 patients who presented HBs antigenemia at some phase of therapy, whether they had showed biochemical evidence of LD or not. Thus, 103 records were analyzed: 66 HBsAg-positive patients, including 51 with LD, and 37 HBsAg-negative patients with LD.

TABLE 13-1.—PERIODS OF HBsAg ACQUISITION IN THE 66
HBsAg-POSITIVE PATIENTS AND PERIODS OF APPEARANCE OF
LIVER DYSFUNCTION IN 37 HBsAg-NEGATIVE PATIENTS

	D1	T1	D2	T2	D3	T3
HBsAg-positive patients						
Patients admitted						
to each period	66	61	26	10	4	1
Mean duration of periods						
in months	12	34	18	33	32	2
Range	1–56	0–110	1–86	1–65	10–56	–
HBsAg-negative patients						
Patients admitted						
to each period	37	31	14	6	0	0
Mean duration of periods						
in months	14	24	14	33	. . .	. . .
Range	2–59	0–86	2–34	22–51	. . .	. . .

HBsAg-Positive Patients

Of the 66 patients admitted to D1, 61 entered T1, 26 were
readmitted to D2, 10 were retransplanted (T2), 4 were readmitted to D3, and 1 received a third transplant (T3). The mean duration of the periods ranged from 12 to 34 months (Table 13–1).

HBs ANTIGENEMIA.—HBsAg made its appearance during a
dialysis period in 37 patients (11.3% of patients at risk) and during a transplant period in 29 patients (13.7% of patients at risk;
Table 13–2).

Time of appearance.—Table 13–3 shows that 62% of the patients who acquired HBsAg in the course of a transplant period
did so during the first postoperative year, and 84% of the patients acquiring it in dialysis became positive in the course of
the first year of therapy.

TABLE 13-2.—TIME OF FIRST
HBsAg DETECTION

PERIOD	PATIENTS AT RISK	PATIENTS ACQUIRING HBsAg
D1	267	27 (10%)
T1	185	28 (15%)
D2	59	10 (17%)
T2	26	1 (4%)
D3	10	0
Total	547	66 (12%)

TABLE 13-3.—LATENCY OF HBs ANTIGENEMIA
APPEARANCE IN THE 66 HBsAg-POSITIVE
PATIENTS AND LATENCY OF LIVER
DYSFUNCTION APPEARANCE IN THE 37 HBsAg-
NEGATIVE PATIENTS

YEAR	D1	T1	D2	T2	D3
HBsAg-positive patients					
1st	23	17	8	1	0
2d	4	6	2	0	0
3d	0	3	0	0	0
4th	0	1	0	0	0
5th	0	1	0	0	0
Total	27	28	10	1	0
HBsAg-negative patients					
1st	7	10	4	3	0
2d	3	1	1	0	0
3d	0	4	0	1	0
4th	1	1	0	0	0
5th	0	0	0	0	0
6th	0	0	0	1	0
Total	11	16	5	5	0

Duration.—The duration of HBs antigenemia did not exceed
one year in 42 (64%) of the 66 patients, and it exceeded three
years in 22 patients (33%, Table 13-4). It should be stressed
that six patients died while being HBsAg carriers during the
first year of therapy, so some of them should have remained
HBsAg-positive had they not died of intercurrent diseases.

Thirty-eight patients were followed for a sufficient length of
time to demonstrate HBsAg negativation: 30 lost HBsAg after
1-4 months, 4 after 7-8 months, 2 after 10-12 months and 2

TABLE 13-4.—DURATION OF
HBs ANTIGENEMIA

DURATION (YR)	PATIENTS ACQUIRING HBsAg	PATIENTS AS HBsAg CARRIERS
<1	42	6
1-2	1	1
2-3	1	0
3-4	5	1
4-5	4	3
5-6	12	2
6-7	1	0
Total	66	13

TABLE 13–5.—PREVALENCE OF HBs ANTIGENEMIA AND LIVER DYSFUNCTION IN THE 267 PATIENTS ADMITTED TO THE DIALYSIS-TRANSPLANTATION PROGRAM FROM 1969 TO 1976

PERIOD	PATIENTS ADMITTED TO THE PROGRAM (a)	HBsAg-POSITIVE PATIENTS (b)	HBsAg-POSITIVE PATIENTS WITH HEPATITIS (c)	HBsAg-NEGATIVE PATIENTS WITH HEPATITIS (d)	HBsAg-POSITIVE OR NEGATIVE PATIENTS WITH HEPATITIS (c+d)
1969–70	55	1	1	2	3
1971–72	58	38	31	6	37
1973–74	74	22	14	6	20
1975–76	80	5	5	23	28
Total	267	66	51	37	88

after 47–53 months. Those last two patients presently contain no HBsAg after two and three years. Eight patients thus became HBsAg-negative after being in a carrier state for longer than six months. Of the 38 individuals followed for a sufficient length of time, HBsAg disappeared in 17 during a transplant period under immunosuppressive therapy; the last 21 remained on dialysis.

In summary, 66 (25%) of the 267 patients admitted to the dialysis-transplantation program acquired HBsAg, but 55% of the HBsAg-positive patients became HBsAg-negative within four months, even during immunosuppressive therapy. However, 32 patients who retained their HBsAg for time intervals exceeding six months would be considered chronic carriers, although 8 (25%) of them lost their HBsAg after 7–53 months.

Prevalence.—The prevalence of HBs antigenemia showed important fluctuations from 1969 to 1976 (Table 13–5). A hepatitis B epidemic developed in our unit during 1971–72, when 38 (66%) of the patients admitted acquired HBsAg. In 1973–74, HBsAg incidence dropped to 30% and reached the low level of 6% in 1975–76, probably as a consequence of the various prophylactic measures described previously.

In June 1977, our dialysis unit was taking care of 56 patients, 5 (9%) of whom carried HBsAg, while 11 (13%) of the 86 patients followed at the transplant clinic were HBsAg-positive. All 16 individuals were chronic carriers after four to seven years. The reintroduction of HBV into our dialysis unit is presently taking place through readmission of chronic HBsAg carriers after failure of their graft, with the transplant clinic acting as the main reservoir of virus in our system.

TABLE 13–6.—TYPES OF HEPATITIS IN THE 66 HBsAg-POSITIVE PATIENTS

LIVER FUNCTION	DURATION OF FOLLOW-UP SINCE HBsAg ACQUISITION (MO)	HBsAg-POSITIVE PATIENTS	CHRONIC HBsAg CARRIERS	DEATHS DUE TO HEPATITIS	RECOVERIES FROM HEPATITIS
Normal	30 (2–70)	15	6	—	—
Acute hepatitis	42 (1–91)	31	12	0	31
Intermittent hepatitis	64 (45–70)	8	6	0	8
Chronic hepatitis	44 (6–72)	12	8	3	4
Total		66	32	3	43

HBs ANTIBODY. – The sera of 38 HBsAg-positive patients were screened for anti-HBs, and 19 patients were found to be chronic carriers. Of the 19 individuals who were not carriers, anti-HBs was detected in 11. In the 19 chronic carriers, anti-HBs was found in two sera of the same patient.

THE THREE FORMS OF LD IN HBsAg-POSITIVE PATIENTS. – In the 66 HBsAg-positive patients, 15 (6 chronic HBsAg carriers) never demonstrated biochemical evidence of LD at any time, while 51 (26 chronic HBsAg carriers) showed acute, intermittent or chronic LD (Table 13–6).

Acute hepatitis. – Acute hepatitis ran a 1- to 12-week course in half of the cases. Biochemical evidence of LD was accompanied by the usual clinical manifestations of the disease, but no fulminating course was recorded.

The 31 patients with acute hepatitis included 12 chronic HBsAg carriers. In 11 of these patients, LD and HBs antigenemia appeared simultaneously. In the 12th patient, liver function became abnormal 52 months after HBsAg acquisition, but this acute hepatitis followed within a short time after CMV seroconversion; anti-CMV titers rose from 1/16 to 1/4000.

Intermittent hepatitis. – Eight individuals exhibited several bouts of LD without clinical manifestations; six were chronic HBsAg carriers. In two cases, one episode was coincident with CMV seroconversion, whereas in three other patients seroconversion was conspicuously absent. Four patients experienced two episodes of hepatitis, two had three episodes, one had four and one had six. In seven cases, the episodes followed HBsAg acquisition, and hepatitis preceded it in one patient. The free intervals between LD episodes ranged from 6 to 60 months.

In a chronic HBsAg carrier with a renal transplant 14 months old cholestatic hepatitis appeared, characterized by jaundice, pruritus and increased alkaline phosphatase serum levels (Fig. 13–1). Twenty months after surgery, azathioprine withdrawal was followed by the immediate disappearance of LD. After 22 months without azathioprine, the serum creatinine level was found to be rising slowly but steadily, and cyclophosphamide therapy was instituted. This was followed by prompt recurrence of LD, and cyclophosphamide was withdrawn after eight weeks. Six weeks later, bilirubin, transaminase and alkaline phosphatase serum levels were still elevated. The role of azathioprine in the onset of this cholestatic hepatitis was suggested by the

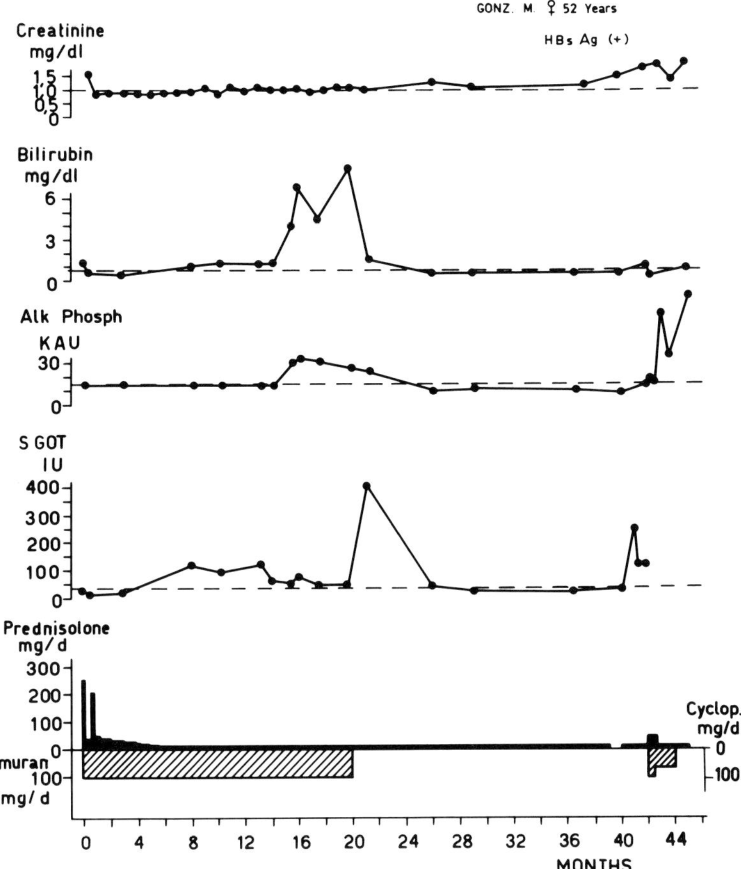

Fig. 13–1.—This 52-year-old woman with analgesic nephropathy is a chronic HBsAg carrier, who was followed for up to 45 months after cadaver kidney transplantation. Abbreviations: *Alk. Phosph. KAU* = serum level of alkaline phosphatase in King-Armstrong units; *SGOT IU* = serum level of transaminase (oxaloacetic) in international units; *cyclop.* = cyclophosphamide.

prompt recovery that followed azathioprine withdrawal, but the relapse precipitated by another, chemically unrelated, immunosuppressive drug may cast some doubt on this assumption.

None of the eight patients with intermittent hepatitis developed portal hypertension during follow-up periods extending from 45 to 70 months after HBsAg acquisition (Table 13–6).

Chronic hepatitis.—In 12 patients, including eight chronic HBsAg carriers, liver function was found to be persistently abnormal for periods exceeding one year. In three of these patients, LD constituted the main cause of death. Portal hypertension was observed in three individuals. Signs of LD disappeared spontaneously in four patients who might be considered as having recovered from liver disease 9 to 14 months later.

In three patients, chronic hepatitis developed two to seven months before the acquisition of HBsAg. In another, signs of LD appeared simultaneously with HBs antigenemia. In the eight other individuals, hepatitis started 1 to 48 months after HBsAg acquisition.

LIVER HISTOPATHOLOGY. — Autopsy was performed in 16 of the 66 HBsAg-positive patients (Table 13–7), including 15 kidney-graft recipients. Most of the microscopic pictures of the liver were difficult to interpret, owing to the circumstances preceding death: widespread tuberculosis, visceral mycoses, acute pancreatitis, *Pneumocystis carinii* or CMV pneumonites, congestive heart failure, cerebrovascular accident or septicemia.

In two patients, death occurred during severe jaundice with widespread hemorrhagic syndrome, and the liver showed mi-

TABLE 13–7. — HISTOPATHOLOGY OF THE LIVER IN 16 HBsAg-POSITIVE AND 9 HBsAg-NEGATIVE PATIENTS WITH HEPATIC DYSFUNCTION

	BIOCHEMICAL AND CLINICAL PICTURE				
HISTOPATHOLOGY	NORMAL LIVER FUNCTION	ACUTE HEPATITIS	INTERMITTENT HEPATITIS	CHRONIC HEPATITIS	TOTAL
HBsAg-positive patients					
Normal or nonsuggestive*	4	4	0	1	9
Acute hepatitis	0	0	0	0	0
Chronic hepatitis	2	2	1	2	7
Cirrhosis	0	0	0	0	0
Total	6	6	1	3	16
HBsAg-negative patients					
Normal or nonsuggestive*	. . .	4	0	0	4
Acute hepatitis	. . .	0	0	0	0
Chronic hepatitis	. . .	2	0	1	3
Cirrhosis	. . .	0	0	2†	2
Total	. . .	6	0	3	9

*Lesions absent or not suggestive of viral hepatitis (steatosis, dextran thesaurismosis, cysts, cholestasis in acute pancreatitis, bacterial hepatitis and granulomas in generalized tuberculosis and in schistosomiasis).

†Besides cirrhosis, in one of those two patients who died from acute leukemia after 10 years of immunosuppressive therapy (two transplants), the liver showed leukemic infiltration.

croscopic evidence of chronic hepatitis. With the exception of these two cases, Table 13–7 demonstrates a poor correlation between the biochemical or clinical picture and the microscopic lesions of the liver. For instance, of six patients with persistently normal liver function two showed lesions typical of chronic hepatitis. On the other hand, the histologic pictures of acute viral hepatitis and cirrhosis were never observed. Finally, of three patients whose hepatic function had been persistently abnormal for more than 12 months, only two showed the typical picture of chronic hepatitis.

HBsAg-Negative Patients

Of the 37 HBsAg-negative patients with LD, 6 remained on dialysis, 25 received one transplant, and 6, two renal transplants (Table 13–1). The mean durations of successive periods of therapy were similar to those observed in HBsAg-positive patients: 14–33 months.

Time characteristics of hepatitis. — *Time of appearance.* — Eleven of the 16 patients whose hepatitis occurred while on dialysis and 13 of the 21 hepatitis patients observed during a transplant period developed the disease during the first year of therapy (Table 13–3).

Duration. — In the HBsAg-positive patients, three patterns of LD were observed: acute, intermittent and chronic. The mean duration of the observation periods following the onset of LD was 21 months (range of 2 to 92 months).

Prevalence. — The prevalence of LD in HBsAg-negative patients varied considerably during the course of the eight-year program. In relation to the numbers of individuals admitted to this program, the incidence ranged between 4% and 10% from 1969 to 1974, but rose to 29% for the 1975–76 period (Table 13–5). In 1975–76, 82% (23 of 28) of the hepatitis cases occurred in HBsAg-negative patients, whereas this fraction reached only 23% (14 of 60) between 1969 and 1974.

Potential viral etiology of hepatitis. — Of the 37 HBsAg-negative individuals with LD, 17 developed CMV seroconversion (Table 13–8). Nine of those 17 patients were also screened for anti-HBs. As anti-HBs was present in two of them, HBV could have been an alternative cause of hepatitis, whereas CMV was probably the culprit in the other seven cases. On the other

TABLE 13-8.—POSSIBLE RESPECTIVE ROLES OF CYTOMEGALOVIRUS AND TYPE B HEPATITIS VIRUS IN THE ETIOLOGY OF HEPATIC DYSFUNCTION IN 267 PATIENTS ADMITTED TO THE DIALYSIS-TRANSPLANTATION PROGRAM FROM 1969 TO 1976

	ACUTE HEPATITIS	INTERMITTENT HEPATITIS	CHRONIC HEPATITIS	TOTAL
Positive CMV-seroconversion *(a)*	10	5	2	17
Negative CMV-seroconversion *(b)*	2	1	2	5
Unknown CMV-seroconversion *(c)*	10	0	5	15
HBsAg-negative patients *(a+b+c)*	22	6	9	37
HBsAg-positive patients *(d)*	31	8	12	51
Total *(a+b+c+d)*	53	14	21	88

hand, in five patients LD was not accompanied by CMV seroconversion (Table 13-8). Three of these individuals were also screened and found to contain no anti-HBs. In the 15 remaining HBsAg-negative individuals with LD, anti-CMV titers were not done (Table 13-8), but in three of those patients who had elaborated anti-HBs, HBV could have been responsible for hepatitis.

THE THREE FORMS OF HEPATITIS.—*Acute hepatitis.*—Acute hepatitis occurred during the dialysis therapy in 13 patients and during a transplant period in 9. The mean time interval between the admission of the patients into the program and the appearance of hepatitis was 17 months (range of 1 to 49 months). Five of the 22 patients developed jaundice, with fever and digestive symptoms. In ten patients, CMV seroconversion occurred. In two cases, anti-CMV titers remained unchanged, and anti-CMV titers were not measured in ten patients.

Intermittent hepatitis.—The initial biochemical abnormalities of LD appeared during dialysis in two patients and during a transplant period in four. Time intervals from the admission into the program to the first evidence of LD ranged from 4 to 114 months (mean of 31 months). Three of the six individuals with intermittent hepatitis experienced jaundice and fever. No patients died from hepatic failure. CMV seroconversion occurred during an LD episode in five patients, and was never observed in one.

Figure 13-2 illustrates the course of one of these patients. The renal graft was well tolerated during the first postoperative year, but several episodes of fever and LD were noted. During the 16th month, persistent fever and the appearance of jaundice led to azathioprine withdrawal. Within 20 days, fever and jaun-

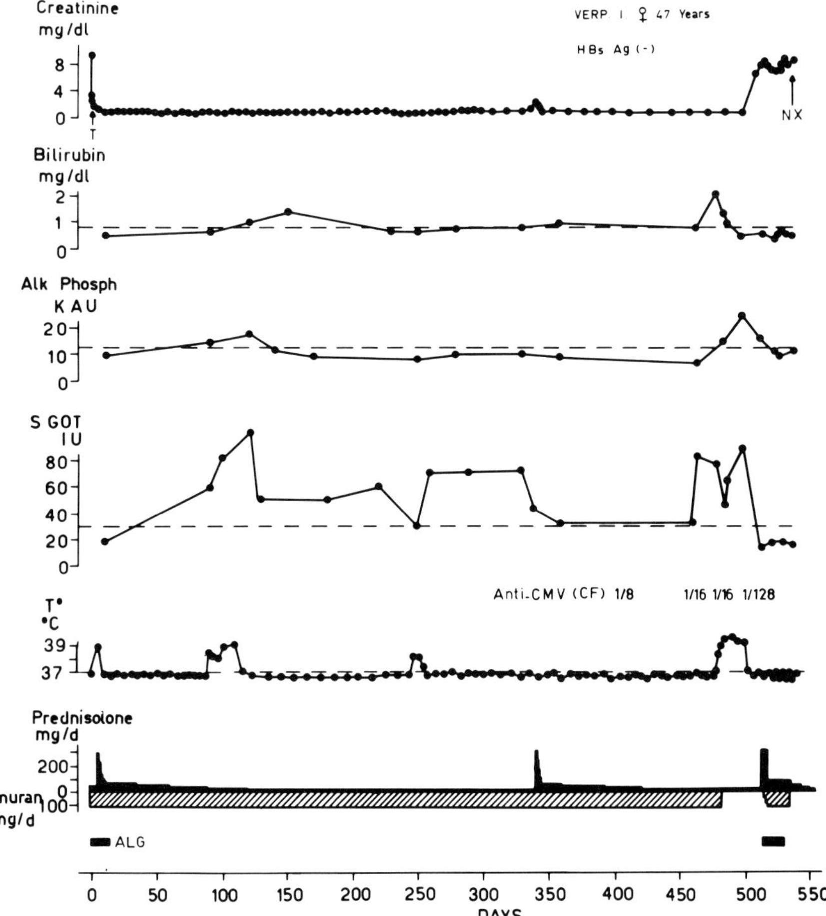

Fig. 13–2.—This HBsAg-negative 42-year-old woman with chronic glomerulone-phritis was followed for up to 560 days after cadaver kidney transplantation. Abbreviations: *Alk. Phosph. KAU* = serum level of alkaline phosphatase in King-Armstrong units; *SGOT IU* = serum level of transaminase (oxaloacetic) in international units. *ALG* = antilymphocyte globulin.

dice disappeared, anti-CMV titers rose from $^{1}/_{8}$ to $^{1}/_{128}$ and acute graft rejection supervened. Despite reinstitution of azathioprine, increase in corticoid doses and antilymphocyte globulin administration, the patient was readmitted to dialysis; now, 22 months later, liver function is normal and anti-CMV titers remain elevated.

Chronic hepatitis.—This serious form of hepatitis was observed in nine patients, one on dialysis and eight during a transplant period. The initial biochemical signs of LD appeared after time intervals ranging from 3 to 105 months (mean of 29 months) following admission.

Five of those nine patients experienced persistent jaundice with weight loss and lassitude, but without fever. One patient apparently recovered after a 14-month course, with liver function remaining normal 9 months afterward. In three cases, hepatitis led to death with jaundice and widespread hemorrhages after courses of 15 to 21 months. In three other patients, death was due to CMV pneumonitis, bacterial endocarditis and acute leukemia, respectively; but portal hypertension occurred after courses of 17 to 34 months in all three cases. In the 8th patient, chronic hepatitis is still present after a 40-month course, with intermittent jaundice, lassitude, weight loss and portal hypertension (Fig. 13–3). In the last case, liver function was found to be abnormal in the early postoperative period of renal transplantation, and remained so by the 9th postoperative month. In three patients, azathioprine was withdrawn for periods ranging from 4 to 28 months, but this did not result in any change in the course of liver disease.

In four patients, anti-CMV titers were assessed regularly, two of them showed seroconversion. The course of one of those patients is depicted in Figure 13–3. Three of the nine HBsAg-negative patients with chronic hepatitis also contained no anti-HBs, and two of them showed no CMV seroconversion, so in those two individuals hepatitis was probably caused by an agent distinct from HBV and CMV.

CMV was considered to be responsible for at least three of the nine cases of chronic hepatitis occurring in HBsAg-negative individuals: CMV seroconversion was observed in the absence of anti-HBs in two, while the third died from CMV pneumonitis, which was verified at autopsy.

LIVER HISTOPATHOLOGY.—As in HBsAg-positive patients, the nine autopsies performed on HBsAg-negative individuals with LD (two on dialysis and seven graft recipients) yielded microscopic pictures of the liver that were difficult to interpret, owing to the various circumstances leading to death: septicemia, cerebrovascular accident, visceral mycoses, CMV pneumonitis, rupture of aneurysmal aorta and acute leukemia. Table 13–7 demonstrates, however, a better correlation between microscopic

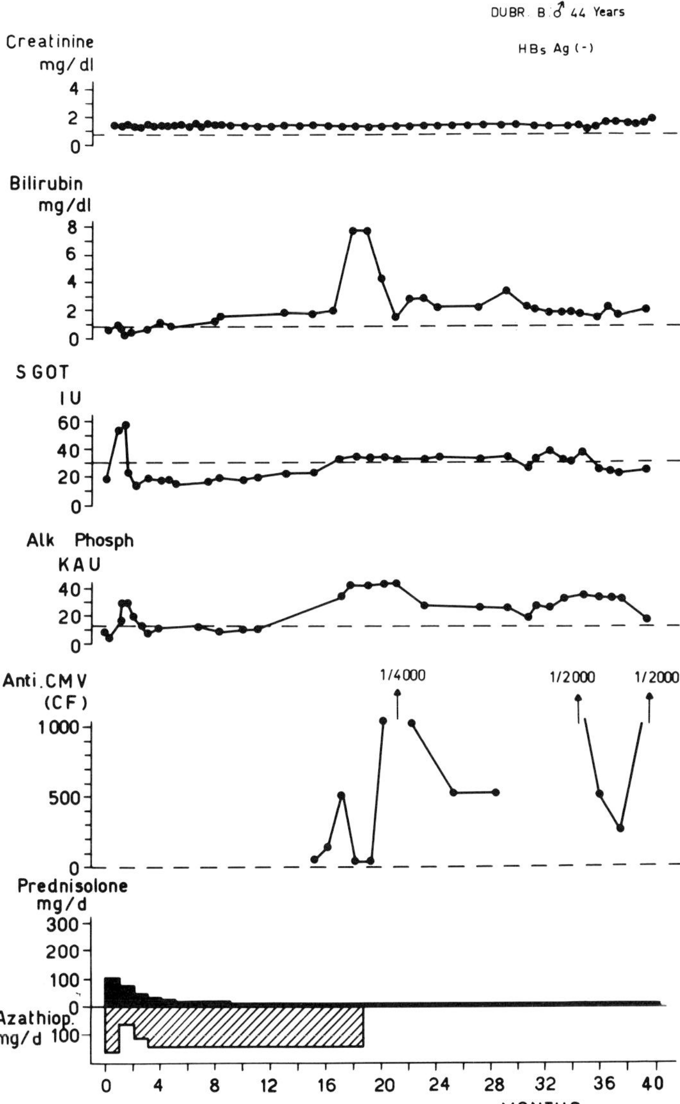

Fig. 13–3.—This HBsAg-negative 44-year-old man with polycystic kidneys was followed for up to 41 months after cadaver kidney transplantation. Abbreviations: *SGOT IU* = transaminase (oxaloacetic) serum level in international units; *Alk. Phosph. KAU* = alkaline phosphatase serum level in King-Armstrong units; *anti-CMV (CF)* = anti-CMV titer as determined by complement fixation; *Azathiop.* = azathioprine.

lesions and clinical or biochemical manifestations of liver disease. Of six patients with a history of acute hepatitis, lesions of chronic hepatitis were observed in two; but in the three patients with clinical and biochemical chronic hepatitis, microscopic examination of the liver demonstrated chronic hepatitis in one and cirrhosis in the two other patients. The first of these patients died from CMV pneumonitis, the second from acute leukemia and the third from hepatic failure.

Discussion

Eighty-eight (33%) of our 267 patients showed evidence of LD. In 53 of those individuals, hepatic abnormalities were transient, but in 21 cases the biochemical and often the clinical courses of liver disease were chronic, and contributed to death in nine patients. Potential causes of LD in patients treated by dialysis and transplantation may be of circulatory, toxic or microbiologic origin. Circulatory factors could be ruled out in most cases, but hepatotoxic drugs, especially azathioprine, could be incriminated.

DRUG HEPATOTOXICITY

The hepatotoxicity of azathioprine has been clearly demonstrated in dogs,[30, 65] although LD was often present only during the initial period of azathioprine administration and usually disappeared thereafter. Azathioprine hepatotoxicity has been reported in a few graft recipients,[43, 64, 83] but as several other factors might also have been operative, these reports are far from convincing.

In one of our patients with persistent LD (Fig. 13–1), azathioprine withdrawal was followed by prompt disappearance of LD; but in this chronic HBsAg carrier, cyclophosphamide administration induced immediate recurrence of liver disease. Rather than a direct toxic action of the immunosuppressive drugs on the liver, this would suggest some disruption in the equilibrium between host and virus.[19, 21, 22, 29]

In another HBsAg-negative patient (Fig. 13–2), azathioprine withdrawal was followed by prompt disappearance of LD but also by CMV seroconversion and by acute rejection of the graft, which had been well tolerated up to that time. In this case, immunosuppressive therapy might have prevented virus elimination, as described in murine CMV infection.

Other drugs, such as oral contraceptives, isoniazid, rifampycin, methyldopa, semisynthetic penicillinase, and resistant penicillins, have also been incriminated as causes of LD in dialyzed and transplanted individuals,[6, 23, 35, 67] but they seemed to play no role in the LD of most of our patients.

Nonviral Infections

Some acute nonviral infections, such as bacterial hepatitis during the course of septicemia, or chronic infections, such as tuberculosis and schistosomiasis, may lead to LD[5]; but such infections were clearly demonstrated in only four patients with liver disease. It should be stressed that three of these individuals had been HBsAg carriers.

Hepatitis B

Due to the high prevalence of HBsAg in patients in dialysis units,[27, 28, 38, 40, 51, 63, 69, 70] HBV is usually considered the main cause of LD occurring in kidney graft recipients.[4, 26, 47, 50, 66] This opinion is not shared by all investigators, however, because a high prevalence of hepatitis often has been observed in this particular population with clear-cut absence of HBs antigenemia.[2, 3, 7, 9, 15, 16, 25, 34, 36, 42, 45, 59, 67, 74, 80]

The present analysis demonstrates that the majority of hepatitis cases in our program occurred between 1969 and 1974 in HBsAg-positive patients. This situation was radically reversed in 1975–76, a period in which hepatitis was recorded in five HBsAg-positive and 23 HBsAg-negative patients. This resulted, of course, from the marked decrease in the prevalence of HBs antigenemia in our unit but, unexpectedly, it was not accompanied by any decrease in the incidence of hepatitis. Factors distinct from HBV must therefore have been responsible for most cases of hepatitis observed in 1975–76 and possibly also during the preceding years, because some HBsAg carriers were demonstrated to be also strongly anti-CMV-positive. Among our 66 HBsAg-positive patients, 15 had persistently normal liver function while 31 developed transient hepatic abnormalities, with chronic hepatitis occurring in 12 patients and leading to death in 3. On the other hand, 9 HBsAg-negative patients developed chronic hepatitis, which contributed to death in 6.

Furthermore, microscopic lesions of the liver correlated poorly with the clinical course of the disease in HBsAg-positive patients, whereas correlation was better for chronic hepatitis occurring in HBsAg-negative patients. Cirrhosis of the liver was demonstrated only in this latter group. On the contrary, Ton That *et al.,*[73] who performed 19 liver biopsies in dialyzed chronic HBsAg carriers, reported microscopic evidence of chronic hepatitis in 16 of these patients. In the Necker Hospital series (450 dialyzed patients with 42 liver biopsies), 9 of the 20 chronic HBsAg carriers presented chronic active hepatitis, whereas patients who had eliminated HBsAg did not show this lesion.[63] Of our own 14 autopsied HBsAg-positive graft recipients, microscopic examination of the liver revealed chronic hepatitis in seven; five of those patients had been chronic HBsAg carriers. Since our pathologic material was obtained from transplanted patients undergoing immunosuppressive therapy, its comparison with the biopsy material obtained by Ton That *et al.*[73] and by Soulier and Jungers[63] from dialyzed patients is impossible, because immunosuppression could alter the course of liver disease. In a previous paper, we reported regression of LD during the early postoperative period in eight kidney transplant recipients.[20]

CYTOMEGALOVIRUS

During the past years, many reports stressed the important role of CMV in the morbidity of renal graft recipients.[1-3, 7, 15, 16, 25, 31, 34, 36, 42, 45, 78, 80] Various pathogenic mechanisms were proposed to explain the high prevalence of CMV infection during the early postoperative course of renal transplantation, such as transmission from ward personnel[34] or from donor to recipient,[8, 32, 34] but studies on murine CMV infection strongly suggest that allogenic stimulation and immunosuppressive therapy are both important. In mice, latent CMV infection was activated either by histoincompatible skin graft[82] or by cyclophosphamide administration.[44] Moreover, CMV was activated in vitro by co-cultivation of infected B-lymphocytes with histoincompatible mouse embryo cells, whereas co-cultivation of lymphoid cells from infected mice with embryo cells from highly inbred histocompatible donors failed to activate CMV.[48] After kidney transplantation in humans, CMV infection was reported to occur more frequently in recipients who were preoperatively CMV-seropositive than in seronegative recipients.[34, 49] Besides, CMV titers remain elevated for several years, while this is never observed in patients who are not submitted to immunosuppressive therapy.[71] These findings would also support the concept of reactivation of latent CMV infection in kidney graft recipients.

In renal transplant recipients, CMV infection may be asymptomatic.[81] It may also produce pneumonitis,[1, 15, 31, 56, 78] encephalitis,[57] acute febrile illness with leukopenia and transplant crisis[34, 41, 61] or hepatitis, with or without the hematologic picture of infectious mononucleosis.[81]

Within a group of 81 kidney graft recipients whose anti-CMV titers had been assessed monthly,[77] 51 showed seroconversion. In 22 individuals, seroconversion remained *asymptomatic*. In four cases, it was followed by *rejection crisis,* as described by Simmons *et al.*[61] In four other patients, seroconversion was followed by permanent *proteinuria.* In 19 patients, CMV seroconversion preceded or accompanied biochemical and sometimes clinical evidence of *hepatic dysfunction.* Since five of those individuals had also been HBsAg carriers, HBV could be incriminated, but CMV could be considered as responsible for liver disease in 16 of 81 kidney recipients. Within the same group of 81 patients, we recorded 12 cases of chronic hepatitis, with 6 possibly caused by CMV.[77]

In the present series, hepatitis was coincidental with CMV seroconversion in 17 cases. In two of these patients, hepatitis ran a chronic course. In a third case of chronic hepatitis, anti-CMV titers were not available, but the patient died from CMV pneumonitis, which was confirmed at autopsy.

Our experience is thus similar to that of many investigators:[2, 3, 7, 15, 16, 25, 34, 36, 42, 45, 80] CMV may well be responsible for LD in many kidney graft recipients. Besides, if 21 (7%) of the patients with kidney transplants who were surveyed in the present report developed chronic hepatitis, nine of these were persistently HBsAg-negative patients and CMV could reasonably be incriminated in three, although, according to Toghill *et al.*,[72] CMV would not produce chronic disease of the liver.

Within this group of 21 patients, chronic hepatitis contributed to death in three HBsAg-positive and in six HBsAg-negative patients. Our observations are thus at variance with the recent report of Pirson et al.,[50] who recorded 10 deaths from liver disease among 61 HBsAg-positive kidney recipients, and 2 deaths from liver disease among 60 HBsAg-negative recipients. The presence of HBs antigenemia in a given patient with LD does not necessarily prove that HBV is responsible for the observed hepatic disease, because in the course of our own dialysis-transplantation program, LD was still observed in 30% of our patients despite a marked fall in the prevalence of HBs antigenemia. Moreover, only 25% of HBsAg-positive blood donors demonstrated a rise in transaminase serum levels, and up to 20% healthy HBsAg carriers have been observed in some Far East populations.[62] Finally, London et al. recorded more marked and longer increases in transaminase serum levels in HBsAg-positive than in HBsAg-negative hemodialyzed patients;[40] the overall mortality, however, was identical in both groups and no patient died from liver disease. This latter observation would cast some doubt on the major role attributed to HBV in the mortality of kidney graft recipients.[50]

OTHER VIRUSES

Besides hepatitis A and hepatitis B viruses, the occurrence of hepatitis C virus has been proposed as a factor in liver disease.[17, 18, 24, 53, 79] Posttransfusion and postinoculation hepatites were reported in cases where HAV, HBV, EBV and CMV could be excluded.[17, 18, 24, 33, 53] Similar data were obtained in endemic hepatitis in Costa Rica.[79] As is the case with hepatitis B, hepatitis C could presumably become chronic.[24, 33] An epidemic of EBV hepatitis was described in a hemodialysis unit,[14] while seroepidemiologic studies conducted in 15 dialysis units excluded HAV as a significant cause of LD in dialyzed patients.[68]

Mosley et al. reported in detail on three patients with a history of multiple self-injections who experienced three or four bouts of acute hepatitis.[46] Some LD episodes occurring in a single patient were allegedly due not only to HAV or HBV but also to HCV, and possibly to a fourth unidentified virus. Patients treated by hemodialysis and kidney transplantation are exposed to numerous blood transfusions and drug injections. They would consequently be particularly prone to develop multiple episodes of LD caused by different viruses in the course of follow-up periods extending up to ten years, as reported here.

Summary

Liver dysfunction was observed in 33% of patients treated by hemodialysis and kidney transplantation. Fifty-eight percent of these cases of hepatitis occurred in patients with past or present HBs antigenemia, and 77% of HBsAg-positive patients showed evidence of LD. However, during the course of a program conducted from 1969 to 1976 and involving 267 patients, the decrease in the prevalence of HBs antigenemia observed during the last two years did not lead to any reduction in LD incidence.

In a small number of patients, potentially hepatotoxic drugs could be incriminated, but in our experience azathioprine never appeared to be involved. In a few patients, LD was due to granulomatous disease of the liver, such as tuberculosis and schistosomiasis.

Twenty-one (7%) of the 267 patients at risk developed chronic hepatitis, which contributed to death in nine patients. In 12 cases (three deaths), this form of hepatitis occurred in HBsAg-positive patients, and in nine cases (six deaths), in HBsAg-negative patients. In three of these latter individuals, cytomegalovirus could be incriminated.

Routine monthly screening for CMV in kidney recipients confirmed the high incidence of this viral infection in such patients. Studies on murine CMV infection have demonstrated that this infection can be enhanced by histoincompatible graft or by cyclophosphamide in a model that is very close to the kidney recipient. As in mice, CMV infection in kidney recipients apparently results from reactivation of a latent infection. It seems to play a major role in the LD observed and could apparently lead to chronic hepatitis and even to cirrhosis of the liver.

Finally, the occurrence of LD in HBsAg-, anti-HBs- and anti-CMV-negative patients would suggest the responsibility of other viruses for the pathogenesis of liver disease in patients treated by hemodialysis and kidney transplantation. Besides Epstein-Barr virus, other viruses, such as hepatitis C virus, should be thoroughly scrutinized.

Acknowledgments

This work was supported by the Fonds de la Recherche Scientifique Médicale (contract no. 1208) and by the Fondation Universitaire Alice et David van Buuren in Brussels.

References

1. Andersen, H. K., and Spencer, E. S.: Cytomegalovirus infection among renal allograft recipients, Acta Med. Scand. 186:7, 1969.
2. Armstrong, D., Balakrishnan, S. L., Steger, L., Yu, B., and Stenzel, K. H.: Cytomegalovirus infections with viremia following renal transplantation, Arch. Intern. Med. 127:111, 1971.
3. Armstrong, J., Evans, A., Rao, N., and Ho, M.: Viral infections in renal transplant recipients, Infect. Immun. 14:970, 1976.
4. Aronoff, A., Gault, M. H., Huang, S. N., Lal, S., Wu, K. T., Moinuddin, M. D., Spence, L., and MacLean, L. D.: Hepatitis with Australia antigenemia following renal transplantation, Can. Med. Assoc. J. 108:43, 1973.
5. Beeson, P. B., and McDermott, W.: *Textbook of Medicine* (14th ed.; Philadelphia: W. B. Saunders Co., 1975).
6. Berger, M., and Potter, D. E.: Pitfall in diagnosis of viral hepatitis on haemodialysis unit, Lancet 2:95, 1977.
7. Berne, T. V., Chatterjee, S. N., Craig, J. R., Redeker, A. G., and Payne, J. E.: Hepatic dysfunction in recipients of renal allografts, Surg. Gynecol. Obstet. 141:171, 1975.
8. Betts, R. F., Freeman, R. B., Douglas, R. G., Jr., Talley, T. E., and Rundell, B.: Transmission of cytomegalovirus infection with renal allograft, Kidney Int. 8:387, 1975.
9. Briggs, W. A., Lazarus, J. M., Birtch, A. G., Hampers, C. L., Hager, E. B., and Merrill, J. P.: Hepatitis affecting hemodialysis and transplant patients, Arch. Intern. Med. 132:21, 1973.
10. Chatterjee, S. N.: Hepatitis and renal transplants, N. Engl. J. Med. 296:1171, 1977.
11. Chatterjee, S. N., Payne, J. E., Bischel, M. D., Redeker, A. G., and Berne, T. V.: Successful renal transplantation in patients positive for hepatitis B antigen, N. Engl. J. Med. 291:62, 1974.
12. Claes, G., Blohme, I., and Engeset, J.: Simplifications in the use of continuous perfusion for renal preservation, Transplant. Proc. 6:261, 1974.
13. Collins, G. M., Bravo-Shugarman, M., and Terasaki, P. I.: Kidney preservation for transportation. Initial perfusion and 30 hours' ice storage, Lancet 2:1219, 1969.
14. Corey, L., Stamm, W. E., Feorino, P. M., Jabryan, J. A., Weseley, M. B., Gregg, M. B., and Solangi, K.: HBsAg negative hepatitis in a hemodialysis unit, N. Engl. J. Med. 293:1273, 1975.
15. Coulson, A. S., Lucas, Z. J., Condy, M., and Cohn, R.: Forty-day fever. An epidemic of cytomegalovirus disease in a renal transplant population, West. J. Med. 120:1, 1974.
16. Craighead, J. E., Hanshaw, J. B., and Carpenter, C. B.: Cytomegalovirus infection after renal allotransplantation, J.A.M.A. 201:725, 1967.
17. Dienstag, J. L., Alaama, A., Mosley, J. W., Redeker, A. G., and Purcell, R. H.: Etiology of sporadic hepatitis B surface antigen – negative hepatitis, Ann. Intern. Med. 87:1, 1977.
18. Dienstag, J. L., Feinstone, S. M., Purcell, R. H., Wong, D. C., Alter, H. J., and Holland, P. V.: Non-A, non-B post-transfusion hepatitis, Lancet 1:560, 1977.
19. Dudley, F. J., Fox, R. A., and Sherlock, S.: Cellular immunity and hepatitis – associated Australia antigen liver disease, Lancet 1:723, 1972.

20. Dusart, D., De Roy, G., Thiry, L., Clinet, G., and Toussaint, C.: L'hépatite de dialyse. Effets de la greffe rénale, Acta Gastroenterol. Belg. 35:357, 1972.
21. Eddleston, A. L. W. F., and Williams, R.: Inadequate antibody response to HBAg or suppressor T-cell defect in development of active chronic hepatitis, Lancet 2:1543, 1974.
22. Edgington, T. S., and Chisari, F. V.: Immunological aspects of hepatitis B virus infection, Am. J. Med. Sci. 270:213, 1975.
23. Evans, D. B., Millard, P. R., and Herbertson, B. M.: Hepatic dysfunction associated with renal transplantation, Lancet 2:929, 1968.
24. Feinstone, S. M., Kapikian, A. Z., Purcell, R. H., Alter, H. J., and Holland, P. V.: Transfusion associated hepatitis not due to viral hepatitis type A or B, N. Engl. J. Med. 292:767, 1975.
25. Fiala, M., Payne, J. E., Berne, T. V., Moore, T., Henle, W., Montgomerie, J., Chatterjee, N. S., and Guze, L.: Epidemiology of cytomegalovirus infection after transplantation and immune depression, J. Infect. Dis. 132:421, 1975.
26. Fine, R. N., Malekzadeh, M. H., Pennisi, A. J., Uittenbogaart, C. H., Ettenger, R. B., Landing, B. H., and Wright, H. T. Jr.: HBs antigenemia in renal allograft recipients, Ann. Surg. 185:411, 1977.
27. Fine, R. N., Malekzadeh, M., and Wright, H. T.: Hepatitis B in a pediatric hemodialysis unit, J. Pediatr. 86:349, 1975.
28. Garibaldi, R. A., Forrest, J. N., Bryan, J. A., Hansow, B. F., and Dismukes, W. E.: Hemodialysis – associated hepatitis, J.A.M.A. 225:384, 1973.
29. Giustino, V., Dudley, F. J., and Sherlock, S.: Thymus-dependent lymphocyte function in patients with hepatitis-associated antigen, Lancet 2:850, 1972.
30. Haxhe, J. J., Alexandre, G. P. J., and Kestens, P. J.: The effect of imuran and asazerine on liver function tests in the dog, Arch. Int. Pharmacodyn. Ther. 168:366, 1967.
31. Hill, R. B., Jr., Rowlands, D. T., Jr., and Rifkind, D.: Infectious pulmonary disease in patients receiving immunosuppressive therapy for organ transplantation, N. Engl. J. Med. 271:1021, 1964.
32. Ho, M., Suwansirikul, S., Dowling, J. N., Youngblood, L. A., and Armstrong, J. A.: The transplanted kidney as a source of cytomegalovirus infection, N. Engl. J. Med. 293:1109, 1975.
33. Hoofnagle, J. H., Gerety, R. J., Tabor, E., Feinstone, S. M., Barker, L. F., and Purcell, R. H.: Transmission of non-A, non-B hepatitis, Ann. Intern. Med. 87:14, 1977.
34. Howard, R. J., Kalis, J. M., Balfour, H. H., Jr., Marker, S. M., Simmons, R. L., and Najarian, J. S.: Viral infections in kidney donors and recipients: a prospective study, Transplant. Proc. 9:113, 1977.
35. Ireland, P., Rashid, A., Von Lichtenberg, F., Cavallo, T., and Merrill, J. P.: Liver disease in kidney transplant patients receiving azathioprine, Arch. Intern. Med. 132:29, 1973.
36. Kanich, R. E., and Craighead, J. E.: Cytomegalovirus infection and cytomegalic inclusion disease in renal homotransplant recipients, Am. J. Med. 40:874, 1966.
37. Kinnaert, P., Vereerstraeten, P., Toussaint, C., and Van Geertruyden, J.: Nine years experience with internal arteriovenous fistulas for haemodialysis: a study of some factors influencing the results, Br. J. Surg. 64:242, 1977.
38. London, W. T., Difigli, A. M., Sutnick, A. I., and Blumberg, B. J.: An epidemic of hepatitis in a chronic hemodialysis unit. Australia antigen and differences in host response, N. Engl. J. Med. 281:571, 1969.
39. London, W. T., Drew, J. S., Blumberg, B. S., Grossman, R. A., and Lyons, P. J.: Association of graft survival with host response to hepatitis B infection in patients with kidney transplants, N. Engl. J. Med. 296:241, 1977.
40. London, W. T., Drew, J. S., Lustbader, E. D., Werner, B. G., and Blumberg, B. S.: Host responses to hepatitis B infection in patients in a chronic hemodialysis unit, Kidney Int. 12:51, 1977.

41. Lopez, C., Simmons, R. L., Mauer, S. M., Najarian, J. S., and Good, R. A.: Association of renal allograft rejection with virus infections, Am. J. Med. 56:280, 1974.
42. Luby, P., Burnett, W., Hull, A., Ware, A., Shorey, J., and Peters, P.: Relationship between cytomegalovirus and hepatic function abnormalities in the period after renal transplant, J. Infect. Dis. 129:511, 1974.
43. Malekzadeh, M. H., Grushkin, C. M., Wright, H. T., and Fine, R. N.: Hepatic dysfunction after renal transplantation in children, J. Pediatr. 81:279, 1972.
44. Mayo, D. R., Armstrong, J. A., and Ho, M.: Reactivation of murine cytomegalovirus by cyclophosphamide, Nature 267:721, 1977.
45. Millard, P. R., Herbertson, B. M., Nagington, J., and Evans, D. B.: The morphological consequences and the significance of cytomegalovirus infection in renal transplant patients, Q. J. Med. 42:585, 1973.
46. Mosley, J. W., Redeker, A. G., Feinstone, S. M., and Purcell, R. H.: Multiple hepatitis viruses in multiple attacks of acute viral hepatitis, N. Engl. J. Med. 296:75, 1977.
47. Nagington, J., Cossart, Y. E., and Cohen, B. J.: Reactivation of hepatitis B after transplantation operations, Lancet 1:558, 1977.
48. Olding, L. B., Jensen, F. C., and Oldstone, M. B. A.: Pathogenesis of cytomegalovirus infection. I. Activation of virus from bone marrow-derived lymphocytes by in vitro allogenic reaction, J. Exp. Med. 141:561, 1975.
49. Pien, F. D., Smith, T. F., Anderson, C. F., Webel, M. L., and Taswell, H. F.: Herpesviruses in renal transplant recipients, Transplantation 16:489, 1973.
50. Pirson, Y., Alexandre, G. P. J., and van Ypersele de Strihou, C.: Long-term effect of HBs antigenemia on prognosis of renal transplantation, N. Engl. J. Med. 296:194, 1977.
51. Polakoff, S., Cossart, Y., and Tillett, H.: Hepatitis in dialysis units in the United Kingdom, Br. Med. J. 3:94, 1972.
52. Ponticelli, C., De Vecchi, A., Cantaluppi, A., Tarantino, A., and De Franchis, R.: Hepatitis and renal transplantation, N. Engl. J. Med. 296:1170, 1977.
53. Prince, A. M., Brotman, B., Grady, G. F., Kuhns, W. J., Hazzi, C., Levine, R. W., and Millian, S. J.: Long-incubation post-transfusion hepatitis without serological evidence of exposure to hepatitis B virus, Lancet 2:241, 1974.
54. Purcell, R. H., Feinstone, F. M., and Kapikian, A. Z.: in Greenwalt, T. J., and Jameson, G. A. (eds.): *Transmissible Disease and Blood Transfusion* (New York: Grune & Stratton, 1975), p. 11.
55. Rashid, A., Sengar, D., Couture, R., Jindal, S., and Harris, J.: Hepatitis and renal transplantation, N. Engl. J. Med. 296:1170, 1977.
56. Rifkind, D., Goodman, N., and Hill, R. B., Jr.: Significance of cytomegalovirus infection in renal transplant recipients, Ann. Intern. Med. 66:1116, 1967.
57. Schneck, S. A.: Neuropathological features of human organ transplantation. I. Probable cytomegalovirus infection, J. Neuropathol. Exp. Neurol. 24:415, 1965.
58. Sever, J. C.: Application of a microtechnique to viral serological investigations, J. Immunol. 88:320, 1962.
59. Shons, A. R., Simmons, R. L., Kjellstrand, C. M., Buselmeier, T. J., and Najarian, J. S.: Renal transplantation in patients with Australia antigenemia, Am. J. Surg. 128:699, 1974.
60. Shons, A. R., Simmons, R. L., Kjellstrand, C. M., and Najarian, J. S.: Hepatitis and renal transplants, N. Engl. J. Med. 296:1169, 1977.
61. Simmons, R. L., Lopez, C., Mauer, S. M., Park, B., Najarian, J. S., and Good, R. A.: Viral infections and rejection crises in transplanted patients, in *International Course on Transplantation Lyon 1973* (Villeurbanne: Simep, 1974), pp. 51–58.
62. Soulier, J. P.: Données essentielles concernant l'antigène HB, in Mery, J. Ph. (ed.): *Hépatite à virus B et hémodialyse* (Paris: Flammarion, 1975), pp. 11–18.
63. Soulier, J. P., and Jungers, P.: L'hépatite à virus B dans les centres d'hémodialyse, in Grunfeld, J. P. (ed.): *Actualités Néphrologiques de l'Hôpital Necker 1976* (Paris: Flammarion, 1976), pp. 411–44.

64. Sparberg, M., Simon, N., and Del Greco, F.: Intrahepatic cholestasis due to azathioprine, Gastroenterology 57:439, 1969.
65. Starzl, T. E., Marchioro, T. L., Porter, K. A., Taylor, P. D., Faris, T. D., Herrmann, T. J., Hlad, C. J., and Waddell, W. R.: Factors determining short- and long-term survival after orthoptic liver homotransplantation in the dog, Surgery 58:131, 1965.
66. Steiness, I. B., and Skinhøj, P.: Hepatitis associated antigen: elimination from a dialysis unit and persistence in renal transplant recipients, Acta. Pathol. Microbiol. Scand. [B] 79:721, 1971.
67. Strom, T. B., and Merrill, J. P.: Hepatitis B, transfusions and renal transplantation, N. Engl. J. Med. 296:225, 1977.
68. Szmuness, W., Dienstag, J. L., Purcell, R. H., Prince, A. M., Stevens, C. E., and Levine, R. W.: Hepatitis type A and hemodialysis. A seroepidemiologic study in 15 U.S. centers, Ann. Intern. Med. 87:8, 1977.
69. Szmuness, W., Prince, A. M., Grady, G., Mann, M., Levine, R., Friedman, E., Jacobs, M., Josephson, A., Ribot, S., Shapiro, F., Stenzel, K., Suki, W., and Vyas, G.: Hepatitis B infection. A point-prevalence study in 15 U.S. hemodialysis centers, J.A.M.A. 227:901, 1974.
70. Tacquet, A., Lelievre, G., and Wambergue, F.: Résultats d'une enquête sur l'hépatite à virus B dans les centres d'hémodialyses français. Fréquence, aspects cliniques et évolutifs, in Mery, J. Ph. (ed.): *Hépatite à Virus B et Hémodialyse* (Paris: Flammarion, 1975), pp. 19–31.
71. The, T. H., Andersen, H. K., Spencer, E. S., and Klein, G.: Antibodies against cytomegalovirus-induced early antigens (CMV-EA) in immunosuppressed renal-allograft recipients, Clin. Exp. Immunol. 28:502, 1977.
72. Toghill, P. J., Williams, R., and Stern, H.: Cytomegalovirus infection in chronic liver disease, Gastroenterology 56:956, 1969.
73. Ton That, H., Duffaut, M., Orfila, C., Durand, D., Dupuy, P., Rumeau, J. L., and Suc, J. M.: Hépatite des dialysés chroniques. Corrélation anatomobiologiques, rapport entre l'antigène Australia et les résultats de l'immunofluorescence directe des biopsies hépatiques, in Mery, J. Ph. (ed.): *Hépatite à Virus B et Hémodialyse* (Paris: Flammarion, 1975), pp. 33–44.
74. Torisu, M., Yokoyama, T., Amemyia, H., Kohler, P. F., Schroter, G., Martineau, G., Penn, I., Palmer, W., Halgrimson, C. G., Putnam, C. W., and Starzl, T. E.: Immunosuppression liver injury, and hepatitis in renal, hepatic and cardiac homograft recipients: with particular reference to the Australia antigen, Ann. Surg. 174:620, 1971.
75. Toussaint, C., Kinnaert, P., Vereerstraeten, P., Buchin, R., Tagnon, A., and Van Geertruyden, J.: Sémiologie de la crise de rejet du premier trimestre de la greffe rénale. Influence de l'administration de globuline antilymphocytaire, in *Cours International de Transplantation Lyon 1971* (Villeurbanne: Simep, 1972), pp. 221 ff.
76. Toussaint, C., Thiry, L., Kinnaert, P., Clinet, G., Vereerstraeten, P., and Van Geertruyden, J.: Prognostic significance of hepatitis B antigenemia in kidney transplantation, Nephron 17:335, 1976.
77. Toussaint, C., Thiry, L., Vereerstraeten, P., Kinnaert, P., Cappel, R., Dupont, E., and Van Geertruyden, J.: Clinical aspects of infections due to herpesviruses in renal transplant recipients, in *International Course on Transplantation and Clinical Immunology, Lyon 1977* (Amsterdam: Excerpta Medica, 1978), in press.
78. Vereerstraeten, P., De Koster, J. P., Vereerstraeten, J., Kinnaert, P., Van Geertruyden, J., and Toussaint, C.: Pulmonary infections after kidney transplantation, Proc. Eur. Dial. Transplant Assoc. 11:300, 1975.
79. Villarejos, V. M., Kirsten, A., Visona, P. H., Eduarte, C. A., Provost, P. J., and Hilleman, M. R.: Evidence for viral hepatitis other than type A or type B among persons in Costa Rica, N. Engl. J. Med. 293:1350, 1975.
80. Ware, A. J., Luby, J. P., Eigenbrodt, E. H., Long, D. L., and Hull, A. R.: Spectrum of liver disease in renal transplant recipients, Gastroenterology 68:755, 1975.

81. Weller, T. H.: The cytomegaloviruses: ubiquitous agents with protean clinical manifestations, N. Engl. J. Med. 285:203, 267, 1971.
82. Wu, B. C., Dowling, J. N., Armstrong, J. A., and Ho, M.: Enhancement of mouse cytomegalovirus infection during host-versus-graft reaction, Science 190:56, 1975.
83. Zarday, Z., Veith, F. J., Gliedman, M. L., and Soberman, R.: Irreversible liver damage after azathioprine, J.A.M.A. 222:690, 1972.

PART IV

CURRENT ISSUES IN NEPHROLOGY

14

Use of Angiotensin Antagonists in Experimental and Human Renovascular Hypertension

MORTON H. MAXWELL, M.D.

University of California, and Hypertension Division,
Cedars-Sinai Medical Center, Los Angeles, California

The availability of specific inhibitors of the renin-angiotensin system has permitted a direct approach to studying the role of this system in various pathologic states.[80] In this chapter, I shall present a summary of the use of angiotensin antagonists in experimental and human renovascular hypertension, with the aim of answering the question: Is renovascular hypertension renin-mediated? I shall also assess the present and possible future role of angiotensin antagonists in the diagnosis of human renovascular hypertension.

Renin-Angiotensin Metabolism and Sites of Action of Angiotensin Antagonists

Renin, a proteolytic enzyme formed in the kidney, enters the bloodstream, where it acts on its substrate, angiotensinogen, an α-globulin synthesized by the liver, to produce the decapeptide,

Some of the studies reported in this article were supported by USPHS RR-865 and the University Medical Research Foundation.

297

angiotensin I (A-I). Although A-I has been considered biologically inactive, i.e., a prohormone, studies with converting enzyme
inhibitors have suggested that the decapeptide can stimulate
the release of catecholamines from the adrenal medulla,[76] act on
the central nervous system to increase blood pressure and induce thirst,[25, 87] and act on the same receptor site as angiotensin
II (A-II) in isolated smooth muscle.[68] A-I is hydrolyzed in the
pulmonary circulation by a converting enzyme, which cleaves
off the carboxyl-terminal dipeptide, His-Leu, to form the octa-
peptide, A-II. A-II is the most potent endogenously produced
vasoconstrictor, has a positive inotropic action on heart muscle
and has important effects on the sympathetic and central nervous systems.[29, 85] Removal of the N-terminal aspartyl residue of
A-II by aminopeptidases yields the heptapeptide, (des-asp^1) angiotensin II, or angiotensin III (A-III). It is possible that A-III,
which has little vascular action, is the primary stimulus for aldosterone release from the adrenal glands.[5, 28, 77, 78] The remaining by-products of angiotensin breakdown appear to be physio-
logically inert.

It is apparent that there are several sites for selective inhibition of the renin-angiotensin system.[69] Several types of antago-

Fig. 14–1. — Renin-angiotensin metabolism and sites of action of angiotensin antagonists.

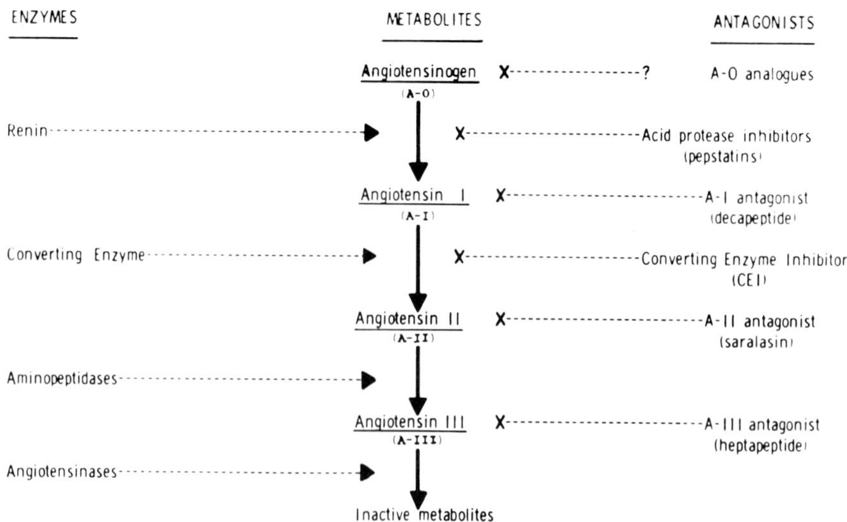

nists that have been discovered are shown in Figure 14–1. (1) *Pepstatins* inhibit acid proteases, including the proteolytic action of renin[66, 67]; since pepstatins are not specific for renin and have not been used in experimental or clinical renovascular hypertension, they will not be considered further. (2) *A-I analogues* have been designed that compete with A-I at its receptor sites.[68, 74] The presently available A-I antagonists are 100 times less potent than their comparable A-II analogues in pressor assays,[59] and they have not been used in studying renovascular hypertension. (3) Small peptides, originally isolated from snake venom,[23, 71] have been found to inhibit the conversion of A-I to A-II.[3, 24, 34] These *converting enzyme inhibitors* (CEI) also inhibit the breakdown of bradykinins, and have been called bradykinin-potentiating factors (BPF). There is considerable controversy in the interpretation of these two simultaneous effects when CEI is utilized in studying experimental or clinical hypertension.[99] The most widely used CEI in testing experimental and clinical hypertension has been SQ 20881. (4) *A-II antagonists* have been shown to inhibit the vascular, enzymatic and central nervous system (CNS) effects of both A-I and A-II.[69] It is believed that the C-terminal amino acid of A-II carries the code necessary for receptor binding.[9] Substitution in position 8 with aliphatic amino acids produces specific competitive antagonists of A-II.[45, 84] Additional variations in position 1 increase resistance to degradative enzymes. Sar^1-Ala^8-angiotensin II (saralasin), first described by Pals *et al.*,[75] has been the most widely used A-II antagonist in the study of hypertension.

The majority of studies of renovascular hypertension, experimental or clinical, have used saralasin or other 1,8-substituted A-II analogues. A smaller number have used CEI. Before the development of synthetic analogues of A-II, a number of studies were performed using immunization with renin[18, 96] or angiotensin.[14, 21, 41, 51] Because of differences in methodology and lack of specificity of these antibodies as compared with currently available angiotensin antagonists,[72, 93] these earlier studies will not be included in this review.

Peripheral and Renal Vein Renin Measurements

Before the synthesis of specific angiotensin analogues, the contribution of the renin-angiotensin system to renovascular hypertension could be judged only by the measurement of peripheral renin activity (PRA) and renal vein renin values. As is the case in chronic experimental renovascular hypertension,[73] in human renovascular hypertension PRA levels often may be within so-called normal limits.[42] This apparent dilemma led to the theory that although renovascular hypertension is initiated by increased renin secretion, a different mechanism is involved in its chronic phase.[11, 73] Rapid lowering of blood pressure following nephrectomy or a corrective vascular operation in unilateral renal artery stenosis, however, indicates that it is renal-mediated, even in its chronic form.

In a recent study in our laboratory of chronic two-kidney renovascular hypertension in the dog, the animal model that most closely resembles the human disorder, we found that even when PRA had returned to within control levels, all hypertensive animals demonstrated significantly increased ipsilateral renal renin secretion that greatly exceeded the combined renin secretion from both kidneys prior to renal artery constriction.[50] Since animal and human studies have demonstrated progressive increases in vascular responsiveness to renin and angiotensin over a prolonged period of time,[19, 48, 65, 86] we interpreted these results to indicate that both the acute[61] and chronic[50] phases of renovascular hypertension in the dog are renal-dependent and probably mediated through a renin mechanism.

In human renovascular hypertension, PRA levels have been found to be elevated in only 56% of 109 cases.[58] Therefore, in recent years renal vein renin value determinations have been widely used to identify the functional significance of renal artery stenosis, i.e., to identify the hypertensive patient most likely to benefit from a corrective operation. Because the numerical definitions of abnormal renal vein renin ratios used by different investigators varied widely[35, 39, 89, 95] and were based largely on retrospective observations of patients in whom an arbitrary renal vein renin ratio was itself used as an indication for operative intervention, we designed prospective studies to analyze the symmetry of renal vein renin values in large populations of patients with essential hypertension[63] and with unilateral renal artery stenosis.[62] In a sample of 227 patients with mild to moderate essential hypertension,[63] the cumulative renal vein renin ratios approximated half of a bell-shaped probability curve (Fig. 14-2). The widely used critical renal vein renin ratio of 1.5 was

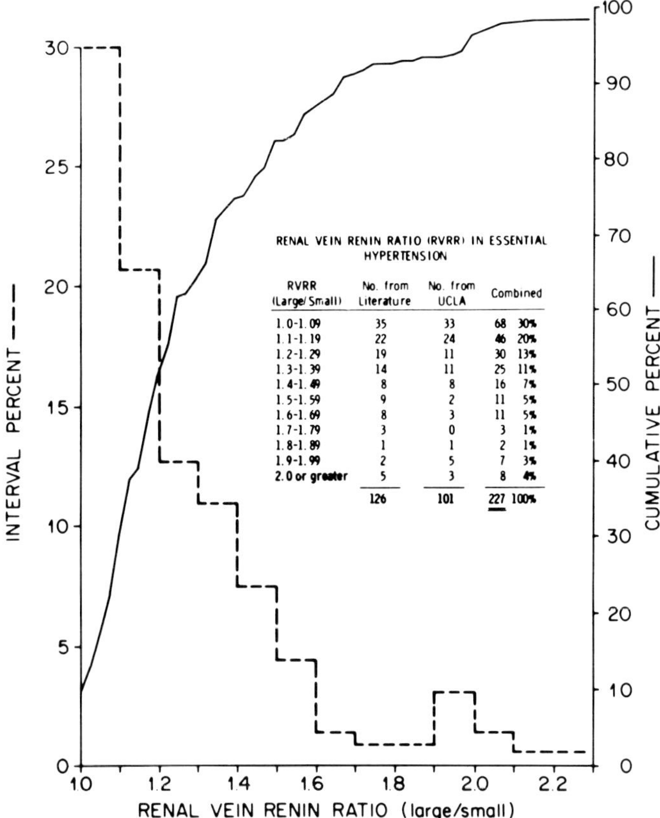

RVRR (Large/Small)	No. from Literature	No. from UCLA	Combined	
1.0-1.09	35	33	68	30%
1.1-1.19	22	24	46	20%
1.2-1.29	19	11	30	13%
1.3-1.39	14	11	25	11%
1.4-1.49	8	8	16	7%
1.5-1.59	9	2	11	5%
1.6-1.69	8	3	11	5%
1.7-1.79	3	0	3	1%
1.8-1.89	1	1	2	1%
1.9-1.99	2	5	7	3%
2.0 or greater	5	3	8	4%
	126	101	227	100%

Fig. 14–2. – Frequency distribution of renal vein renin ratios *(RVRR)*, large-small, in patients with essential hypertension. Dashed line indicates interval percentages for each *RVRR*, derived from inset table. Solid line indicates cumulative percent for each *RVRR*. (From Maxwell, M. H., *et al.*: Renal vein renin in essential hypertension, J. Lab. Clin. Med. 86:901, 1975. Used by permission.)

located at the 81% confidence level, i.e., 19% of patients with essential hypertension had renal vein renin ratios greater than 1.5. This statistical analysis showed that a renal vein renin ratio of 2.0 or higher falls beyond the 95% confidence level, and may therefore be considered abnormal in patients with essential hypertension.

PRA and renal vein renin levels were then analyzed in 66 patients with unilateral renal artery stenosis, *all of whom underwent corrective surgery regardless of renin results.*[62] Fifty-three percent of those with confirmed renovascular hypertension (marked reduction of elevated blood pressure following corrective surgery) had renal vein renin ratios of less than 2.0, i.e., within the 95% confidence level for the large control group with essential hypertension.[63] Renal vein renin ratios thus represent a continuum in both populations, with no arbitrary value lower than 2.0 being statistically discriminative. Thirty-four patients with clearly lateralizing renin data benefited by operation,[62] but 23 additional patients with nonlateralizing data also benefited (Fig. 14–3). No proposed scheme or mathematical equation for

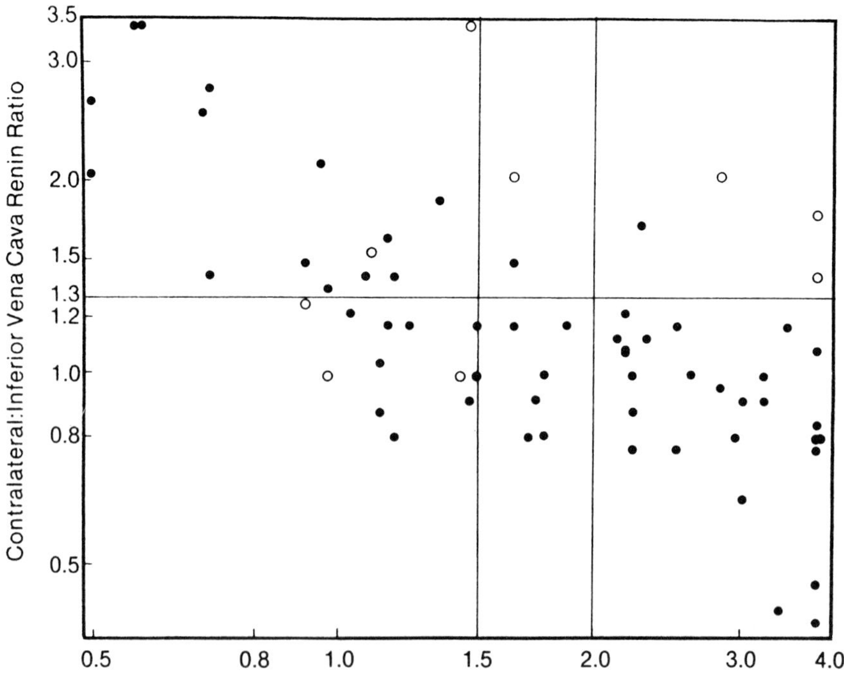

Fig. 14–3. – Predictive value of renin ratios in 66 hypertensive patients with unilateral renal artery stenosis. Lines are placed at proposed discrimination ratios of 1.5 and 2.0 on the horizontal axis, and at 1.3 on the vertical axis. Closed circles represent cured-improved patients (no. = 57). Open circles represent operative failures (no. = 9). All patients with both ipsilateral hypersecretion (renal vein renin ratio of 1.5 or higher) and contralateral suppression (contralateral-caval ratio of 1.3 or lower) (no. = 34) were cured or improved by operation. The nine operative failures and an additional 23 patients cured or improved by operation appear in all other sections of the figure. (Maxwell, M. H., *et al.*: Predictive value of renin determinations in renal artery stenosis, J.A.M.A. 238:2617, 1977. Copyright 1977, American Medical Association. Used by permission.)

TABLE 14-1.—OPERATIVE RESULTS VERSUS RENAL VEIN RENIN RATIOS IN HYPERTENSIVE PATIENTS WITH UNILATERAL STENOSIS OF A MAIN RENAL ARTERY

	NO. OF PATIENTS	PATIENTS WITH LATERALIZING RENAL VEIN RENIN RATIOS*		PATIENTS WITHOUT LATERALIZING RENAL VEIN RENIN RATIOS*	
		CURED/ IMPROVED	FAILED	CURED/ IMPROVED	FAILED
Summary of literature review†	412	267	19	64	62
Present data	66	36	4	21	5
Totals	478	303 (326)	23	85 (152)	67

*Each author's own definition of lateralizing was used to construct the table. In terms of renal vein renin ratios (ipsilateral-contralateral), that definition varied from 1.4 to 2.5 in the 21 studies reviewed. We used 1.5 in the present data.

†All patients underwent vascular repair or nephrectomy. Excluded from the review were operative deaths, known anatomical failures, patients with lesions other than unilateral stenosis of a main renal artery and patients from small series (less than nine cases). Details of the literature are published elsewhere.[54]

renin data analysis[26, 35, 39, 89, 92, 95, 101] detected more than 75% of those with proved renovascular hypertension.

Data gathered from a critical review of the pertinent medical literature[54] together with our own results are shown in Table 14-1. These data confirm the prognostic value of a high renal vein renin ratio in the presence of unilateral renal artery stenosis, but they also underscore the fact that many subjects with potentially curable renovascular hypertension would be denied an operation if one were to rely solely on renin values. They again raise the legitimate question: Is renovascular hypertension renin-dependent in those patients who benefit from surgery despite nonlateralizing renal vein renin ratios?

Use of Angiotensin Antagonists

EXPERIMENTAL RENOVASCULAR HYPERTENSION

The administration of 8-substituted A-II analogues or CEI in patients with experimental renovascular hypertension prevents the initial rise in blood pressure,[4, 10, 17, 31, 75, 86] confirming the fact that the acute-onset phase of hypertension is renin-dependent.

The two-kidney model of chronic experimental hypertension (one renal artery constricted, with the contralateral kidney untouched) most resembles the human disorder. In this model, interpretation of published data is complicated by apparent species differences; variations of methodology (method and degree of renal artery constriction, anesthetized versus unanesthetized animals); sodium-fluid balance; type, dose and duration of the angiotensin antagonist used; degree of change in or level of absolute blood pressure that is defined as hypertension; and duration of time required following renal artery constriction for definition of chronic (versus acute) hypertension.

A detailed analysis of these studies is beyond the scope of this chapter. At present, there seems to be general agreement that in the rat, two-kidney hypertension is responsive to A-II blockade, but that in the rabbit and dog, pressor mechanisms other than the renin-angiotensin system may play an important role in sustaining the elevated blood pressure.[16] It should be noted that in animals with two-kidney renovascular hypertension who are resistant in the sodium-replete state, angiotensin antagonists may significantly lower blood pressure following sodium depletion,[30, 49, 82, 98] apparently unmasking a renin dependence of the hypertension. This same phenomenon occurs in human renovascular hypertension (see below).

Human Renovascular Hypertension

The first use of an 8-substituted A-II analogue in humans was reported by Brunner *et al.* in 1973.[7] This group administered infusions of saralasin to 12 patients with very severe or malignant hypertension of varying etiologies; they noted a significant fall in blood pressure in eight patients with high PRA levels, whereas there was no change in blood pressure in the four patients with normal or low PRA. In a more detailed analysis of the same 12 patients,[8] they demonstrated in one subject that modest sodium depletion potentiated the vasodepressor response to saralasin, whereas in another patient a saline infusion blocked the vasodepressor response. That same year Donker and Leenen reported a vasodepressor response to saralasin infusion in two subjects with unilateral renovascular hypertension, in one of whom sodium depletion markedly augmented the drop in blood pressure.[20]

In 1975, Streeten *et al.* reported on the use of saralasin as a screening procedure for renin-mediated hypertension.[91] In normal control subjects, saralasin infusion did not change the blood pressure, and it blocked the hypertensive action of A-II but not that of norepinephrine. Among 60 consecutive patients with hypertension studied in the sodium-deplete state, saralasin infusion lowered the blood pressure in 16, all of whom had either high PRA levels or renal artery stenosis. In the same year, our investigative group described the saralasin bolus test (rapid intravenous injection) administered to 21 hypertensive patients in the salt-deplete state (Fig. 14–4).[57] An unequivocal vasodepressor response was noted in 13 patients, of whom 11 had renovascular hypertension with normal or high PRA levels and two had high-renin essential hypertension. Blood pressure was un-

Fig. 14–4.—Response to saralasin bolus test in 21 patients with hypertension. Patients were studied 16 hours after the oral administration of furosemide (sodium-replete state). Patients with renovascular hypertension *(RVH)* exhibited a vasodepressor response to saralasin injection, regardless of PRA level, whereas only two patients with high renin essential hypertension *(EH)* responded. (From Marks, L. S., Maxwell, M. H., and Kaufman, J. J.: Saralasin bolus test. Rapid procedure for renin-mediated hypertension, Lancet 2:784, 1975. Used by permission.)

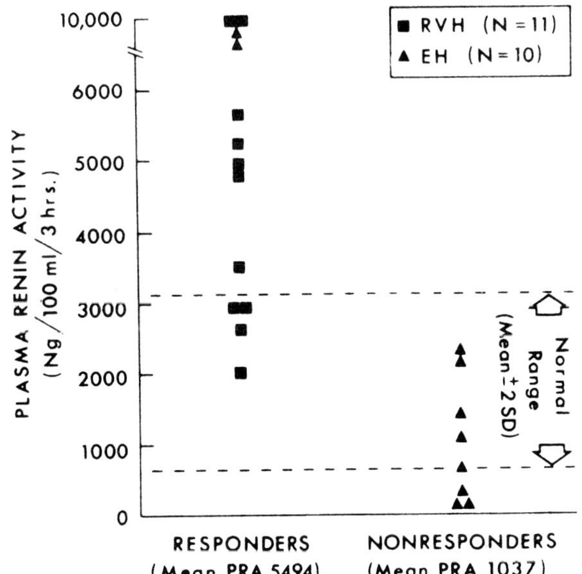

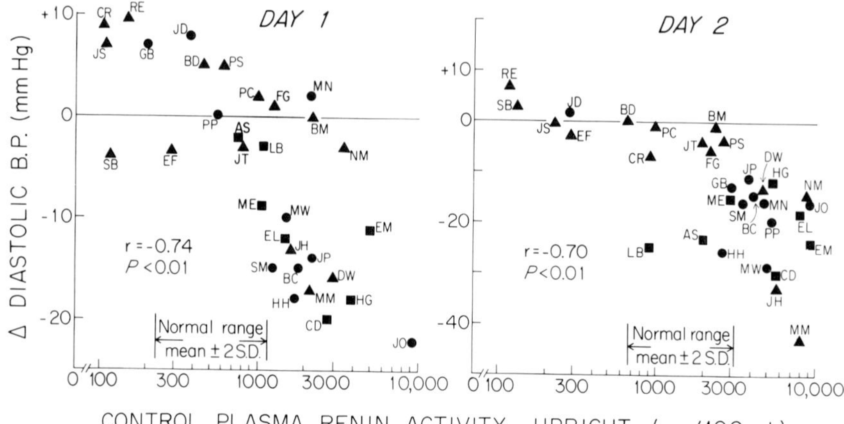

Fig. 14–5.—Changes in diastolic blood pressure *(B.P.)* after a bolus injection of saralasin versus control upright plasma renin activity. Seven patients who failed to respond in the normal sodium state (day 1) showed a vasodepressor response after sodium depletion (day 2). Note the change in the scale of the vertical axis between day 1 and day 2. Triangles are essential hypertension; circles are unilateral and squares are bilateral renal artery stenosis. (From Marks, L. S., Maxwell, M. H., and Kaufman, J. J.: Renin, sodium, and vascular response to saralasin in renovascular and essential hypertension, Ann. Intern. Med. 87:176, 1977. Used by permission.)

changed in eight patients with low- or normal-renin essential hypertension. In the salt-replete state prior to furosemide diuresis, only seven patients responded to saralasin. Importantly, in all patients blood pressure response to saralasin bolus (10 mg) correlated with blood pressure response to subsequent infusion of saralasin (10 μg/kg/min).

We subsequently extended our observations to 32 patients,[56] each of whom was studied before (day 1) and after (day 2) mild sodium depletion (146 mEq $\pm$ 19 SEM) achieved by the oral administration of furosemide (1 mg/kg body weight) the evening before the test (Fig. 14–5). A blood-pressure-lowering effect of saralasin was observed in 16 of 17 patients with renovascular hypertension on day 2, but in only 10 of the 17 on day 1. Of 15 patients with essential hypertension, only the four with high PRA levels exhibited a vasodepressor response on day 2; three of these responded similarly on day 1. Changes in blood pressure after saralasin injection correlated with control PRA levels ($p <$ 0.01, $r = -0.74$), in agreement with others.[2, 6, 12, 33] The average net sodium loss between the two test days was greater for patients responding to saralasin on day 2 (170 mEq) than for those not responding (129 mEq) ($p < 0.05$); however, there was no correlation between blood pressure response and either net sodium loss or urinary sodium excretion at the time of testing. It was again demonstrated in this larger patient population that the bolus and infusion blood pressure changes were closely correlated in both normal and sodium-deplete states ($p < 0.01$, $r = 0.89$) (Fig. 14–6). Four of the 16 patients with renovascular hypertension who responded to saralasin infusion had nonlateralizing renal vein renin data.

These results clearly establish the superiority of saralasin testing to renal vein renin levels in detecting both unilateral and bilateral renovascular hypertension. Our single nonresponder with confirmed renovascular hypertension (J.D. in Fig. 14–5) also had low stimulated PRA levels and nonlateralizing renal vein renin values;[56] this patient and another similar pa-

Fig. 14–6.—Comparison of changes in diastolic blood pressure *(B.P.)* on day 2 after a bolus injection (10 mg) and during a sustained infusion (10 μg/kg/min) of saralasin in all 32 patients. There is a high degree of correlation in blood pressure response between the two methods of testing. (From Marks, L. S., Maxwell, M. H., and Kaufman, J. J.: Renin, sodium, and vascular response to saralasin in renovascular and essential hypertension, Ann. Intern. Med. 87:176, 1977. Used by permission.)

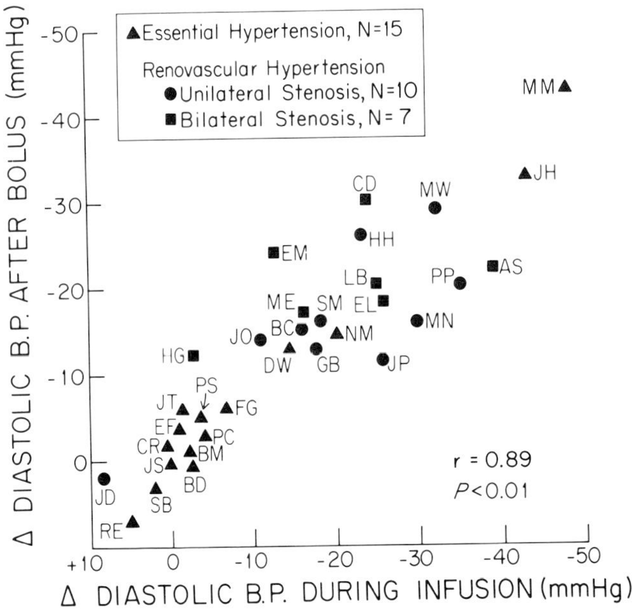

tient, both of whom apparently had non-renin-mediated renovascular hypertension, are described in detail elsewhere.[55] Strikingly similar results were reported simultaneously by Wilson *et al.*[100] Their protocol for furosemide-induced diuresis prior to the saralasin infusion was identical with ours. In patients with demonstrated renal artery stenosis, all 11 with "proven renovascular hypertension" (benefited by surgery) had a vasodepressor response to saralasin, as did seven of eight patients with "highly probable renovascular hypertension" (lateralization of renal vein renin values and differential renal function studies) and 13 of 16 with "probable renovascular hypertension" (lateralization of only one functional study). Six of the 11 patients with proven renovascular hypertension had nonlateralization of one or both functional tests. Positive saralasin responses occurred in only two of ten patients with essential hypertension (PRA values not given) and in none of five patients with low-renin hypertension. Streeten *et al.* reported saralasin responsiveness in seven patients with surgically proved renovascular hypertension,[90] and Baer *et al.* noted positive saralasin test results in ten subjects with probable renovascular hypertension (renal artery stenosis with lateralizing renal vein renin values).[2]

Is Human Renovascular Hypertension Renin-Dependent?

These combined data show that a vasodepressor response to an angiotensin inhibitor is a reliable way to diagnose renin-mediated, largely renovascular hypertension, and further indicate that chronic renovascular hypertension is renin-mediated. As mentioned above, we and others[2, 6, 12, 33, 56] have demonstrated a correlation between blood pressure change after saralasin injection and control PRA level, with correlation coefficients of approximately -0.7. Why is this correlation coefficient not closer to 1.0? Part of the difference may be accounted for by small inaccuracies in blood pressure measurements and laboratory variability in renin determinations, although in a large-population sample these errors should cancel out. An analysis of 140 saralasin bolus tests, stratifying patients by etiologies (essential versus renovascular hypertension), makes it apparent that the correlation between blood pressure change after saralasin injection and control PRA level is significantly greater in patients with essential hypertension ($r = -0.79$) than in those with renovascular hypertension ($r = -0.53$). This difference is largely explained by the proportion of patients with renovascular hypertension who demonstrate a vasodepressor response to saralasin despite "normal" PRA levels, whereas patients with essential hypertension do not respond unless they are in the high-renin category. These findings support the position that increased vascular responsiveness to angiotensin, with normal or only slightly increased PRA levels, maintains the elevated pressure in cases of renovascular hypertension[2, 6, 11, 50, 86] and explains the paradox of normal PRA values in a significant number of these patients. Circulating levels of PRA may not reflect increased activity or concentration of angiotensin at various receptor sites.

Figure 14–7 depicts the *ratio* of mean arterial pressure changes (Δ MAP) after saralasin administration as compared with the *ratio* of changes in PRA level (Δ PRA). There are 140 data points, regardless of the directional changes in either pa-

Fig. 14–7. – Changes in mean arterial pressure *(MAP)* versus changes in PRA levels following saralasin bolus test in patients with hypertension of various etiologies. Blood pressures were obtained at the time of PRA sampling. Changes are designated by ratios, with 1.0 representing no change from control values.

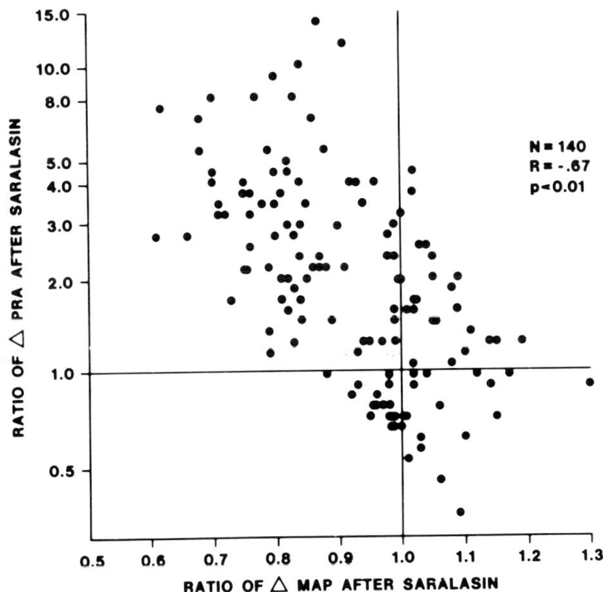

rameter. There is a correlation between these two parameters, i.e., the greater the percent change in MAP, the greater the percent change in PRA in the opposite direction. This correlation suggests that the dynamic equilibrium of renin release is different in those patients who manifest a vasodepressor response to saralasin (renin-mediated hypertension) than in those who do not. It has been shown in cases of chronic experimental and human renovascular hypertension that regardless of circulating PRA levels, the involved kidney has increased juxtaglomerular cell granulation,[37] renin content[94] and renin secretion.[70] It is not unreasonable that in these kidneys there would be a greater sensitivity of renin release in response to changes in blood pressure and intrarenal blood flow/distribution.

Another practical consideration is apparent from Figure 14–7. The maximum blood pressure decrease in response to saralasin administration is approximately 40% lower than the control value, or a ratio of 0.6; whereas in the patients who respond to saralasin, the PRA value often increases by five- to tenfold. The minute-to-minute variability of blood pressure recordings sometimes makes it difficult to stratify an individual patient with an equivocal decrease in blood pressure as a true saralasin responder. The change in PRA values in these cases is at least as sensitive as the change in blood pressure. In an attempt to best stratify patients subjected to the saralasin test, a stepwise, linear discriminant analysis was performed, using the data from 34 patients with essential hypertension and 37 patients with renovascular hypertension. Variables used were: presaralasin PRA level in erect and supine positions, supine PRA level 30 minutes after saralasin bolus injection, and ratios of systolic and diastolic pressures (postsaralasin pressures/control pressures). When each of these variables was considered separately, the best discrimination was achieved using postsaralasin PRA levels alone, which resulted in misclassification of seven patients with essential hypertension (false positive tests) and four with renovascular hypertension (false negative tests), or 15.5% of the total population. The second best single variable was the diastolic ratio, which resulted in misclassification of 21% of the population. Adding the diastolic ratio to the postsaralasin PRA value eliminated only one of the four misclassified patients with renovascular hypertension, for a total misclassification of ten patients, or 11% of the entire population.

The important point is that in response to saralasin administration, the PRA value increases to a much higher level in patients with renovascular hypertension than in those with essential hypertension. In using this test criterion, the critical, absolute value of postsaralasin PRA used to stratify patients would have to be determined by individual laboratories, depending on their own renin methodology and control values. Once this is done, however, the absolute level of postsaralasin PRA, regardless of presaralasin control values, may be a more accurate index of a positive or negative saralasin response than are changes in blood pressure.

Renin-Sodium Interrelations and the Use of Angiotensin Antagonists

The interrelation between the renin-angiotensin-aldosterone system and sodium-fluid volume is well known.[47] Sodium-fluid overload can suppress PRA and attenuate or prevent a vasodepressor response to angiotensin antagonists.[31] Conversely, sufficient sodium depletion in normotensive animals[15, 40, 83, 88] and in humans[36, 53, 81] results in angiotensin dependence of blood pressure, with vasodepressor responses to angiotensin inhibitors. Gavras *et al.* demonstrated that even patients with low levels of renin and essential hypertension may become responsive to saralasin injections after protracted sodium depletion.[32] Case *et al.* reported that saralasin administration resulted in vasodepressor responses in 64% of sodium-depleted patients with normal-renin hypertension.[12] Is it possible, therefore, that a vasodepressor response to saralasin in some patients may represent a homeostatic response to volume depletion and low cardiac output rather than signifying a particular subset of hypertension? This could theoretically result in false positive saralasin tests.

Net sodium losses in animals sufficient to cause an unequivocal fall in blood pressure during saralasin or CEI infusion[15, 40, 83, 88] were several times greater per body weight than the 150 mEq ± 19 SEM resulting from furosemide, 1 mg/kg body weight, used by us and others.[2, 56, 100] In normal human subjects, even with cumulative sodium losses of more than 200 mEq, saralasin[53, 81] or CEI[36] infusion caused a vasodepressor response *only in the upright position*. The four low-renin essential hypertension patients reported by Gavras *et al.* had a cumulative sodium loss of 383 mEq,[32] itself resulting in a more significant decrease in blood pressure in the supine position than did the saralasin infusion; a marked decrease in blood pressure during saralasin infusion occurred only in patients in the standing position. In the report of Case *et al.*, the patients were tested in the prolonged seated posture.[12] In the presence of sodium depletion, the added stimulus of a further decrease of effective plasma volume resulting from the upright or seated position may be sufficient to result in angiotensin dependence of blood pressure.

From the currently available data, the supine posture and modest sodium depletion (100–200 mEq) provide optimal discriminant value of the saralasin test,[56] as well as reduce the partial agonistic effect of this drug.[97]

Present and Future Roles of Angiotensin Antagonists in the Diagnosis of Renovascular Hypertension

The Cooperative Study of Renovascular Hypertension showed that the use of the rapid-sequence intravenous urogram and the radioisotope renogram results in a misclassification of approximately 25% of patients with renal artery stenosis.[60] More important, neither these tests nor the renal arteriogram serves to assess the functional significance of the renal artery lesions, i.e., differentiate between renal artery stenosis and renovascular hypertension.[64] Peripheral and renal vein renin values are highly accurate prognostic indices of operative success when they are positive, but they fail to diagnose almost 50% of patients with potentially curable renovascular hypertension.[54, 58, 62] It is possible that the sensitivity of renal vein renin values could be improved by simultaneous sampling of renal veins and replicate sampling.[38, 63]

When saralasin is administered during a state of modest sodium depletion with the patient in the supine position, there appear to be almost no false negative test results in patients with renovascular hypertension.[2, 56, 90, 100] In our experience, there are also very few false positive test results, in that the patients with essential hypertension who respond to saralasin are those with high renin levels and who, therefore, presumably have renin-mediated hypertension. A larger series of patients with essential hypertension will have to be studied to determine the true incidence of false positive results.

Potential complications of saralasin testing appear to relate entirely to the effect of the drug on blood pressure, either untoward hyper-[1, 12, 13, 44] or hypotensive[22, 52, 79] episodes, although no serious sequelae have been reported in more than 3000 patients.[43] The immediate, transient elevation of blood pressure following saralasin administration that may occur when the patient is sodium replete can be attenuated or prevented by prior sodium depletion,[97] and hypotensive episodes have been reported only in patients receiving concomitant antihypertensive drugs, particularly vasodilators.[79]

The saralasin bolus technique has many characteristics of an ideal test for screening hypertensive populations.[56, 57, 97] It is

Fig. 14–8. — Currently used decision tree for diagnosis of renovascular hypertension: selection of patients for arteriography. (From Franklin, S. S., and Maxwell, M. H.: Clinical workup for renovascular hypertension, Urol. Clin. North Am. 2:301, 1975. Used by permission.)

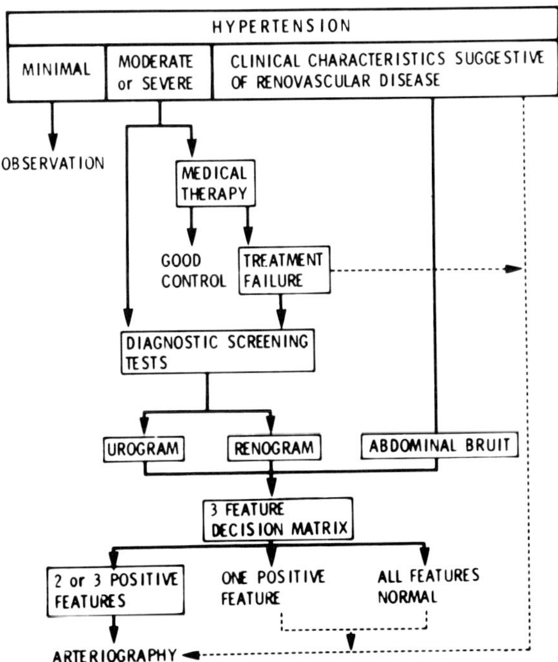

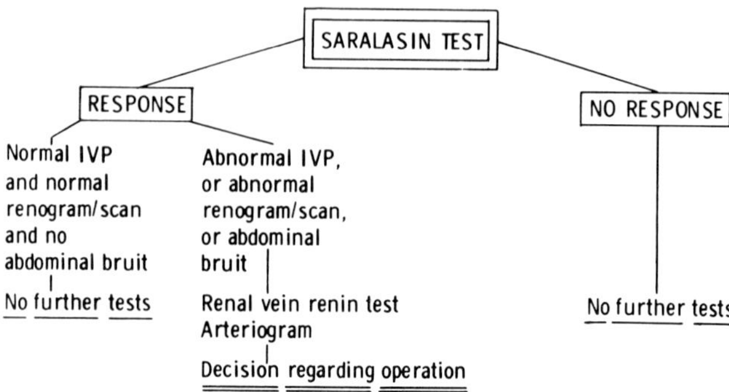

Fig. 14–9.—Potential decision tree for diagnosis of renovascular hypertension. *IVP*, intravenous pyelogram.

rapid, simple, safe, inexpensive, easy to interpret and may be performed as an office procedure. Figure 14–8 shows the standard decision matrix in screening patients for renovascular hypertension,[27] based upon the results of the Cooperative Study of Renovascular Hypertension.[64] Figure 14–9 shows a potential decision matrix for the future. In this scheme, all hypertensive patients suspected of having renovascular hypertension would undergo a bolus test of saralasin (or another angiotensin analogue) as a first procedure. Only if the results were positive would it be necessary to proceed to further, more complicated testing.

References

1. Anderson, G. H., Jr., Streeten, H. P., and Dalakos, T. G.: Pressor response to 1-sar-8-ala-angiotensin II (saralasin) in hypertensive subjects, Circ. Res. 40:243, 1977.
2. Baer, L., Parra-Carrillo, J. Z., Radichevich, J., and Williams, G. A.: Detection of renovascular hypertension with angiotensin II blockade, Ann. Intern. Med. 86:257, 1977.
3. Bakhle, Y. S.: Inhibition of angiotensin I converting enzyme by venom peptides, Br. J. Pharmacol. 43:252, 1971.
4. Bing, J., and Nielsen, K.: Role of the renin system in normo- and hypertension, Acta Pathol. Microbiol. Scand. [A] 81:254, 1973.
5. Blair-West, J. R., Coghlan, J. P., Denton, D. A., Funder, J. W., Scoggins, B. A., and Wright, R. D.: Effect of the heptapeptide (2–8) and hexapeptide (3–8) fragments of angiotensin II on aldosterone secretion, J. Clin. Endocrinol. 32:575, 1971.
6. Brown, J. J., Brown, W. C. B., Fraser, R., Lever, A. F., Morton, J. J., Robertson,

J. I. S., Rosei, E. A., and Trust, P. M.: The effects of saralasin, an angiotensin II antagonist, on blood pressure and the renin-angiotensin-aldosterone system in normal and hypertensive subjects, Aust. N. Z. J. Med. (Suppl. 3) 6:47, 1976.

7. Brunner, H. R., Gavras, H., Laragh, J. H., and Keenan, R.: Angiotensin II blockade in man by sar[1]-ala[8]-angiotensin II for understanding and treatment of high blood pressure, Lancet 2:1045, 1973.

8. Brunner, H. R., Gavras H., Laragh, J. H., and Keenan, R.: Hypertension in man: Exposure of the renin and sodium components using angiotensin II blockade, Circ. Res. (Suppl. 1) 34–35:35, 1974.

9. Bumpus, F. M., and Khosla, M. C.: Angiotensin analogs as determinants of the physiologic role of angiotensin and its metabolites, in Genest, J., Koiw, E., and Kuchel, O. (eds.): *Hypertension – Physiopathology and Treatment* (New York: McGraw-Hill, 1977), p. 183.

10. Bumpus, F. M., Sen, S., Smeby, R. R., Sweet, C., Ferrario, C. M., and Khosla, M. C.: Use of angiotensin II antagonists in experimental hypertension, Circ. Res. 32:150, 1973.

11. Caravaggi, A. M., Bianchi, G., Brown, J. J., Lever, A. F., Morton, J. J., Powell-Jackson, J. D., Robertson, J. I. S., and Semple, P. F.: Blood pressure and plasma angiotensin II concentration after renal artery constriction and angiotensin infusion in the dog, Circ. Res. 38:315, 1976.

12. Case, D. B., Wallace, J. M., Keim, H. J., Sealey, J. E., and Laragh, J. H.: Usefulness and limitations of saralasin, a partial competitive agonist of angiotensin II, for evaluating the renin and sodium factors in hypertension patients, Am. J. Med. 60: 825, 1976.

13. Case, D. B., Wallace, J. M., Keim, H. J., Weber, M. A., Drayer, J. I. M., White, R. P., Sealey, J. E., and Laragh, J. H.: Estimating renin participation in hypertension: Superiority of converting enzyme inhibitor over saralasin, Am. J. Med. 61:790, 1976.

14. Christlieb, A. R., Biber, T. U. L., and Hickler, R. B.: Studies on the role of angiotensin in experimental renovascular hypertension: Immunologic approach, J. Clin. Invest. 48:1506, 1969.

15. Coleman, T. G., and Guyton, A. C.: The pressor role of angiotensin in salt deprivation and renal hypertension in rats, Clin. Sci. Mol. Med. 48:45s, 1975.

16. Davis, J. O.: The pathogenesis of chronic renovascular hypertension, Circ. Res. 40: 439, 1977.

17. Davis, J. O.: The use of blocking agents to define the function of the renin-angiotensin system, Clin. Sci. Mol. Med. 48:3, 1975.

18. Deodhar, S. D., Haas, E., and Goldblatt, H.: Production of antirenin to homologous renin and its effect on experimental renal hypertension, J. Exp. Med. 119:425, 1964.

19. Dickinson, C. J., and Yu, R.: Mechanisms involved in the progressive pressor response to very small amounts of angiotensin in conscious rabbits, Circ. Res. 21:157, 1967.

20. Donker, A. J. M., and Leenen, F. H. H.: Infusion of angiotensin II analogue with unilateral renovascular hypertension, Lancet 2:1535, 1974.

21. Eide, I.: Renovascular hypertension in rats immunized with angiotensin II, Circ. Res. 30:149, 1972.

22. Fagard, R., Amery, A., and Timmermans, U.: Severe hypotension during infusion of saralasin (Letter), Lancet 1:1136, 1976.

23. Ferreira, S. H., Bartelt, D. C., and Greene, L. J.: Isolation of bradykinin-potentiating peptides from *Bothrops jaracara* venom, Biochemistry 9:2583, 1970.

24. Ferreira, S. H., Greene, L. J., Alabaster, V. A., Bakhle, Y. S., and Vane, J. R.: Activity of various fractions of bradykinin-potentiating factor against angiotensin converting enzyme, Nature 225:379, 1970.

25. Fitzsimmons, J. T.: The effect on drinking of peptide precursors and of shorter chain peptide fragments of angiotensin II injected into the rat's diencephalon, J. Physiol. 214:295, 1971.

26. Foster, J. H., Dean, R. H., Pinkerton, J. A., and Rhamy, R. K.: Ten years experience with the surgical management of renovascular hypertension, Ann. Surg. 177:755, 1973.

27. Franklin, S. S., and Maxwell, M. H.: Clinical workup for renovascular hypertension, Urol. Clin. North Am. 2:301, 1975.

28. Freeman, R. H., Davis, J. O., Lohmeier, T. E., and Spielman, W. S.: [Des-Asp^1] angiotensin II: Mediator of the renin-angiotensin system? Fed. Proc. 36:1766, 1977.

29. Ganong, W. F.: The renin-angiotensin system and the central nervous system, Fed. Proc. 36:1771, 1977.

30. Gavras, H., Brunner, H. R., Thurston, H., and Laragh, J. H.: Reciprocation of renin dependency with sodium volume dependency in renal hypertension, Science 188:1316, 1975.

31. Gavras, H., Brunner, H. R., Vaughan, E. D., and Laragh, J. H.: Angiotensin-sodium interaction in blood pressure maintenance of renal hypertensive and normotensive rats, Science 180:1369, 1973.

32. Gavras, H., Ribeiro, A. B., Gavras, I., and Brunner, H. R.: Reciprocal relations between renin dependency and sodium dependency in essential hypertension, N. Engl. J. Med. 295:1278, 1976.

33. Geyskes, G. G., Boer, P., Vos, J., and Dorhout Mees, E. J.: Renin dependency of blood pressure, Lancet 1:1049, 1976.

34. Green, L. J., Camargo, A. C. M., Krieger, E. M., Steward, J. M., and Ferreira, S. H.: Inhibition of the conversion of angiotensin I to II and potentiation of bradykinin by small peptides present in *Bothrops jaracara* venom, Circ. Res. (Suppl. 2) 30–31:62, 1972.

35. Gunnels, J. C., McGuffin, W. L., Johnsrude, I., and Robinson, R. R.: Peripheral and renal venous plasma renin activity in hypertension, Ann. Intern. Med. 71:555, 1969.

36. Haber, E., Sancho, J., Re, R., and Barger, A. C.: The role of the renin-angiotensin system in cardiovascular homeostasis in normal man, Clin. Sci. Mol. Med. 48:495, 1975.

37. Hartroft, P. M.: Juxtaglomerular cells, Circ. Res. 12:525, 1963.

38. Horvath, J. S., Baxter, C. R., Sherbon, K., Smee, I., Roche, J., Uther, J. B., and Tiller, D. J.: An analysis of errors found in renal vein sampling for plasma renin activity, Kidney Int. 11:136, 1977.

39. Hussain, R. A., Gifford, R. W., and Stewart, B. H.: Differential renal venous renin activity in diagnosis of renovascular hypertension, Am. J. Cardiol. 32:707, 1973.

40. Johnson, J. A., and Davis, J. O.: Effects of a specific competitive antagonist of angiotensin II on arterial pressure and adrenal steroid secretion in dogs, Circ. Res. (Suppl. 1) 32:159, 1973.

41. Johnston, C. I., Hutchinson, J. S., and Mendelsohn, F. A.: Biological significance of renin angiotensin immunization, Circ. Res. (Suppl. 2) 26:215, 1970.

42. Kaplan, N. M.: *Clinical Hypertension* (New York: Medcom, 1973).

43. Keenan, R.: Personal communication.

44. Keim, J. H., Drayer, J. I., Case, D. B., Lopez-Oversero, J., Wallace, J. M., Weber, M. A., and Laragh, J. H.: A role for renin in rebound hypertension and encephalopathy after infusion of saralasin acetate (sar^1-ala^8-angiotensin II), N. Engl. J. Med. 295:1175, 1976.

45. Khairallah, P. A., Toth, A., and Bumpus, F. M.: Analogs of angiotensin II. II. Mechanism of receptor interactions, J. Med. Chem. 13:181, 1970.

46. Kirkendall, W. M., Fitz, A. E., and Lawrence, M. S.: Renal hypertension: Diagnosis and surgical treatment, N. Engl. J. Med. 276:479, 1967.

47. Laragh, J. H.: Vasoconstriction — volume analysis for understanding and treating

hypertension: The use of renin and aldosterone profiles, Am. J. Med. 55:261, 1973.
48. Laragh, J. H., Cannon, P. J., and Ames, R. P.: Interaction between aldosterone secretion, sodium and potassium balance and angiotensin activity in man, Can. Med. Assoc. J. 90:248, 1964.
49. Lohmeier, T. E., and Davis, J. O.: Renin-angiotensin-aldosterone system in experimental renal hypertension in the rabbit, Am. J. Physiol. 230:311, 1976.
50. Lupu, A. N., Maxwell, M. H., and Kaufman, J. J.: Mechanisms of hypertension during the chronic phase of one-clip, two-kidney model in the dog, Circ. Res. (Suppl. 1) 40:I-57, 1977.
51. MacDonald, G. J., Louis, W. J., Renzini, V., Boyd, G. W., and Peart, W. S.: Renal-clip hypertension in rabbits immunized against angiotensin II, Circ. Res. 27:197, 1970.
52. MacGregor, G. A.: Hypotension during angiotensin blockade with saralasin (Letter), Lancet 2:181, 1975.
53. MacGregor, G. A., and Dawes, P. M.: Agonist and antagonist effects of sar^1-ala^8-angiotensin II in salt-loaded and salt-depleted normal man, Br. J. Clin. Pharmacol. 3:483, 1976.
54. Marks, L. S., and Maxwell, M. H.: Renal vein renin. Value and limitations in the prediction of operative results, Urol. Clin. North Am. 2:311, 1975.
55. Marks, L. S., Maxwell, M. H., and Kaufman, J. J.: Non-renin-mediated renovascular hypertension: A new syndrome? Lancet 1:615, 1977.
56. Marks, L. S., Maxwell, M. H., and Kaufman, J. J.: Renin, sodium, and vascular response to saralasin in renovascular and essential hypertension, Ann. Intern. Med. 87:176, 1977.
57. Marks, L. S., Maxwell, M. H., and Kaufman, J. J.: Saralasin bolus test. Rapid procedure for renin-mediated hypertension, Lancet 2:784, 1975.
58. Marks, L. S., Maxwell, M. H., Varady, P. D., Lupu, A. N., and Kaufman, J. J.: Renovascular hypertension: Does the renal vein renin ratio predict operative results? J. Urol. 115:365, 1976.
59. Marshall, G. R.: Structure-activity relations of antagonists of the renin-angiotensin system, Fed. Proc. 35:2494, 1976.
60. Maxwell, M. H.: Cooperative study of renovascular hypertension. Current status, Kidney Int. 8:s-153, 1975.
61. Maxwell, M. H., Lupu, A. N., Viskoper, R. V., Aravena, L. A., and Waks, U. A.: Mechanisms of hypertension during the acute and intermediate phases of the one-clip, two-kidney model in the dog, Circ. Res. 25:I-24, 1977.
62. Maxwell, M. H., Marks, L. S., Lupu, A. N., Cahill, P. J., Franklin, S. S., and Kaufman, J. J.: Predictive value of renin determinations in renal artery stenosis, J.A.M.A. 238:2617, 1977.
63. Maxwell, M. H., Marks, L. S., Varady, P. D., Lupu, A. N., and Kaufman, J. J.: Renal vein renin in essential hypertension, J. Lab. Clin. Med. 86:901, 1975.
64. Maxwell, M. H., and Varaday, P. D.: Cooperative study of renovascular hypertension. Clinical characteristics, diagnostic tests and results of surgery, Contr. Nephrol. 3:1, 1976.
65. McCubbin, J. W., Demoura, R. S., Page, I. H., and Olmstead, K.: Arterial hypertension elicited by subpressor amounts of angiotensin, Science 149:1391, 1965.
66. McKown, M. M., Workman, R. J., and Gregerman, R. I.: Pepstatin inhibition of human renin, J. Biol. Chem. 249:7770, 1974.
67. Miller, R. P., Poper, C. J., Wilson, C. W., and DeVito, E.: Renin inhibition by pepstatin, Biochem. Pharmacol. 21:2941, 1972.
68. Needleman, P., Johnson, E. M., Jr., Vine, W., Flanigan, E., and Marshall, G. R.: The pharmacology of antagonists of angiotensin I and II, Circ. Res. 31:862, 1972.
69. Needleman, P., and Marshall, G. R.: Angiotensin antagonists: Overview and projection, Fed. Proc. 35:2486, 1976.
70. Omae, T., Masson, G. M. C., and Page, J. H.: Release of pressor substances from

renal grafts originating from rats with renal hypertension, Circ. Res. 9:441, 1961.
71. Ondetti, M. A., Williams, N. J., Sabo, E. F., Pluscec, J., Weaver, E. R., and Kocy, O.: Angiotensin-converting enzyme inhibitors from the venom of *Bothrops jaracara.* Isolation, elucidation of structure, and synthesis, Biochemistry 10:4033, 1971.
72. Oster, P., Bauknecht, H., and Hackenthal, E.: Active and passive immunization against angiotensin II in the rat and rabbit. Evidence for a normal regulation of the renin-angiotensin system, Circ. Res. 37:607, 1975.
73. Page, I. H., and McCubbin, J. W. (eds.): *Renal Hypertension* (Chicago: Year Book Medical Publishers, Inc., 1968).
74. Paiva, A. C. M., Nouaitheta, V. L. A., Miyamoto, M. E., Mendes, G. B., and Paiva, T. B.: Neurospecific angiotensin antagonists. (8-valine)-, (8-isoleucine)-, and chlorambucil-des-1-aspartic, 8-valine-angiotensin, J. Med. Chem. 16:6, 1973.
75. Pals, D. T., Masucci, F. D., Sipos, F., and Denning, G. S., Jr.: A specific competitive antagonist of the vascular action of angiotensin II, Circ. Res. 29:664, 1971.
76. Peach, M. J.: Adrenal medulla, in Page, I. H., and Bumpus, F. M. (eds.): *Angiotensin* (New York: Springer-Verlag, 1974), p. 400.
77. Peach, M. J., and Ackerly, J. A.: Angiotensin antagonists and the adrenal cortex and medulla, Fed. Proc. 35:2502, 1976.
78. Peach, M. J., and Chiu, A. T.: Stimulation and inhibition of aldosterone biosynthesis in vitro by angiotensin II and analogs, Circ. Res. (Suppl. 1) 34–35:7, 1974.
79. Pettinger, W. A., and Mitchell, H. C.: Renin release, saralasin and the vasodilator-beta-blocker drug interaction in man, N. Engl. J. Med. 292:1214, 1975.
80. *Pharmacology of Angiotensin Antagonists—Symposium,* Cochairman: Needleman, P., and Marshall, G. R., Fed. Proc. 35:2486, 1976.
81. Posternak, L., Brunner, H. R., Gavras, H., and Brunner, D. B.: Angiotensin II blockade in normal man: Interaction of renin and sodium in maintaining blood pressure, Kidney Int. 11:197, 1977.
82. Romero, J. C., Holmes, D. R., and Strong, C. G.: The effect of high sodium intake and angiotensin antagonist in rabbits with severe and moderate hypertension induced by constriction of one renal artery, Circ. Res. 40:I-17, 1977.
83. Samuels, A. I., Miller, E. D., Fray, J. C. S., Haber, E., and Barger, A. C.: Renin-angiotensin antagonists and the regulation of blood pressure, Fed. Proc. 35:2512, 1976.
84. Schoelkens, B. A.: Comparative pharmacology of new specific angiotensin antagonists, Clin. Sci. Mol. Med. 48:19s, 1975.
85. Severs, W. B., and Daniels-Severs, A. E.: Effects of angiotensin on the central nervous system, Pharmacol. Rev. 25:415, 1973.
86. Skulan, T. W., Brousseau, A. C., and Leonard, K. A.: Accelerated induction of two-kidney hypertension in rats and renin-angiotensin sensitivity, Circ. Res. 35:734, 1974.
87. Solomon, T. A., Cavero, I., and Buckley, J. P.: Inhibition of arterial pressor effects of angiotensin I and II, J. Pharm. Sci. 63:511, 1974.
88. Spielman, W. S., and Davis, J. O.: The renin-angiotensin system and aldosterone secretion during sodium depletion in the rat, Circ. Res. 35:615, 1974.
89. Stockigt, J. R., Noakes, C. A., Collins, R. D., Schambelan, M., and Biglieri, E. G.: Renal-vein renin in various forms of renal hypertension, Lancet 1:1194, 1972.
90. Streeten, D. H. P., Anderson, G. H., and Dalakos, T. G.: Angiotensin blockade: Its clinical significance, Am. J. Med. 60:817, 1976.
91. Streeten, D. H. P., Anderson, G. H., Freiberg, J. M., and Dalakos, T. G.: Use of an angiotensin II antagonist (saralasin) in the recognition of "angiotensinogenic" hypertension, N. Engl. J. Med. 292:657, 1975.
92. Strong, C. G., Hunt, J. C., Sheps, S. G., Tucker, R. M., and Bernatz, P. E.: Renal venous renin activity: Enhancement of sensitivity of lateralization by sodium depletion, Am. J. Cardiol. 27:602, 1971.

93. Thurston, H., and Swales, J. D.: Comparison of angiotensin II antagonist and antiserum infusion with nephrectomy in the rat with two-kidney Goldblatt hypertension, Circ. Res. 35:325, 1974.
94. Tobian, L., Janeck, J., and Tomboulian, A.: Correlation between granulation of juxtaglomerular cells and extractable renin in rats with experimental hypertension, Proc. Soc. Exp. Biol. Med. 100:94, 1959.
95. Vaughan, E. D., Buhler, F. R., and Laragh, J. H.: Renovascular hypertension: Renin measurements to indicate hypersecretion and contralateral suppression, estimate renal plasma flow, and score for surgical curability, Am. J. Med. 55:402, 1973.
96. Wakerlin, G. E.: Antibodies to renin as proof of the pathogenesis of sustained renal hypertension, Circulation 17:653, 1958.
97. Waks, U. A., Maxwell, M. H., Marks, L., Zawada, E. T., and Kaufman, J. J.: Pressor response to saralasin (1-sar-8-ala-angiotensin II) bolus injection in hypertensive patients, Circulation, in press.
98. Watkins, B. E., Davis, J. O., Hanson, R. C., Lohmeier, T. E., and Freeman, R. H.: Incidence and pathophysiological changes in chronic two-kidney hypertension in the dog, Am. J. Physiol. 231:954, 1976.
99. Williams, G. H.: Angiotensin-dependent hypertension — potential pitfalls in definition, Editorial, N. Engl. J. Med. 296:684, 1977.
100. Wilson, H. M., Wilson, J. P., Slaton, P. E., Foster, J. H., Liddle, G. W., and Hollifield, J. W.: Saralasin infusion in the recognition of renovascular hypertension, Ann. Intern. Med. 87:36, 1977.
101. Winer, B. M., Lubbe, W. F., Simon, M., and Williams, G. A.: Renin in the diagnosis of renovascular hypertension: Activity in renal and peripheral vein plasma, J.A.M.A. 202:121, 1967.

15

Experimental Immune Glomerulonephritis Induced in the Rat by Mercuric Chloride

P. DRUET, M.D., K. AYED, M.D., J. BARIETY, M.D., J. F. BERNAUDIN, M.D., E. DRUET, J. F. GIRARD, M.D., N. HINGLAIS, M.D., AND C. SAPIN

Unité de Recherches sur la Pathologie Rénale et Vasculaire (INSERM U 28), ERA 48 CNRS, and Centre de Transfusion Sanguine, Hôpital Broussais, Paris, France.

It is now evident that both experimental and human immune glomerulonephritis (GN) are mediated either by antiglomerular basement membrane (GBM) antibodies or by circulating immune complexes (IC) that become deposited in the glomerular capillary wall.[12] Numerous agents are able to induce the formation of IC with subsequent GN. However, the agents responsible for human GN mediated by anti-GBM antibodies are still unknown. Influenza virus A_2[46] and certain toxic agents such as hydrocarbons[49] have been suggested as causes on the basis of epidemiologic data. On the other hand, several toxic agents, e.g., mercury[30] and gold salts,[24] are able to induce human GN similar to that mediated by IC.

In 1971, we demonstrated the induction of GN with extra-membranous deposits in approximately 30% of Wistar rats that had received subcutaneous injections of mercuric chloride for seven to nine months.[1] The antigen responsible has not yet been

321

0084-5957/79/080321-22$3.75

identified. Subsequently, when the experimental procedure was extended, a reduction in the incidence of GN was observed. This suggested the involvement of a genetic factor, and a further study of the response of several different strains of rats, both inbred and not inbred, was undertaken.

The experimental rats received, in most instances, 0.2 mg $HgCl_2$ per 100 gm body weight three times a week for two months. Renal biopsies were performed 15, 30 and 60 days after the beginning of the injections. These renal biopsies were studied by immunofluorescence using a fluoresceinated sheep antirat IgG antiserum in all cases and, in some, antirat C_3, IgM[36] and albumin[5] antisera. When the animals were killed, usually at two months (sometimes at 15 days), various organs were studied by the same method (lung, heart, bronchus, spleen, liver, adrenal gland and intestine). Some of the samples were examined under both the optical and the electron microscope. Generally, 24-hour urinary protein excretion was measured before the kidney biopsy or just before killing the animal. The control rats received the same volume of distilled water (0.1 ml/100 gm body weight) adjusted to the same pH.[4]

Immune Glomerular Disease in the Brown-Norway (BN) Rat

The results of studies by immunofluorescence have shown that the rats of the BN strain consistently respond to the injection of $HgCl_2$ by developing a glomerular disease. The latter takes place in two stages. The first is caused by anti-GBM antibodies,[37] and the second has characteristics suggestive of an IC-mediated GN.

FIRST STAGE

Demonstration of Participation of Anti-GBM Antibodies

In the 15 eight-week-old BN rats (ten females and five males) injected with $HgCl_2$, renal biopsy on the 15th day revealed, by immunofluorescence using the sheep antirat IgG antiserum, a parietal, regular, intense and linear pattern of fixation in all the loops of all the glomerular capillary walls (Fig. 15–1). A similar but less intense staining was noted with the antirat C_3 anti-

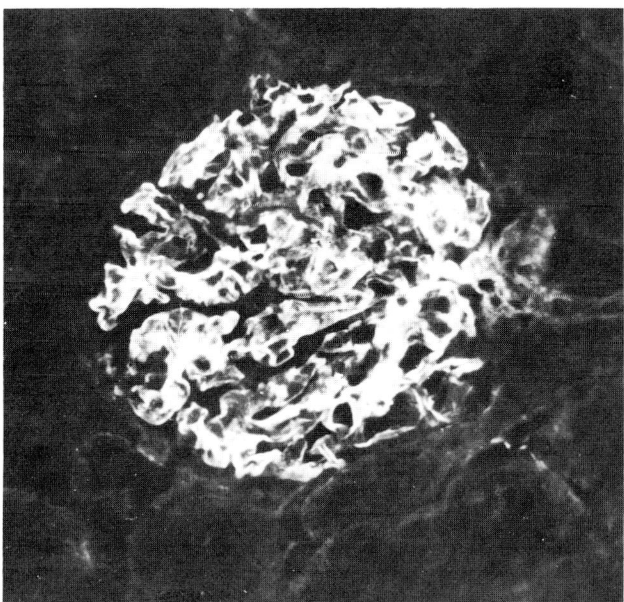

Fig 15–1. – Kidney cryostat section from a BN rat injected with mercuric chloride for 15 days. Staining was with a fluoresceinated antirat IgG antiserum. Note the linear and continuous labeling along all the loops of all the glomerular capillary walls (×700).

serum. When the antirat IgM antiserum was used, the pattern of fixation was not so well defined. Proteinuria in the ten female rats was moderate, not exceeding 90 mg/24 hours. In order to confirm that anti-GBM antibodies were responsible for the pattern observed, the rats were killed and the antibodies were eluted from the kidneys at an acid pH.[26] The eluate thus obtained, tested by indirect immunofluorescence on kidney sections from normal rats, fixed itself in a linear pattern on the glomerular capillary walls, on the tubular basement membranes and on the arterioles. The eluted antibodies, when injected intravenously into a normal rat, became fixed on the glomerular capillary wall. Similar results were obtained, in vitro and in vivo, with IgG isolated from the sera of these rats.[37]

The kidneys of these rats, studied under the optical microscope, did not show any well-defined glomerular lesions. The well-known tubular lesions were observed in all the rats.[19] The kidneys of nine BN rats injected with mercuric chloride were examined under the electron microscope. The samples were taken between the 12th and 16th days after the beginning of the injections. The kidneys of five normal BN rats were used as controls. In the rats that had received $HgCl_2$, the following abnormalities were found: endothelial lesions, abnormal deposits, modifications of the epithelial cells and an abnormally high number of circulating monocytes. These modifications were not consistent from one rat to another, or even from one glomerulus to another. Some of the glomeruli were normal. Some endothelial cells appeared to be separated from the GBM by a clear space, sometimes quite wide, containing a heterogeneous granular substance. The cytoplasm of these detached cells did not show any significant alterations. The compact, abnormal deposits, slightly electron dense, were observed largely in these pathologic subendothelial areas. When particularly abundant, they were also seen in the mesangial regions. The epithelial cells were voluminous, rich in ergastoplasm, with pedicels extending throughout the length of the GBM, and filled with microvilli. Finally, there were numerous intracapillary monocytes, sometimes in close contact with the detached basement membrane. When the deposits were particularly abundant, the monocytes were filled with very dense inclusions, probably containing phagocytosed material. Polymorphonuclear cells were much more rare. No rupture of the GBM was observed, nor was there any endo- or extracapillary proliferation. The kidneys of the control rats did not show any of these features.

The lesions encountered are more like those appearing during the initial phase of GN induced by anti-GBM heteroantibodies[16, 38] than those in GN induced by anti-GBM autoantibodies.[16, 32] The latter process results in severe proliferative and destructive lesions. The isolated detachment of the endothelial cells has already been described in the literature as the most constant and characteristic alteration caused by the interaction of the antibodies with the GBM. The preferential, early afflux of polymorphonucleated cells occurring at the onset of the fixation of the heteroantibodies[38] was not observed in the present experimental group, but the very early phase is difficult to observe experimentally. On the other hand, the later afflux of monocytes in GN induced by heteroantibodies was also detected in the GN induced by anti-GBM antibodies subsequent to $HgCl_2$ administration. The nature of the deposits observed in these cases and their similarity with those appearing during the heterologous phase of heteroimmune GN are difficult to explain. In the latter case, the deposits seem more discontinuous, or consisting of a fibrillar material having the same periodicity as fibrin.[16] This remains to be confirmed. The alterations of epithelial cells are not very characteristic and probably reflect the extensive modifications in the permeability of the GBM.

In order to more accurately determine the date of appearance of the anti-GBM antibodies, 12 BN rats were injected with $HgCl_2$ and kidney biopsy specimens were taken on days 2, 6, 8, 10, 11 and 13. The specimens were taken from two different rats on each occasion, and the same animals were killed on day 15. A linear pattern of fixation was observed in all the rats killed and, in the rats with kidney biopsy specimens taken, as early as the 8th day.

These data demonstrate that a toxic agent such as $HgCl_2$ is consistently able to induce the formation of anti-GBM antibodies in eight-week-old BN rats. It is likely that the mercury salt acts by modifying a component of the basement membrane, thus rendering it antigenic. The affinity of mercury salts for SH groups is well known and might be the cause of this phenomenon. Recently, the same observations were made in rabbits injected with $HgCl_2$ in a similar experimental procedure.[35]

Study of Proteinuria and Complement Level

In the first experimental series, the proteinuria on the 15th day was moderate. In other rats, daily determination of proteinuria was undertaken. Serum complement (CH50) was measured in these animals on days 0, 10 and 15, and then once a week for two months.[31] A total of 29 male BN rats were studied in this manner. Two new facts were ascertained. (1) Nine rats died early, seven before day 8 and two before day 10, i.e., before or at the time of fixation of the antibodies. These rats died from anuria and acute renal failure. This high mortality is probably due to the greater sensitivity of the males during mercury poisoning.[25] It is possibly also partly due to the new experimental conditions. In this protocol, the rats remained isolated in metabolic cages. (2) Among the 20 other rats, 8 showed moderate proteinuria (20–70 mg/24 hours) and 12 had a proteinuria of more than 70 mg. In four of the latter rats, the proteinuria reached or exceeded 1 gm/24 hours. In all cases the proteinuria was maximum

TABLE 15–1.–PROTEINURIA AND SERUM
COMPLEMENT LEVEL IN BN RATS
INJECTED WITH $HgCl_2$

NO. OF RATS	$HgCl_2$ INJECTED (mg/100 gm)	PROTEINURIA* (mg/24 hr)	CH50† (UNITS/ml)
12	0.2	0 – 1,515	200 – 50
8	0.2	20 – 70	36 – 73
12	0	4 – 20	40 – 60‡

*Maximum proteinuria output (extreme values).
†Minimum CH50 level (extreme values).
‡CH50 level in control BN rats (extreme values).

between the 11th and 20th days, and then decreased. Among
these 20 rats, only four survived; in these the proteinuria disappeared and did not recur. The 16 other rats died even though, in
most cases, the proteinuria was decreasing. The kidney was
examined in two of these animals; there were no glomerular lesions, but extensive tubular lesions were present.

Among the 20 rats that were alive after day 10, there was a
drop in the CH50 level in 11 of the 12 rats that had demonstrated proteinuria (Table 15 – 1). This decrease was quite marked in
nine cases in which the CH50 level was between 25 and 0. In 11

TABLE 15–2.–DAY OF MAXIMUM
PROTEINURIA OUTPUT AND MINIMUM
CH50 LEVEL IN BN RATS INJECTED
WITH $HgCl_2$

MAXIMUM PROTEINURIA OUTPUT		MINIMUM CH50 LEVEL	
(mg/24 hr)	DAY	UNITS/ml	DAY
200	12	25	10
340	25	32	20
400	11	50	10
540	11	30	10
600	18	0	15
600	16	0	15
880	17	0	12
900	21	17	20
1,000	21	0	20
1,050	18	0	20
1,200	21	0	20
1,515	22	25	20

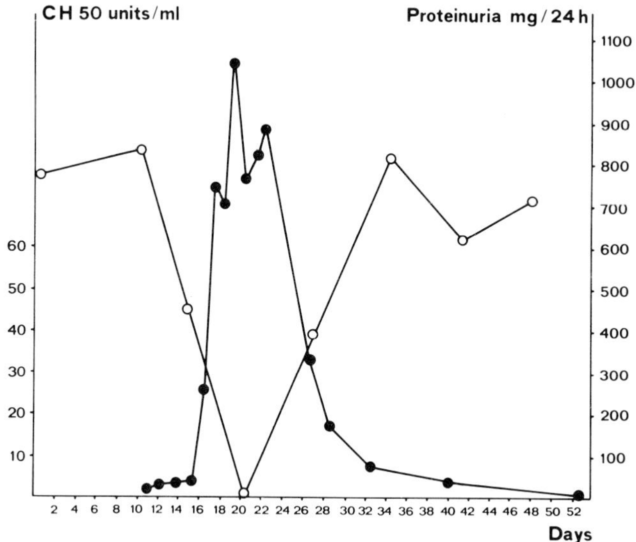

Fig. 15–2. – Evolution of proteinuria *(solid circles)* and of the CH50 level *(open circles)* in a BN rat injected with mercuric chloride.

cases, the decrease in complement level preceded the occurrence of proteinuria by 24 to 48 hours (Table 15 – 2). The CH50 level returned to normal and remained so until the end of the experiment. Figure 15 – 2 shows the course of proteinuria and CH50 level in a typical rat.

These results confirm our previous observations and show that in certain animals, even in the absence of proliferative GN, pronounced but temporary proteinuria may occur. It is tempting to relate the proteinuria to the ultrastructural modifications observed, and to establish a connection between the decrease in the level of complement and the occurrence of anti-GBM antibodies. A possible sequence of events could be: formation of anti-GBM antibodies; fixation and activation of the complement as confirmed by the fixation of the anti-rat C_3 antiserum and by the decrease in the CH50 level; ultrastructural lesion of the capillary wall; and, finally, proteinuria. Further sequential studies and the effect of prior decomplementation may provide arguments to substantiate this hypothesis. These observations can be compared with those of the heterologous phase of GN induced in the rat by intravenous injection of anti-GBM antibodies.[43]

Genetic Study

The fact that all the eight-week-old BN rats developed anti-GBM antibodies following injection of $HgCl_2$, whereas such a phenomenon was not observed in standard non-inbred Wistar rats, suggested the involvement of a genetic factor. For this reason, other inbred strains (Lewis, Wistar AG, August, PVG/c) and non-inbred strains of rats (Sprague-Dawley) were also tested. Under the same experimental conditions, which were studied on days 15, 30 and 60, these rats did not produce anti-GBM antibodies. The rats of the Lewis strain were studied after they were injected with a double dose of $HgCl_2$ (0.4 mg/100 gm body weight). Even under these conditions, no anti-GBM antibodies were observed. In order to establish the genetic implication of this model, segregants were bred from the sensitive strain (BN) and from one of the resistant strains (Lewis). F_1 and F_2 hybrids as backcrosses between F_1 hybrids and Lewis parents were submitted to the same experimental procedure. The Ag-B (or H-1) of these segregants was determined by the hemagglutination technique[20] using alloantisera prepared according to Soulillou.[40] The animals underwent kidney biopsies on the 15th day. The production of anti-GBM antibodies was judged by the linear pattern observed by immunofluorescence.

It was found (Table 15–3) that under these conditions the F_1 hybrids, whether male or female, produced anti-GBM antibodies, but in lesser amounts than did the BN rats, as assessed by

TABLE 15–3.—ANTI-GBM ANTIBODIES
OBSERVED IN THE VARIOUS
SEGREGANTS BRED FROM BN AND
LEWIS STRAINS OF RATS INJECTED
WITH $HgCl_2$

RAT STRAIN	Ag-B HAPLOTYPE	POSITIVE RATS/ RATS TESTED
(Lew × BN) F_1	1/3	17/17
(Lew × BN) F_2	1/1	0/22
	1/3	19/31
	3/3	8/14
(Lew × BN) F_1	1/1	0/27
× Lew	1/3	9/20
Lew/BN	3/3	0/8

the intensity of the fluorescence. It was, moreover, interesting to note that these rats showed no proteinuria and that their CH50 levels remained normal. The results noted in the F_1 hybrids and in the backcrosses revealed that: (1) the rats that responded were found only among the heterozygous or homozygous rats possessing the Ag-B (Ag-B$_3$) or the H-1 (H-1^n) of the BN strain. The homozygous animals for the Ag-B (Ag-B$_1$) or the H-1 (H-1^l) from the Lewis strain were resistant. (2) Only a certain percentage of the rats bearing the Ag-B from the BN strain responded, whether they were heterozygous or homozygous. The statistical analyses are compatible with a genetic control depending on two or three genes. One of these genes is linked to the major histocompatibility complex.[13] The polygenic nature of this control was confirmed by the fact that congenic Lewis BN rats with the Ag-B haplotype of the BN strain are resistant. The difference in sensitivity between the two strains could be partially due to the absence of the antigen in the Lewis strain. The experiments carried out with the eluates from the kidney of $HgCl_2$ injected BN rats showed that the Lewis strain fixed these antibodies, as revealed by indirect immunofluorescence. Similarly, preliminary experiments carried out with $^{203}HgCl_2$ have shown that the metabolism of the mercury salt is the same in Lewis as in BN rats.

Benacerraf and McDevitt[3] and Biozzi et al.[6] have demonstrated the role of genetic factors, particularly the *Ir* genes, in the immune response to certain antigens. A genetic basis for certain experimental diseases has thus been found. This has been well demonstrated in the cases of experimental allergic encephalomyelitis in the rat[18, 44] and Heymann's autoimmune GN.[41] It is interesting to note that in the latter experimental disease, the sensitive strain is the Lewis strain,[14] whereas the BN strain is resistant. On the other hand, the fact that the BN strain easily and consistently produces antitubular basement membrane antibodies possibly reflects the facility with which this strain produces anti-BM antibodies.[42]

Influence of the Dose of $HgCl_2$

As the dose of 0.2 mg/100 gm body weight three times a week sometimes caused a high early mortality due to acute tubular renal insufficiency, lower doses of $HgCl_2$ were injected. The 15 rats receiving 0.10 or 0.05 mg/100 gm body weight three times a week responded in the same way as those injected with 0.2 mg $HgCl_2$.

SECOND STAGE

Kidney biopsy specimens taken from ten BN rats at a later stage (day 30 or 60) have made it possible to demonstrate a considerable modification of the pattern, observed by immunofluorescence, in which the response sometimes occurs before the first month but is always preceded by the appearance of anti-GBM antibodies. At this second stage, in five rats out of the ten studied, the fluoresceinated antirat IgG antiserum became fixed on the glomerular capillary walls in a well-defined granular pattern (Fig. 15–3, A). The linear pattern often persisted but became attenuated. In the five other rats, no definite glomerular granular pattern was observed; a considerable linear fixation persisted in these cases, which possibly could have masked the granular pattern. Among the ten rats studied, a granular fixation was observed at this stage, with the antirat IgG antiserum in the walls of the small arteries of the kidney (Fig. 15–3, B). No granular fixation was found in the tubular basement membrane. Serial biopsy specimens taken from these animals showed that the granular pattern occurred subsequent to the linear pattern. The granular pattern may be observed as early as the 15th day, but it was not observed on the 10th day. At this stage, only the linear pattern of fixation could be found. The serum complement level, measured in four of these rats, remained normal. Protein excretion levels measured at the end of the experiment were within the normal range in nine rats; one animal showed a proteinuria of 100 mg/24 hours. The presence of extramembranous deposits, suggested on the basis of the immunofluorescence findings, was confirmed by light and electron microscopic study. The latter examination established that in two rats that did not show a granular pattern by immunofluorescence, there were, nevertheless, extramembranous deposits; in the three other rats, there were no visible deposits. It was verified in one rat that the granular pattern observed in the small arteries of the kidney corresponded to the presence of electron-dense deposits.

The effect of the dose of $HgCl_2$ an the onset of this second stage

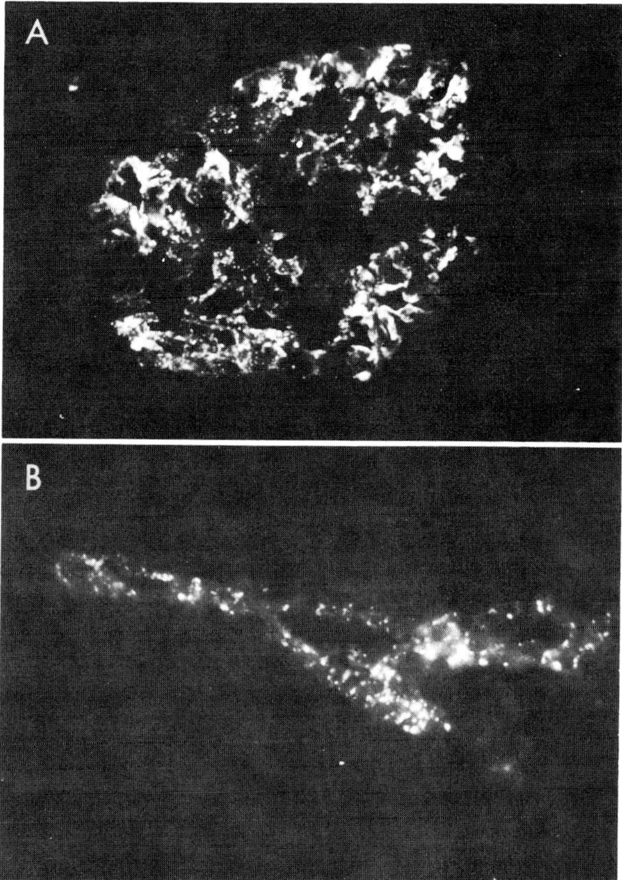

Fig. 15–3.—Kidney cryostat section from a BN rat injected with mercuric chloride for two months. Staining was with a fluoresceinated antirat IgG antiserum. Note the discontinuous and granular pattern of fixation on the glomerular tuft (×400) (**A**) and on the wall of a small renal artery (×450) (**B**).

was investigated (Table 15 – 4). The dosage of 0.2 mg three times a week for two months is sufficient for a granular pattern to occur in the glomerular capillaries and/or in the small arteries. On the other hand, with one injection per week for two weeks, no fixation of the antirat IgG antiserum was observed at the 8th week, but a linear fixation throughout the length of the glomerular capillaries was noted as early as the 15th day.

Until now, it has not been possible to identify the antigen re-

TABLE 15-4.—PATTERN OF FIXATION OBSERVED WITH THE FLUORESCEINATED ANTIRAT IgG ANTISERUM IN BN RATS INJECTED WITH VARIOUS DOSES OF $HgCl_2$

$HgCl_2$ INJECTED		PATTERN OF FIXATION*			
DOSE (PER WK, mg/100 gm)	DURATION (WK)	TWO WK GBM	EIGHT WK GBM	ARTERIES	INTERSTITIUM
0.6	8	10/10 L	10/10 L		
			5/10 G	10/10 G	0/10
0.2	8	5/5 L	3/3 L		
			2/3 G	3/3 G	2/3 G
0.6	2	6/6 L	5/5 L		
			4/5 G	1/5 G	0/5
0.2	2	5/5 L	0/5	0/5	0/5
0.2	1	3/5 L	0/5	0/5	0/5

*L = linear; G = granular.

sponsible for this second stage. The eluate obtained from rat kidneys showing a granular fixation could not be used because linear fixation of the antirat IgG antiserum always persisted. It is, nevertheless, tempting to imagine that the same antigen is responsible for both stages. First of all, a BM antigen is responsible for the formation of antibodies, so the circulating antigen may become complexed with the circulating antibodies. The IC then formed may be responsible for the second stage. It has been proved that GBM antigens may be present in normal serum in humans.[28] It is possible that antigens are liberated subsequent to the fixation of the antibodies on the GBM. This mechanism may be responsible for the granular glomerular deposits observed during the evolution of GN induced by anti-GBM heteroantibodies.[47]

Brown-Norway Control Rats

Fifty-seven BN control rats (15 males and 42 females) from 8 to 24 weeks old were studied. These rats were injected at the same intervals as the rats that had received $HgCl_2$, but with distilled water only, adjusted to the same pH as the $HgCl_2$ solution.[4] No linear or granular fixation of the antirat IgG antiserum was observed in these rats on the glomerular tuft or on the small arteries. On the other hand, in 12 of these rats, a segmental and focal fixation was noted, most likely in the mesangium. This type of fixation is easily distinguishable from the fixations already described in the rats receiving $HgCl_2$. These observations have already been made in other rat strains.[11, 15] They seem to be more frequent in older animals, but the reason for this has not been clarified.

Extraglomerular Localizations

In the kidney, during the first stage of the disease anti-GBM antibodies were detected only in the glomerular capillary walls. In a few cases (5 of 15), however, much lighter staining was observed on the tubular basement membranes with the antirat IgG antiserum. At the second stage, a granular pattern was frequently noted in the wall of the arteries. This fact led us to investigate extrarenal localizations.

EXTRARENAL LOCALIZATIONS OF ANTI-GBM ANTIBODIES

The in vivo distribution of anti-GBM antibodies in rats receiving $HgCl_2$ has been compared with antibodies eluted in vitro from the kidneys of rats injected with $HgCl_2$. To do this, the eluted antibodies were incubated with frozen sections of normal organs and then exposed to the fluoresceinated antirat IgG antiserum. Under these conditions, all of the basement membranes tested fixed the eluate (Table 15–5), as well as similar structures, such as reticulin. The antibodies, in particular, fixed to the pulmonary alveolocapillary basement membranes. These results are similar to those reported by other authors using anti-GBM heteroantibodies.[7, 22, 34]

In vivo, a linear pattern of fixation, considered as evidence of the presence of anti-BM antibodies, was consistently observed with the rat anti-IgG antiserum on the reticulin of the white splenic pulp (Table 15–5). A similar fixation was observed in numerous other organs.[4] It should be noted: (1) that certain sites recognized in vitro by the eluted antibodies do not fix the circulating antibodies; (2) that the intensity of the fluorescence was always much more pronounced on the glomerular capillary walls and the splenic reticulin; and (3) that the pulmonary alveolar basement membrane and capillaries are only slightly and inconsistently labeled. The latter point can be related to the

TABLE 15–5.–IN VITRO AND IN VIVO LOCALIZATION OF ANTI-GBM ANTIBODIES*

ORGAN TESTED[†]	IN VITRO	IN VIVO
Kidney		
GBM	+	15/15
TBM	+	5/15
Arterioles	+	0/15
BC	+	0/15
Spleen		
WP reticulin	+	15/15
WP arterioles	+	10/15
RP reticulin	±	1/15
Lung		
Alv-cap BM	+	2/14[‡]
Bronchial cap	+	1/14
Bronchial epi BM	+	0/14
Liver		
Portal spaces	+	3/3
Suprahepatic veins	+	3/3
Sinusoïdes	±	0/3
Adrenal		
Capillaries	+	2/2
Intestine		
Epi BM	+	1/2[‡]
Capillaries	+	2/2
Myocardium		
Sarcolemma	+	1/4[‡]
Capillaries	+	3/4

*Localizations were determined in vivo by direct immunofluorescence and in vitro by indirect immunofluorescence, using an eluate from BN rat kidneys.

[†]GBM = glomerular basement membrane; TBM = tubular basement membrane; BC = Bowman's capsule; WP = white pulp; RP = red pulp; cap = capillaries; BM = basement membrane; Alv-cap = alveolocapillary; epi = epithelial.

[‡]The fixations observed were very slight.

greater technical difficulty in localizing the anti-GBM heteroantibodies injected intravenously on the alveolar BM of lung than those on the GBM.[45]

Several hypotheses can be considered: (1) The quantity of antibody induced by the injection of $HgCl_2$ is insufficient. Although the level of circulating antibodies has not been measured, this seems unlikely on the basis of the level of proteinuria observed in certain animals. (2) It is possible that, for anatomical reasons, certain antigenic sites are less easily accessible to antibodies. (3) Finally, the specificity and/or the affinity of the antibodies induced by $HgCl_2$ is possibly different from that of the heteroantibodies induced by immunization with whole GBM mixed with Freund's complete adjuvant. In an attempt to increase the level of circulating antibodies, 17 rats were submitted to a splenectomy and/or binephrectomy on the 15th day. No increase in the frequency of linear fixation on the alveolocapillary basement membrane was observed, nor was there an increase in the intensity of fluorescence in the few positive cases.

EXTRARENAL LOCALIZATIONS OF IMMUNE COMPLEXES

As early as the 15th day and particularly during the first and second months, the presence of granular deposits suggestive of immune complexes was confirmed by immunofluorescence in numerous capillaries or arteries (Table 15–6, Fig. 15–3, B). Here again, only in some animals was granular pulmonary fixation observed. The deposits noted were very scattered, few in number and situated in the pulmonary interstitium. The effect of splenectomy and/or binephrectomy was tested in the same way as for the anti-GBM antibodies. It is striking that under these conditions, three animals developed numerous granular deposits in the pulmonary interstitium. These facts require con-

TABLE 15–6.—EXTRARENAL
LOCALIZATIONS OF GRANULAR
DEPOSITS IN BN RATS INJECTED
WITH $HgCl_2$

ORGANS TESTED	TWO WK	EIGHT WK
Spleen		
White pulp arteries	7/15	4/4
Lung	1/14	0/2
Liver		
Portal spaces	0/3	2/3
Suprahepatic veins	0/3	2/3
Sinusoïdes	0/3	0/3
Adrenal		
Capillaries	0/2	3/3
Intestine		
Capillaries	0/2	2/2
Myocardium		
Capillaries	2/4	2/3

firmation by a larger study. It has been suggested that the favorable effect of binephrectomy in Goodpasture's syndrome[29] may be explained by a "neutralization" of the circulating antibodies complexed to the circulating antigen.[39] The quantity of circulating antigen would increase as a result of the binephrectomy. If this hypothesis is correct, it is not surprising that an increase in circulating IC takes place.

No capillary or arteriolar deposits were detected in the four rats examined on the 10th day following the beginning of the $HgCl_2$ injections or in the control rats studied. Hence, as far as one can judge from the granular pattern of fixation observed by immunofluorescence, there was considerable diffusion of deposits of IC into numerous capillaries within the organism. Similar observations have been made in other diseases where circulating IC is present. These diseases may be either acute, as in acute serum sickness[10] and acute poststreptococcal GN,[33] or chronic, as in chronic serum sickness in the rabbit[8] and disseminated lupus erythematosus.[9, 48] It is still difficult to say whether these deposits have pathologic effects and whether they can cause arteritis.

Results Observed in Other Rat Strains

Other rat strains, both inbred and not inbred, were injected with $HgCl_2$ according to the same experimental procedure (Table 15–7). Certain strains (Lewis, Wistar AG, Sprague-Dawley) did not develop any glomerular disease; they had no proteinuria and no renal fixation was observed with the fluoresceinated sheep antirat IgG antiserum. Rarely, a segmental and focal, probably mesangial, fixation was noted, as in the control and BN rats.

The negative results observed with the Lewis strain have been studied in more detail. Indeed, the Lewis strain is known to consistently develop GN following injection of a brush border antigen from the proximal convoluted tubule.[41] It is tempting to suppose that $HgCl_2$, which has a well-known effect on the proximal convoluted tubule, is able to induce GN by a similar mechanism. In fact, whatever the sex or age (8 or 40 weeks) of the animals and the dose of $HgCl_2$ injected (0.2, 0.3 or 0.4 mg/100 gm body weight), glomerular fixation of the antirat IgG antiserum was never observed. These results are in contradiction with those recently reported by Kelchner *et al.*[23] These authors, using

TABLE 15-7.—PATTERN OF FIXATION OBSERVED BY
IMMUNOFLUORESCENCE* AT EIGHT WEEKS IN VARIOUS
RAT STRAINS

| | | | | GLOMERULAR FIXATIONS | |
| | | | | LINEAR | GRANULAR |
STRAIN	Ag-B	NO. OF RATS AND SEX	HgCl₂ INJECTED‡	(ANTI-GBM)	(IC?)
Lewis (Lew)	1	10 F	0.2	0/10	0/10
		10 F	0	0/10	0/10
		5 M†	0.2	0/5	0/5
		5 M†	0.3	0/5	0/5
		10 M†	0.	0/10	0/10
Wistar AG	2	5 F	0.2	0/5	0/5
		5 F	0	0/5	0/5
Brown Norway	3	5 F, 5 M	0.2	10/10	5/10§
		5 F, 5 M	0	0/10	0/10
PVG/c	5	5 F, 5 M	0.2	0/10	10/10
		5 F, 5 M	0	0/10	0/10
August	5	5 F	0.2	0/5	5/5
		5 F	0	0/5	0/5
Sprague-Dawley	‖	10 F	0.2	0/10	0/10
		10 F	0	0/10	0/10

*Kidney biopsies studied with a fluoresceinated antirat IgG antiserum.
†Ten-month-old rats.
‡Dose expressed in mg/100 gm body weight, three times a week.
§The five other rats had a granular pattern of fixation in the wall of arteries.
‖Non-inbred rats.

the same experimental conditions, observed a parietal, granular
fixation on the glomerular tuft. The eluate obtained from these
kidneys recognizes an antigen from the brush border of the proximal convoluted tubule. In the opinion of the authors, the GN
induced in the Lewis strain by $HgCl_2$ injection would be similar
to that described by Heymann et al.[21]
These conflicting results are difficult to explain. However,
several facts are worth mentioning: The aspects presented by
the aforementioned authors as characteristic of a granular
glomerular fixation are not very convincing. Also, the electron
microscope has not yet been used to confirm the presence of extramembranous deposits. It is surprising that the BN strain
which does not develop a Heymann-type GN,[41] is particularly
sensitive to $HgCl_2$, whereas the Lewis,[14] Sprague-Dawley and
PVG/c[17] strains which easily respond to the injection of tubular
antigen (F × 1A),[14] do not develop any glomerular disease with
$HgCl_2$ (the former two strains) or an immune-type GN, which is

very different with the PVG/c strain. Differences between the Lewis strains used might be a possible explanation for this discrepancy. The rats of the PVG/c and August strains (which both have the same Ag-B) did not produce anti-GBM antibodies on the 15th or the 60th day. These rats did not show significant proteinuria. However, in this experiment, the proteinuria was tested only on the 15th and 60th days. The renal biopsies done during the first and second months render it possible to demonstrate a granular fixation of the antirat IgG antiserum on the

Fig. 15–4.–Kidney cryostat section from a PVG/c rat injected with HgCl$_2$ for two months. Staining with a fluoresceinated antirat IgG antiserum. Note the granular labeling of the mesangial areas (×350) **(A)** and at the base of some proximal convoluted tubules (×350) **(B)**; the glomerular tuft *(arrow)* is not stained.

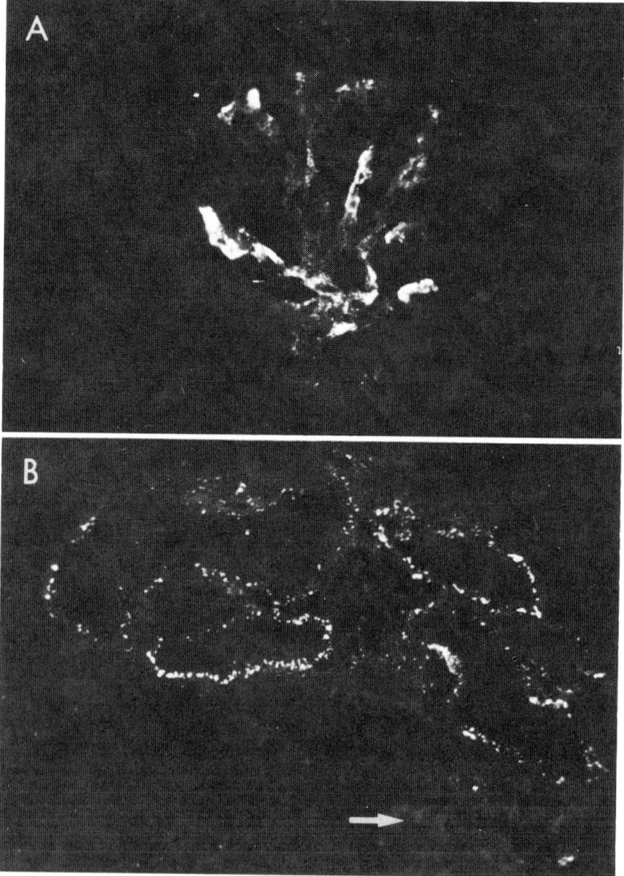

mesangial areas and occasionally on the GBM (Fig. 15–4). In addition, certain rats showed arteriolar deposits and considerable deposits at the base of the proximal convoluted tubules. The rats that showed the most marked tubular deposits were those that had the least glomerular deposits.

In order to try to identify the antigen responsible, the kidneys of these rats were eluted at an acid pH. The eluate contained rat IgG. These immunoglobulins, when tested by indirect immunofluorescence, were not fixed on frozen sections of normal rat kidney. Hence, the antigen still is not identified. It seems unlikely that it is an epithelial antigen of the proximal convoluted tubule, nor is it likely that it is a basement membrane antigen. As Hg^{2+} is known to become fixed on the free SH groups of several serum or tissue proteins, the latter are then liable to play the part of antigen. One important fact is that the same agent can induce various types of GN of which the mechanism seems different depending on the strain tested. Recently, another strain (provided by Dr. Van Es) has been examined. Some animals of this strain developed GN as early as the 15th day, which was characterized by a mixed pattern of fixation, both linear and granular.

Conclusions

It has been confirmed that $HgCl_2$ can induce GN in certain rat strains. The mechanism of this glomerular disease may vary. (1) In BN rats, anti-GBM antibodies were observed in the initial stage. Subsequently, a response suggesting deposits of IC in the glomerular tuft and other organs was observed. It is tempting to assume that complexes of anti-GBM antibodies and GBM antigen are responsible for the second stage. (2) Other strains (PVG/c and August) had essentially mesangial but also tubular deposits. The antigen responsible has not yet been identified, but there is no evidence of a brush border antigen of the proximal convoluted tubule. (3) In another non-inbred strain, mixed GN with both linear and granular fixation patterns was found in only some animals. This suggests that in certain rats, a mechanism similar to that described in BN rats could be involved.

These results are in agreement with those recently described by Roman-Franco et al. in the rabbit.[35] They are, on the other hand, contrary to those reported by Kelchner *et al.* in the Lewis rat strain.[23]

In human pathology, several cases of membranous GN have been described in patients exposed to certain mercury compounds. Mercury salts are used less and less frequently in medicine. They are still included in certain ointments and particularly in local antiseptics, as well as in numerous agricultural products. It is possible that these mercury compounds are responsible for certain IC-type GN. It is difficult to ascertain the role of mercury compounds since the chemical assay of mercury is difficult and inaccurate. The demonstration of the exact mechanism(s) of GN in various species might make it possible to elucidate the mechanism(s) of certain human GN, as suggested by the recent reports of Barr *et al.*[2] and of Lindqvist *et al.*[27] They observed a high prevalence of GN with immune-type deposits in African women who make frequent use of ointments containing mercury salts. In some of these women, linear and granular glomerular fixation patterns were noted. The same glomerular picture was reproduced in two of the three rabbits given the same product.[27] This last point confirms the role of mercury salts in some human GN and suggests that anti-GBM antibodies can in fact be found before or together with an immune complex type of glomerulonephritis.

Acknowledgments

We wish to thank Mrs. D. Moquet for typing and M. P. Teychenne for technical assistance.

References

1. Bariety, J., Druet, P., Laliberte, F., and Sapin, C.: Glomerulonephritis with γ and B1C globulin deposits induced in rats by mercuric chloride, Am. J. Pathol. 65:293, 1971.
2. Barr, R. D., Rees, P. H., Cordy, P. E., Kungu, A., Woodger, B. A., and Cameron, H. M.: Nephrotic syndrome in adult Africans in Nairobi, Br. Med. J. 2:121, 1972.
3. Benacerraf, B., and McDevitt, H. O.: The histocompatibility-linked immune response genes, Science 175:273, 1972.
4. Bernaudin, J. F., Sapin, C., Druet, E., and Druet, P.: Localisation tissulaire des auto-anticorps induits par HgCl₂ chez le rat Brown-Norway, Ann. Immunol. (Paris) 128c: 32, 1977.
5. Bignon, J., Chahinian, G., Feldmann, G., and Sapin, C.: Ultrastructural immunoperoxidase demonstration of autologous albumin in the alveolar capillary membrane and in the alveolar lining material of normal rat, J. Cell. Biol. 64:503, 1975.
6. Biozzi, G., Stiffel, C., Mouton, D., and Bouthillier, Y.: Selection of lines of mice with

high and low antibody responses to complex immunogens, in Benacerraf, B. (ed.): *Immunogenetics and Immunodeficiency.*

7. Blau, M., Day, E. D., Planinsek, T., and Pressman, D.: Specificity and cross localization of anti-kidney antibodies, J. Immunol. 79:334, 1957.

8. Brentjens, J. R., O'Connell, D. W., Pawlowski, I. B., and Andres, G. A.: Extraglomerular lesions associated with deposition of circulating antigen-antibody complexes in kidneys of rabbits with chronic serum sickness, Clin. Immunol. Immunopathol. 3:112, 1974.

9. Brentjens, J., Ossi, E., Albini, B., Sepulveda, M., Kano, K., Sheffer, J., Vasilion, P., Marine, E., Baliah, T., Jockin, H., and Andres, G. A.: Disseminated immune deposits in lupus erythematosus, Arthritis Rheum. 20:962, 1977.

10. Cochrane, C. G., and Koffler, D.: Immune complex disease in experimental animals and man, Adv. Immunol. 16:185, 1973.

11. Couser, W. G., and Stilmant, M. M.: Mesangial lesions and focal glomerular sclerosis in the aging rat, Lab. Invest. 33:491, 1975.

12. Dixon, F. J.: The pathogenesis of glomerulonephritis, Am. J. Med. 44:493, 1968.

13. Druet, E., Sapin, C., Günther, E., Feingold, N., and Druet, P.: Mercuric chloride-induced anti-glomerular basement membrane antibodies in the rat. Genetic control, Eur. J. Immunol. 7:348, 1977.

14. Edgington, T. S., Glassock, R. J., and Dixon, F. J.: Autologous immune complex pathogenesis of experimental allergic glomerulonephritis, Science 155:1432, 1967.

15. Elema, J. D., and Arends, A.: Focal and segmental glomerular hyalinosis and sclerosis in the rat, Lab. Invest. 33:554, 1975.

16. Feldman, J. D.: Pathogenesis of ultrastructural glomerular changes induced by immunologic means, in Grabar, P., and Miescher, P. A. (eds.): *Immunopathology. Proceedings of 3rd International Symposium* (Basel: Benno Schwabe, 1963), p. 263.

17. Fleuren, G. J.: Studies on the pathogenesis and treatment of experimental immune complex glomerulonephritis, Academic thesis, Groningen.

18. Gasser, D. L., Newlin, C. M., Palm, J., and Gonatas, N. K.: Genetic control of susceptibility to experimental allergic encephalomyelitis in rats, Science 181:872, 1973.

19. Gritzka, T. L., and Trump, B. F.: Renal tubular lesions caused by mercuric chloride. Electron microscopic observations: degeneration of the pars recta, Am. J. Pathol. 52:1225, 1968.

20. Günther, E., and Rüde, E.: Genetic complementation of histocompatibility-linked Ir genes in the rat, J. Immunol. 115:1387, 1975.

21. Heymann, W., Hackel, D. B., Harwood, S., Wilson, S. G. F., and Hunter, J. L. P.: Production of nephrotic syndrome in rats by Freund's adjuvant and rat kidney suspensions, Proc. Soc. Exp. Biol. Med. 100:660, 1959.

22. Katz, D. H., Unanue, E. R., and Dixon, F. J.: Nephritogenic properties of cross-reacting kidney-fixing antibodies to heart, spleen and muscle, J. Immunol. 98:260, 1967.

23. Kelchner, J., McIntosh, J. R., Boedecker, E., Guggenheim, S., and McIntosh, R. M.: Experimental autologous immune deposit nephritis in rats associated with mercuric chloride administration, Experientia 32:1204, 1976.

24. Lee, J. C., Dushkin, M., Eyring, E. J., Engleman, E. P., and Hopper, J.: Renal lesions associated with gold therapy: light and electron microscopic studies, Arthritis Rheum. 8:1, 1965.

25. Lehotzky, K.: Protection by estrogenic hormone against nephrotoxicity induced by organic mercury, Int. Arch. Arbeits Med. 30:193, 1972.

26. Lerner, R. A., Glassock, R. J., and Dixon, F. J.: The role of anti-glomerular basement membrane antibody in the pathogenesis of human glomerulonephritis, J. Exp. Med. 126:989, 1967.

27. Lindqvist, K. J., Makene, W. J., Shaba, J. K., and Nantulya, V.: Immunofluorescence and electron microscopic studies of kidney biopsies from patients with nephrotic syndrome, possibly induced by skin-lightening creams containing mercury, East Afr. Med. J. 51:168, 1974.

28. McPhaul, J. J., and Dixon, F. J.: Immunoreactive basement membrane antigens in normal human serum and urine, J. Exp. Med. 130:1395, 1969.
29. Maddock, R. K., Stevens, L. E., Reemtsma, K., and Bloomer, H. A.: Goodpasture's syndrome. Cessation of pulmonary hemorrhage after bilateral nephrectomy, Ann. Intern. Med. 67:1258, 1967.
30. Mandema, E., Arends, A., Van Zeijst, J., Vermeer, G., Van der Hem, G. K., and Van der Slikke, L. B.: Mercury and the kidney, Lancet 1:1266, 1963.
31. Mayer, M. M.: Complement and complement fixation, in Kabat, E. A., and Mayer, M. M. (eds.): *Experimental Immunochemistry* (Springfield, Ill.: Charles C Thomas, Publisher, 1967), pp. 133–240.
32. Muehrcke, R. C., Rudofsky, U., and Steblay, R. W.: Studies on auto-immune nephritis in sheep and rats. III. The pattern and significance of ultrastructural changes in the glomerular lesions, Fed. Proc. 26:743, 1967.
33. Ossi, E., Prezyna, A., Sepulveda, M., Elwood, C., and Andres, G.: Immune deposits in the spleen of a patient with acute poststreptococcal glomerulonephritis (APSGN), Clin. Immunol. Immunopathol. 6:306, 1976.
34. Pressman, D.: The zone of localization of antitissue antibodies as determined by the use of radioactive tracers, J. Allergy 22:387, 1951.
35. Roman-Franco, A. A., Turiello, M., Albini, G., Ossi, E., and Andres, G.: Anti-basement membrane antibody (A-Bm Ab) and immune complexes (Ic) in rabbits injected with mercuric chloride (HgCl$_2$), Kidney Int. 10:549, 1976.
36. Sapin, C., and Druet, P.: Isolation of rat and rabbit IgM from normal serum using anti-human μ antibody polyacrylamide beads immunoadsorbents, J. Immunol. Methods 12:355, 1974.
37. Sapin, C., Druet, E., and Druet, P.: Induction of anti-glomerular basement membrane antibodies in the Brown-Norway rat by mercuric chloride, Clin. Exp. Immunol. 28:173, 1977.
38. Shigematsu, H.: Glomerular events during the initial phase of rat Masugi nephritis, Virchows Arch. (Cell Pathol.) 5:187, 1970.
39. Siegel, R. R.: The basis of pulmonary disease resolution after nephrectomy in Goodpasture's syndrome, Am. J. Med. Sci. 55:565, 1973.
40. Soulillou, J. P., Carpenter, C. B., D'Apice, A. J. F., and Strom, T. B.: The role of non-classical, Fc-receptor associated, Ag-B antigens (Ia) in rat allograft enhancement, J. Exp. Med. 143:405, 1976.
41. Stenglein, B., Thoenes, G. H., and Günther, E.: Genetically controlled autologous immune complex glomerulonephritis in rats, J. Immunol. 115:895, 1975.
42. Sugisaki, T., Klassen, J., Milgrom, F., Andres, G. A., and McCluskey, R. T.: Immunopathologic study of an autoimmune tubular and interstitial disease in the Brown-Norway rats, Lab. Invest. 28:658, 1973.
43. Unanue, E. R., and Dixon, F. J.: Experimental glomerulonephritis. IV. Participation of complement in nephrotoxic nephritis, J. Exp. Med. 119:965, 1964.
44. Williams, R. M., and Moore, M. J.: Linkage of susceptibility to experimental allergic encephalomyelitis to the major histocompatibility locus in the rat, J. Exp. Med. 138:775, 1973.
45. Willoughby, W. F., and Dixon, F. J.: Experimental hemorrhagic pneumonitis produced by heterologous anti-lung antibody, J. Immunol. 104:28, 1970.
46. Wilson, C. B., and Smith, R. C.: Goodpasture's syndrome associated with influenza A$_2$ virus infections, Ann. Intern. Med. 76:91, 1972.
47. Wilson, C. B., and Dixon, F. J.: The renal response to immunological injury, in Brenner, B. M., and Rector, F. C. (eds.): *The Kidney* (Philadelphia: W. B. Saunders Co., 1976), pp. 838–940.
48. Yeo, P. P. B., and Sinniah, R.: Lupus cor pulmonale with electron microscopic and immunofluorescent antibody studies, Ann. Rheum. Dis. 34:457, 1975.
49. Zimmerman, S. W., Groehler, K., and Bierne, G. J.: Hydrocarbon exposure and chronic glomerulonephritis, Lancet 2:199, 1975.

16

Glomerulonephritis and Necrotizing Angiitis

D. DROZ, M.D., L. H. NOEL, M.D.,
M. LEIBOWITCH, M.D., AND C. BARBANEL, M.D.

Hôpital Necker, Paris, France

The term of "necrotizing angiitis" defines a lesion consisting of a fibrinoid necrosis of the arterial, venous or capillary vascular wall associated with a perivascular infiltration of frequently pycnotic polymorphonuclear cells. This lesion can be either localized or disseminated in numerous organs, and the glomerular capillaries are not infrequently affected.

The clinical presentation of necrotizing angiitis is highly variable, depending on the site and extent of the lesions.

Patients and Methods

Twenty-one patients referred to a nephrology clinic between 1970 and 1977 were included in this study. They all presented with extrarenal necrotizing angiitis. At least one kidney specimen was obtained from each of the patients, either by percutaneous biopsy or at the time of postmortem examination.

For light microscopy the specimens were fixed in Duboscq-Brasil liquid, embedded in paraffin and then cut at 2 μm. The following stains were used: hematein-eosin safran, trichrome with light green, silver impregnation according to Wilder's or

Jone's methods, periodic acid-Schiff (PAS) orcein according to Weigert. For each specimen, multiple sections were observed. For immunofluorescence studies, the specimens were frozen in isopentane, cooled by liquid nitrogen and cut at 2 μm using a cryostat. Fluoresceinated antisera against human IgG, IgA, IgM, C3, C1q and fibrin were used (Hyland and Behring-Werke Laboratories). In two cases, the amount of HBsAg was estimated by indirect immunofluorescence, using a specific anti-HBsAg antiserum (Behring-Werke Laboratories).

Serum levels of C3 and C4 were measured by radial immunodiffusion. Circulating immune complexes were measured by precipitation with polyethylene glycol at the final concentration of 3.5%. The serum detection of HBsAg and of antibody anti-HBsAg was made by electroimmunodiffusion and hemagglutination.

Results

Two different types of glomerular lesions were observed. Necrotizing glomerulonephritis, characterized by areas of necrosis in the tufts surrounded by segmental or circumferential epi-

Fig. 16–1.—Segmental necrotic lesion of the glomerular tuft with pycnotic polymorphonuclear cells and epithelial crescent. Masson's trichrome with light green; ×250.

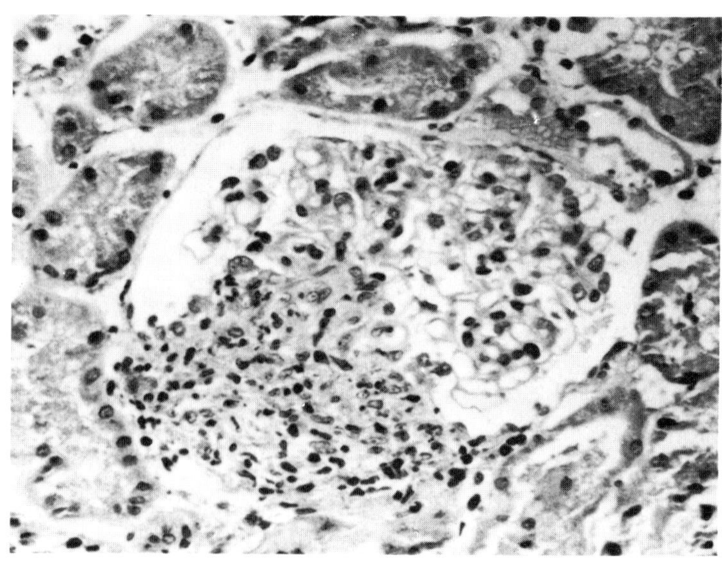

thelial crescents, were found in 18 patients (Fig. 16–1). The necrotic areas contained fibrin deposits, and pycnotic polymorphonuclear cells were common. By immunofluorescence, fibrin alone was detected on crescents in seven of 16 patients and immunoglobulins and/or complement was found in the glomeruli in five of 16 patients.

In the three remaining cases, the lesions were characterized as segmental and proliferative glomerulonephritis without necrotizing areas. In these cases, small endomembranous deposits of IgA and C3 were observed by immunofluorescence.

These 21 patients belong to clinically or biologically distinct entities; 11 had clinical evidence of periarteritis nodosa (PAN), four had Wegener's granulomatosis, one had giant cell temporal arteritis (Horton's disease), one had mixed essential IgG–IgM cryoglobulinemia and four had prominent cutaneous vasculitis characteristic of Gougerot's trisymptomatic purpura (allergic cutaneous angiitis).

PERIARTERITIS NODOSA: 11 CASES

Table 16–1 summarizes the main extrarenal manifestations of PAN for each patient. Table 16–2 indicates the locations of the extrarenal necrotizing angiitis.

Previous allergic manifestations were noted in three patients. An allergic reaction occurred one month before the onset of urinary symptoms in patient 2. In another case (patient 11) the first symptom appeared during a desensitization to candidin for an obstinate eczema. Patient 8 had had asthma since the age of 12, i.e., three years before the first signs of systemic involvement. In two patients, tonsillitis antedated the signs of PAN. The delay between the first signs of the disease and the first renal symptoms was less than three months in six patients and was within three to eight months in the other five. In eight patients, renal involvement was marked by rapidly progressive renal failure associated with proteinuria and hematuria, necessitating chronic hemodialysis in seven. In the three remaining cases (patients 2, 4 and 11), the renal involvement was discovered by routine urinalysis. Preliminary examination revealed severe hypertension in one patient and moderate hypertension in three.

The first renal biopsy (Table 16–3) was performed in five patients during the first month of the renal disease and between

DROZ ET AL.

TABLE 16–1.—EXTRARENAL MANIFESTATIONS OF
PERIARTERITIS NODOSA

| | PATIENT | | | | | | | | | | | |
	1	2	3	4	5	6	7	8	9	10	11	TOTAL
Age	44	60	53	49	59	15	15	47	48	72	26	
Sex	M	F	M	M	F	F	F	M	F	M	M	
Fever	+	+	+	+	0	+	+	+	+	0	+	9/11
Loss of weight	0	+	+	+	0	0	+	+		+	0	6/11
Arthralgia	0	+	+	+	+	+	+	+	+	+	+	10/11
Myalgia	+	0	+	+	0	0	0	+	+	0	0	5/11
Cutaneous symptoms												
Purpura	0			+	0		0	+		+	+	
Others		0	0			0			0			7/11
None	+			+	+		+	0		+	+	
Abdominal pain	+	0	+	+	0	+	0	0	+	+	0	6/11
Nervous system symptoms												
Peripheral	0			+	+	0	+	+	+	+	+	
Central		0	0									7/11
None	0			0	0	0	+	0	0	0	0	
Gastrointestinal bleeding	0	0	+	0	0	0	0	0	0	+	0	2/11
Pulmonary symptoms												
Hemoptysis	0	+		+	+	+	0	+		+		
Others			0						0		0	8/11
None	+	+		+	0	+	+	0		+		
Hepatic symptoms	+	0	+	0	0	0	0	0	0	0	0	2/11
Hypertension	0	0	+	+	+	+	+	0	+		0	6/11
Anemia	+	+	+	+	+	+	+	+	+	+	+	11/11
Leukocytosis	0	+	+	+	+	+	+	+	+	+	0	9/11
Eosinophilia	0	0	+	0	+	+	+	+	+	0	0	6/11
Hypergammaglobulinemia	0	+	+	+	0		0	0	+	0	0	5/11

the first and fourth months in the remaining six. All but two of
the patients (patients 4 and 11) had severe renal insufficiency at
the time of kidney biopsy, and six were already being hemodialyzed.

The types of renal lesions were quite similar, although they

TABLE 16–2.—LOCATIONS OF THE
EXTRARENAL ANGIITIS LESIONS
IN PERIARTERITIS NODOSA

Muscle	6
Skin	3
Nose	1
Diffuse Disseminated	3

varied in intensity from patient to patient. Lesions were characterized by necrotic areas and epithelial crescents in the glomeruli. The crescents involved all the glomeruli in four patients, 50–80% of the glomeruli in four patients and less than 50% of the glomeruli in three patients. Mild proliferation of the mesangial cells was noted in six patients and was sometimes associated with the presence of granulocytes in the glomerular capillary loops. Fibrous segmental lesions of the glomeruli were found in four patients. No deposits were found in seven patients. In contrast, subepithelial deposits or "humps" were observed in four patients, together with mesangial deposits in one. By immunofluorescence, the fixation of the serum against fibrinogen on the crescents remained the most important, although inconstant, feature (Fig. 16–2). In one case (patient 3) C3 was observed in the humps (Fig. 16–3). In another case (patient 10), IgG, C3 and C1q were present on endomembranous deposits (Fig. 16–4). In patient 11, fixation of serum against IgA was observed in the mesangial area, spreading along the capillary wall (Fig. 16–5).

Acute tubular lesions, i.e., necrosis of the tubular epithelium, were present in all but two patients. In six patients a dense interstitial cellular infiltration composed of lymphocytes and plasmocytes was noted. In two patients numerous interstitial cells surrounded the glomeruli. Neither eosinophils nor granulomas were found in the interstitial tissue.

Necrotizing angiitis of the interlobular arteries was seen in four patients. Nonspecific vascular lesions, i.e., arteriosclerosis and/or fibrous endarteritis, were noted in eight patients. By immunofluorescence, deposits of C3 were found in the arteriolar walls in three patients without evidence of necrotic lesions. In patient 9, a fixation of all the studied sera was noted in all the vascular lumina.

The HBs antigen was not found in the kidneys in either of two patients.

IMMUNOLOGIC RESULTS.—The serum levels of C3 and of C4 were normal or high in eight of eight patients and in five of five patients, respectively. The latex test had negative results in seven of nine and slightly positive results in two of nine patients. The Waaler–Rose reaction had negative results in nine of nine patients. Cryoglobulins were detected in one of nine. Circulating immune complexes were found in two of four patients.

TABLE 16–3.—PERIARTERITIS NODOSA RENAL BIOPSY*

| PATIENT | CLINICAL FEATURES | | | | | GLOMERULI | | | | | |
	DELAY BETWEEN ONSET AND RENAL BIOPSY	CREAT mg/100 ml	PROTEINURIA gm/24 hr	RBC/ min	BP	NECROSIS	CRESCENTS (%)	X ENDO	DEPOSITS	FSL	IF
1	10 day		HD		0	++	100	+	0	0	F, crescent
2	0 day	2.0	1	30,000	0	+	20	0	humps, DIC	++	F, crescent
3	15 day	4.5	1.20	50,000	+	++	80	0	Humps	0	F,G, crescent
4	15 day	1.4	2	340,000	+	+	33	+	Humps	0	Negative
5	2 mo		HD		++	+++	100	0	0	0	ND
6	1 mo		HD		0	++	50	+	0	+	Negative
7	3 mo	2.5	0.5	3,700	+	++	80	+ PMN	0	+	ND
8	8 day		HD		0	+++	100	0 PMN	0	0	F, crescent
9	4 mo		HD		0	++	80	0	Humps	0	Negative
10	1 mo		HD		0	++	100	+	0	0	F, crescent, G,C3,C1q, SED
11	4 mo	1.2	1	300,000	0	+	20	+	0	0	F, crescent, A, DIC, C3

*Abbreviations: Creat = serum creatinine, HD = hemodialysis, BP = hypertension, X endo = endocapillary proliferation, FSL = fibrous segmental lesions, DIC = mesangial deposits, IF = immunofluorescence, ND = not done, SED = subendothelial deposit, A = IgA, G = IgG, M = IgM, F = fibrin, ILA = interlobular artery, NA = necrotizing angiitis, FE = fibrous endarteritis, A = arteriolosclerosis, PMN = polymorphonuclear cells, and A° = arterioles.

TABLE 16–3 *continued*

	VESSELS			TUBULOINTERSTITIAL LESIONS		
						INTERSTITIAL CELL
NA	FE	A	IF	ACUTE	FIBROUS	INFILTRATION
0	++	0	0	++	0	++
0	++	+	0	++	+	+
0	++	+	C3, A°	+++	0	+++
0	0	++	C3, A°	0	0	+
ILA	++	0	ND	+++	0	+
ILA	+	+	Negative	+	++	++
ILA	0	0	ND	++	+	+++
0	++	0	M,C3,A°	+++	0	++
ILA	0	0	AGM,C3,C4,F vessels lumen	++	0	+++
0	++	0	Negative	++	0	0
0	+	0	Negative	0	0	0

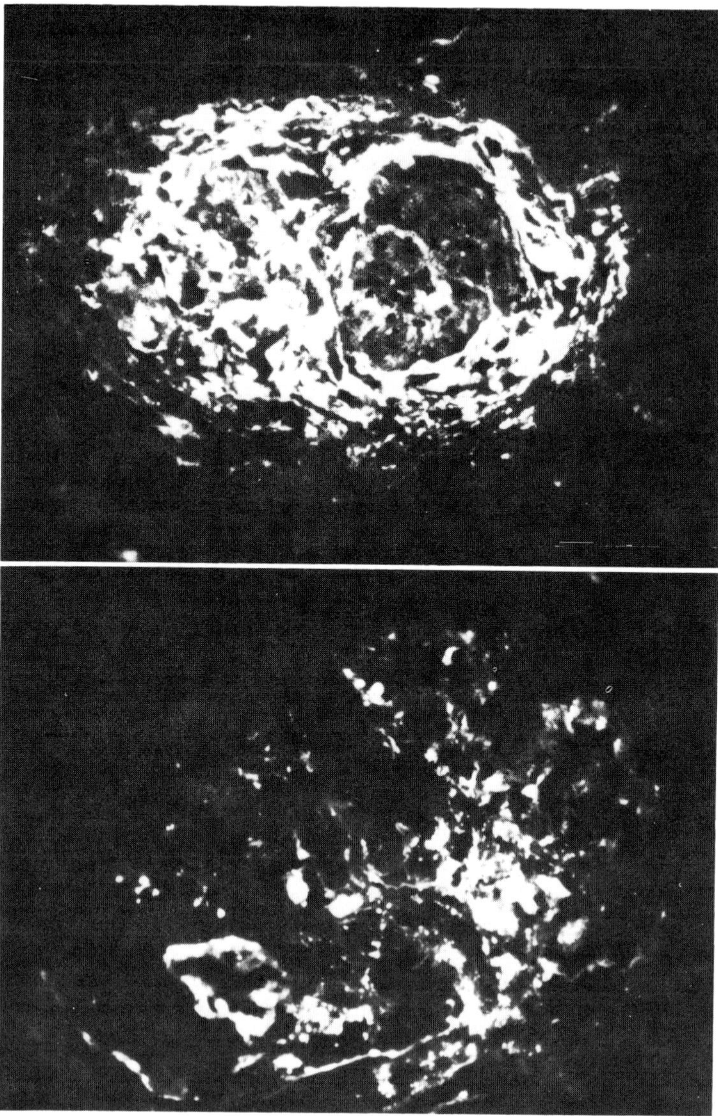

Fig. 16–2 (top).—Immunofluorescence—antifibrinogen serum on epithelial crescent, ×250.

Fig. 16–3 (bottom).—Immunofluorescence—anti-C3 serum on granulous deposits along the capillary walls, ×250.

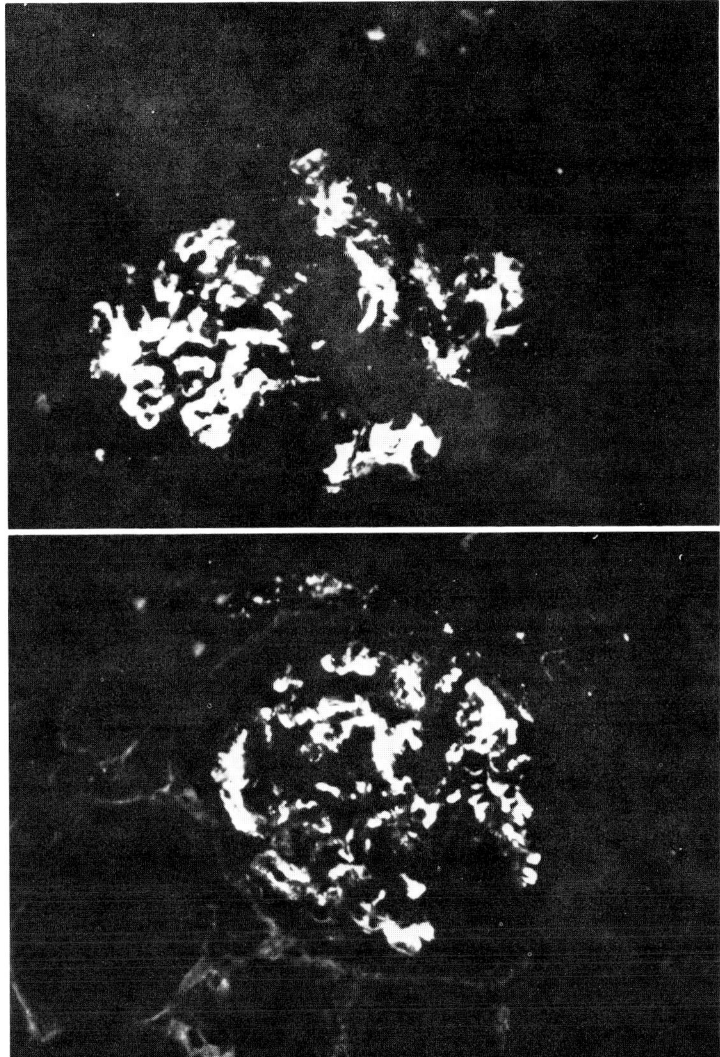

Fig. 16–4 (top). – Immunofluorescence – anti-IgG serum on endomembranous deposits, ×250.

Fig. 16–5 (bottom). – Immunofluorescence – anti-IgA serum on mesangial deposits, ×250.

HBsAg was sought but not found in the serum of eight patients. Anti-HBs antibody was not found in the four cases in which it was sought.

Course. — Five patients, all with severe renal failure, died soon after the beginning of treatment (patients 5, 6, 8, 9 and 10). Death was caused by cardiac arrythmia in two patients, by hemoptysis in one, and by intestinal hemorrhage in another. In one patient the cause of death was not identified. Postmortem examination of the kidney specimen was performed in three cases. No modification in comparison with the first biopsy was found in patients 5 and 8. In contrast, in patient 6 the lesions of necrotizing angiitis were more extensive at the time of death, involving interlobular, arcuate and juxtaglomerular arteries.

Patient 2 had not received any treatment, and the renal insufficiency increased progressively, leading to hemodialysis two years later. No relapse of extrarenal symptoms was observed after the first attack.

Five patients received corticosteroids at an initial dosage of 1–3 mg/kg body weight per day of prednisone, associated in one case (patient 11) with immunosuppressive drugs. In each of these five patients, renal function improved with treatment. Patient 3 died of intestinal hemorrhage two months after the beginning of the treatment. Patient 7 had two relapses with pulmonary and renal involvement nine and 12 months after the initiation of the treatment. A second renal biopsy performed 12 months after the initial specimen showed fibrous lesions of the glomeruli and the interstitium. This patient underwent hemodialysis and had hypertension two years after the onset of renal symptoms.

In three patients renal function has improved. Patient 4, whose initial renal involvement was mild, had a creatinine clearance of 72 ml/minute five years later, without evidence of progressive PAN. Mild hypertension was noted.

Patient 1, whose initial renal failure had been severe, had a creatinine clearance level of 1.8 mg/100 ml six months after the beginning of treatment. A second biopsy performed at that time showed segmental fibrous glomerular lesions and moderate interstitial fibrosis. Fixation of serum against IgM and C3 was observed on the segmental glomerular lesions. A third biopsy was done five years later and showed progression of the fibrous lesions with marked arteriolosclerosis and fibrous endarteritis.

Six years after the first renal symptoms, this patient has hypertension and proteinuria (3 gm/24 hours, creatinine clearance 1.8 mg/100 ml). This patient still receives 0.25 mg/kg/day of prednisone.

A similar course was observed in patient 11, in whom symptoms disappeared. Three years later, renal function is normal and proteinuria, hematuria and hypertension are not noted.

WEGENER'S GRANULOMATOSIS: FOUR CASES

Four patients had Wegener's granulomatosis. The extrarenal symptoms are summarized in Table 16–4. In three patients, pulmonary involvement was prominent with recurrent pneumonia. The first renal symptoms were observed 1, 2, 12 and 18 months, respectively, after the beginning of the disease. In three of these patients, renal involvement was characterized by the rapid appearance of uremia; hemodialysis was required in one case.

Kidney lesions are summarized in Table 16–5. Necrotizing glomerulonephritis with epithelial crescents was observed in each patient. In one case fibrous segmental lesions of the glomeruli were also noted. Intrarenal necrotizing angiitis was found in all of the patients. Interstitial cellular infiltration was observed in three of four patients. Moreover, in two patients large granulomas composed of epithelioid and giant cells were noted surrounding necrotic glomeruli or venules or disseminated in the interstitium.

TABLE 16–4.–WEGENER'S
GRANULOMATOSIS EXTRARENAL
SYMPTOMS

| | PATIENT | | | | TOTAL |
	1	2	3	4	
Fever	+	+	+	+	4/4
Weight loss	+	+	+	+	4/4
Arthritis	0	+	+	+	3/4
Purpura	+	+	0	+	3/4
Central nervous system signs	0	+	0	0	1/4
Pulmonary signs	0	+	+	+	3/4
Upper respiratory tract signs	+	0	0	0	1/4

TABLE 16–5.—WEGENER'S

PATIENT, AGE	DELAY BETWEEN ONSET AND RENAL BIOPSY	SYMPTOMS		CREATININE (mg/100 ml)	NECROSIS
		PROTEINURIA (gm/24 hr)	RBC/MIN		
1, 65	15 day	0.5	100,000	0.8	+
2, 66	6 mo	1	Macroscopic	8.0	+
3, 75	3 mo	1	12,000	4.0	+++
4, 50	15 day	Hemodialysis			+++

*Abbreviations: X endo = endocapillary proliferation, NA = necrotizing angiitis,

The immunofluorescent studies showed fibrinogen in epithelial crescents in three patients and diffuse mesangial deposits o IgA and C3 in one patient.

The serum levels of C3 and C4 were normal in three of three patients. The latex test and the Waaler-Rose reaction had negative results and there were no cryoglobulins in any of three patients. Circulating immune complexes were sought in two patients and found in one. The HBsAg antigen was found in the serum.

Three patients (patients 1, 2 and 3) received corticosteroids, and two also received cyclophosphamides. The remaining patient received only cyclophosphamide. Two patients died soon after initiation of treatment, one of uremia (patient 2) and the second of infectious complications related to the extension of a midline granuloma (patient 1). No follow-up was available for patient 3; patient 4 started hemodialysis six weeks after the beginning of treatment.

Giant Cell Temporal Arteritis (Horton's Disease): One Case

Following one episode of otitis, this 66-year-old woman presented with fever and arthralgias, which regressed under corticosteroid treatment. After six months, fever and arthralgias reappeared, associated with joint and temporal pain. Anemia and leukocytosis were noted. The temporal artery biopsy showed granulomatous arteritis with endarteritis and destruction of elastic fibers. The muscle biopsy showed a typical necrotizing angiitis lesion. At the same time a rapidly progressive renal insufficiency appeared.

GRANULOMATOSIS RENAL BIOPSY*

| GLOMERULI | | | | | INTERSTITIAL | |
CRESCENTS (%)	X ENDO	FSL	NA	INTERSTITIAL GRANULOMA	CELL INFILTRATION	IMMUNO-FLUORESCENCE
25	+	0	+	0	0	IgA, C3 mesangial
30	0	60%	+ +	0	+ +	F, crescents
100	−	0	+ +	+ + +	+ +	0
100	0	0	+	+ +	+ +	F, crescents

FSL = fibrous segmental lesion, and F = fibrin.

Fifteen days later the patient started hemodialysis and the first kidney biopsy was performed. The glomerular lesions were characterized by the presence of necrotic areas and epithelial crescents. A mild mesangial cell proliferation was noted. No glomerular deposit was observed by light microscopy. Diffuse acute tubular necrosis was present. The interstitial cell infiltration was mild. Arteriosclerosis and fibrous endarteritis lesions were noted, but no necrotizing angiitis was found. The immunofluorescence study showed exclusive fixation of antifibrinogen serum on epithelial crescents. The serum levels of C3 and C4 were normal, the latex test and the Waaler–Rose reaction had negative results, and there was no detection of cryoglobulins or the HBs antigen.

The patient received betamethasone (18 mg/day) and cyclophosphamide (150 mg/day). Renal function quickly improved and the serum level of creatinine decreased to 2.2 mg/100 ml four weeks after the initiation of treatment. Two and one-half years later, while the patient was still receiving small doses of steroids, the creatinine clearance was 1.5 mg/100 ml. A second renal biopsy showed fibrous segmental lesions of the glomeruli along with moderate interstitial fibrosis, arteriolosclerosis and fibrous endarteritis. Focal fixation of C3 on the glomeruli was observed.

Mixed IgM – IgG Cryoglobulinemia: One Case

This 48-year-old woman had mixed IgM – IgG cryoglobulinemia, and the clinical picture was similar to that of a diffuse necrotizing angiitis with arthralgias, loss of weight, severe peripheral neuropathy, anemia and eosinophilia. Muscle biopsy showed a typical lesion of necrotizing angiitis. Renal involvement was marked by the appearance of rapidly progressive renal failure requiring hemodialysis.

The first renal biopsy showed necrotic areas surrounded by epithelial crescents involving one third of the glomeruli. Moderate mesangial cell proliferation and thrombi of the intracapillary loops were also observed. Acute tubular necrosis and interstitial edema were present. Some of the juxtaglomerular arterioles were occluded by granulous material. Fibrinoid necrosis of the wall of an arcuate artery without cellular infiltration was observed. Immunofluorescence showed the presence of IgM in some glomerular lumina. The serum level of C3 was normal, and the level of C4 very low (< 5 mg/100 ml). The latex test had positive results (1/5120) and the results of the Waaler–Rose reaction were 1/4096. The serum level of anti-DNA antibodies was normal. The serum level of IgG and IgA was low; and the serum level of IgM was 2.4 gm/L. The polyethylene glycol test had positive results. Neither HBs antigen nor anti-HBs antibody was detected in serum.

One week later the patient died of septic shock. The kidney showed diffuse cortical necrosis with necrosis and thrombosis of vessels of all sizes. C3 and fibrinogen on the vessel walls were detected by immunofluorescence. Necrotizing angiitis lesions were found in liver, spleen and perirenal fat tissue.

GOUGEROT'S TRISYMPTOMATIC PURPURA (ALLERGIC CUTANEOUS ANGIITIS): FOUR CASES

Four patients had infiltrated purpura associated with fever, arthralgias and weight loss. One of them also had gastrointestinal symptoms characterized by nausea, vomiting and rectal bleeding. The skin biopsy showed a typical necrotizing angiitis lesion in each case.

All patients demonstrated renal involvement, and one patient (patient 2) had rapidly progressive renal failure with proteinuria and macroscopic hematuria.

In three patients, the glomerular lesions were characterized by moderate mesangial cell proliferation with neither necrosis nor crescents. In these three patients, immunofluorescence showed IgA and C3 on small endomembranous deposits in all the glomeruli. In contrast, in the fourth case (patient 2), the le-

TABLE 16–6.—TRISYMPTOMATIC GOUGEROT'S PURPURA (ALLERGIC CUTANEOUS ANGIITIS) RENAL BIOPSY

PATIENT, AGE (yr)	DELAY BETWEEN RENAL SIGNS AND RENAL BIOPSY	PROTEINURIA (gm/24 hr)	RBC/MIN	CREATININE (mg/100 ml)	LIGHT MICROSCOPY GLOMERULI	IMMUNOFLUORESCENCE
1, 69	40 day	1–2	84,000	1.0	Focal endocapillary proliferative glomerulonephritis	IgA, C3 diffuse endo-membranous deposits
2, 59	30 day	6	Macroscopic	2.3	Endo-extracapillary proliferative (60%) glomerulonephritis with glomerular necrosis	Fibrin on crescents
3, 47	5 mo	0	50,000	1.0	Focal endocapillary proliferative glomerulonephritis	IgA, C3 diffuse endo-membranous deposits
4, 76	1 mo	1	30,000	1.0	Focal endocapillary proliferative glomerulonephritis	IgA, C3 diffuse small endomembranous deposits

sions were severe: segmental necrosis and crescents were present in 60% of the glomeruli, and a diffuse although moderate mesangial cell proliferation was observed. The presence of fibrinogen on crescents was detected by immunofluorescence. In none of these four cases was there a necrotizing angiitis of intrarenal vessels (Table 16–6).

Serum levels of C3 and C4 and of IgG, IgA and IgM were normal. Cryoglobulins, circulating immune complexes, HBsAg and anti-HBs antibodies were not found. The three patients with mild renal lesions recovered with (two cases) and without (one case) corticosteroid treatment. Patient 2 received 1 mg/kg/day of prednisone for three months and also recovered. No relapse was observed in any of the four patients.

Comments

NOSOLOGIC PROBLEMS

The homogeneity of the glomerular lesions observed in distinct clinical situations is striking. Indeed, the majority of the cases showed a necrotizing glomerulonephritis associated with epithelial crescents. The necrotizing lesion of the tuft was not morphologically different from that observed in skin, muscle or blood vessels: fibrinoid necrosis and polymorphonuclear cell infiltration. The severity of the glomerular lesions, and particularly the degree of extension of the epithelial crescents, correlated with the severity of the initial clinical symptoms.

Such gomerular lesions have been described and documented in the realm of "systemic necrotizing angiitis."[24] This term includes several clinically distinct syndromes characterized by a common histologic lesion, necrotizing angiitis. Since the first description, several classifications have been proposed.[37, 38, 45] In the group of systemic necrotizing angiitis, Zeek has contrasted the classical *PAN* or *Kussmaul-Maier disease* involving the middle-sized arteries with *hypersensitivity angiitis*, which involves the small vessels: arterioles, venules and capillaries. The glomerular lesions we observed are quite similar to those described by Zeek, and identified as a microscopic form of PAN by Davson and Platt.[15, 43, 45] These glomerular lesions are in contrast with those of the macroscopic form, which usually result in glomerular ischemia without glomerulonephritis.[15]

In fact, such a distinction appears artificial, and several studies have been reported where vascular lesions of both types were present in the same patient and even in the same organ.[2] Patient 6 also illustrates this fact: microangiitis found on the kidney biopsy was associated with lesions involving arteries of all diameters at the postmortem examination.

Within the group of systemic necrotizing angiitis, there are two distinct clinical and histological entities: Wegener's granulomatosis[19, 44] and Churg and Strauss allergic angiitis.[10] In both, extravascular granulomatous formations are present. They are necrotic and rich in eosinophils in the Churg – Strauss syndrome and usually composed of epithelioid and giant cells in Wegener's granulomatosis. Kidney involvement is inconstant in Wegener's disease,[6, 25, 40] and seems uncommon in the Churg – Strauss syndrome.[9] In the present series, no patient definitely had Churg – Strauss angiitis, whereas four had Wegener's granulomatosis. These four patients had glomerular lesions identical with those observed in PAN, and only the presence of interstitial granulomas and the constant finding of intrarenal necrotizing angiitis lesions made it possible to distinguish Wegener's disease from PAN in our small group of cases.

The inclusion of Horton's disease in the group of systemic necrotizing angiitis could be questionable, as histologically it is defined by giant cell arteritis without fibrinoid necrosis involving large vessels, especially the temporal artery. However, one case of association between Horton's disease, microscopic necrotizing angiitis and glomerulonephritis has been reported.[34] One other similar case occurred in our series, and it must be emphasized that the glomerular lesions were characterized by a necrotizing glomerulonephritis with crescents, as observed in PAN and in Wegener's disease. It is noteworthy that in our patient with Horton's disease, the lesions that were severe and extensive regressed completely during treatment. The rare reports of an association between systemic necrotizing angiitis, necrotizing glomerulonephritis and Takayashu's disease may also bear discussion.[26]

Since glomerular lesions were found in four patients with necrotizing angiitis of the skin, the borderline between Schönlein-Henoch (SH) purpura (or anaphylactoid purpura) and necrotizing angiitis is less clearly delineated. In fact, these four patients had clinical symptoms identical with those of SH. However, in

SH there is no typical necrotizing angiitis of the skin.[29] Several authors have included the SH syndrome as a form of necrotizing angiitis.[14, 41] In contrast, the glomerular lesions seem more constant, with mesangial deposits of IgA and C3.[5, 30] Indeed, we observed glomerular mesangial deposits of IgA and C3 in one case of typical PAN (patient 11) and in one case of Wegener's granulomatosis (patient 1). It can be concluded that neither the clinical symptoms nor the glomerular patterns seen in immunofluorescence are sufficiently precise to define the limits between Schönlein-Henoch syndrome and systemic necrotizing angiitis.

ETIOLOGY — MECHANISM

Several findings suggest an immunologic mechanism. There are obvious histologic analogies between necrotizing angiitis (NA) and lesions observed in subjects with experimental acute serum sickness[21] and Arthus's phenomenon.[12] In humans, disseminated or more often localized NA lesions may be found in such immunologic disorders as systemic lupus erythematosus,[24] rheumatoid arthritis,[4] Goodpasture's syndrome[3] and mixed cryoglobulinemia.[33] Meltzer *et al.* first reported on two cases of mixed IgM–IgG cryoglobulinemia with diffuse necrotizing angiitis lesions found at autopsy.[32] Since then, other similar observations have been published.[7] We report one such case in which the first renal biopsy showed microangiitis lesions with intraglomerular and intra-arteriolar thrombi and the postmortem examination showed diffuse cortical necrosis.

Fordham *et al.* observed three cases of acute poststreptococcal glomerulonephritis with disseminated necrotizing angiitis lesions at autopsy.[20] Blau *et al.* emphasized the frequency of previous streptococcal infections in children with PAN, and in one of them the onset of the disease coincided with clinical and laboratory evidence of a streptococcal infection.[1] In our patients, the systemic lesions appeared in one patient following tonsillitis with increased antistreptolysin O titer. Moreover, we and others have observed subepithelial deposits of C3 in the glomeruli of patients with PAN.[1] It is known that such glomerular deposits are present in patients with other conditions, such as acute poststreptococcal glomerulonephritis.

Recently, attention has been drawn to the association between

PAN and HBs antigen.[18, 22, 23, 39] In one subject, the HBs antigen, IgM and complement were found by immunofluorescence in the necrotic vessel walls.[22, 23] However, the direct pathogenic role of HBs antigen remains questionable.[42] In none of our patients was HBs antigen found in the serum and, like other authors,[28] we were not able to detect it in the kidney.

A hypersensitivity to drugs or toxic agents, emphasized for the first time by Zeek,[45] is rarely present at the onset of systemic necrotizing angiitis.[31] Sulfonamides, penicillin and methamphetamine have been incriminated, without good evidence.[11] In one of our patients, the signs of PAN followed the injection of penicillin. In another patient, the symptoms of PAN appeared during a desensitization to candidin. These two patients recovered from PAN uneventfully.

Some investigators report a decrease in the serum complement level,[13, 18, 28] an increase in the level of serum IgA, the presence of rheumatoid factor, cryoglobulins[13, 28] and circulating immune complexes[17, 28] in patients with Wegener's granulomatosis.[16, 19] These observations have been noted in patients with PAN[28] as well as Wegener's disease.[8, 27] In our series, with the exception of the case of mixed cryoglobulinemia with diffuse NA lesions, the results of immunologic investigations are unrevealing: prior to treatment, the serum complement level was normal in all of 16 patients, cryoglobulins were present in one of 15, rheumatoid activity was never observed and circulating immune complexes were found in three of ten cases (two PAN and one Wegener). The presence of immunoglobulins and complement in the glomeruli and in the vessels seems uncommon.[24, 28] Moreover, the findings of immunoglobulins and complement must be interpreted cautiously, as it may only reflect hyperpermeability of the involved vascular wall.[35] It is also known that the fixation of C3 and IgM on the kidney arterioles is often observed in patients with arteriosclerosic lesions.

The meager results of the immunologic studies may in some way be explained by either the lack of adequate methodology or inappropriate timing of the samples.

Acknowledgments

We thank Professor Richet and Doctor Morel-Maruger for allowing us access to their observations. Mesdames Atienza,

Adafer, Lallemand and Rioumailhol provided excellent technical assistance. Miss Simon helped us in preparing the manuscript.

References

1. Blau, E. B., Morris, R. F., and Yunis, E. J.: Polyarteritis nodosa in older children, Pediatrics 60:227, 1977.
2. Case records, N. Engl. J. Med. 284:262, 1971.
3. Case records, N. Engl. J. Med. 285:1187, 1971.
4. Case records, N. Engl. J. Med. 285:1250, 1971.
5. Case records, N. Engl. J. Med. 290:1365, 1974.
6. Case records, N. Engl. J. Med. 291:195, 1974.
7. Case records, N. Engl. J. Med. 291:1073, 1974.
8. Case records, N. Engl. J. Med. 297:1164, 1977.
9. Chumbley, L. C., Harrison, E. G., and Deremee, R. A.: Allergic granulomatosis and angiitis (Churg-Strauss syndrome). Report and analysis of 30 cases, Mayo Clin. Proc. 52:477, 1977.
10. Churg, J., and Strauss, L.: Allergic granulomatosis, allergic angiitis and periarteritis nodosa, Am. J. Pathol. 27:277, 1951.
11. Citron, B. P., Halpern, M., McCarron, M., Lunderg, G. D., McCormick, R. Pincus, I. J., Tatter, D., and Haverback, B. J.: Necrotizing angiitis associated with drug abuse, N. Engl. J. Med. 283:1003, 1970.
12. Cochrane, C. G., and Weigle, W. O.: The cutaneous reaction to soluble antigen antibody complexes. A comparison with Arthus phenomenon, J. Exp. Med. 108:591, 1958.
13. Conn, D. L., McDuffie, F. C., Holley, K. E., and Schroeter, A. L.: Immunologic mechanisms in systemic vasculitis, Mayo Clin. Proc. 51:511, 1976.
14. Cream, J. J., Goumpel, J. M., and Peachey, R. D. G.: Schönlein-Henoch purpura in the adult. A study of 77 adults in the anaphylactoid of Schönlein-Henoch, Q. J. Med. 39:461, 1970.
15. Davson, J., Ball, J., and Platt, R.: The kidney in periarteritis nodosa, Q. J. Med. 17: 175, 1948.
16. Deremee, R. A., McDonald, T. J., Harrison, E. G., and Goles, D. T.: Wegener's granulomatosis, anatomic correlates, a proposed classification, Mayo Clin. Proc. 51:777, 1975.
17. Digeon, M., Laver, M., Riza, J., and Bach, J. F.: Detection of circulating immune complexes in human sera by simplified assays with polyethylene glycol, J. Immunol. Methods 16:165, 1977.
18. Duffy, J., Lidsky, M. D., Sharp, J. T., Davis, J. S., Person, D. A., Hollinger, F. B., and Kyung-Whan, Min.: Polyarthritis, polyarteritis and hepatitis B, Medicine 55:19, 1976.
19. Fauci, A. S., and Wolff, S. M.: Wegener's granulomatosis: studies in eighteen patients and a review of the literature, Medicine 52:535, 1973.
20. Fordhan, C. C., III, Epstein, F. M., Huffines, W. D., and Harrington, J. T.: Polyarteritis and acute post-streptococcal glomerulonephritis, Ann. Intern. Med. 61:89, 1964.
21. Germuth, F. G.: A comparative histologic and immunologic study in rabbits of induced hypersensitivity of the serum sickness type, J. Exp. Med. 97:257, 1953.
22. Gocke, D. J., Hsu, K., Morgan, C., Bombardieri, S., Lockshin, M., and Christian, C. L.: Association between polyarteritis and Australia antigen, Lancet 2:1149, 1970.
23. Gocke, D. J., Hsu, K., Morgan, C., Bombardieri, S., Lockshin, M., and Christian, C. L.: Vasculitis in association with Australia antigen, J. Exp. Med. 134:330, 1971.

24. Heptinstall, R. H.: *Pathology of the Kidney* (Boston: Little, Brown and Co., 1974), pp. 601–39.
25. Horn, R. G., Fauci, A. S., Rosenthal, A. S., and Wolff, S. M.: Renal biopsy pathology in Wegener's granulomatosis, Am. J. Pathol. 74:423, 1974.
26. Hosoda, Y., Iri, H., and Wakasugi, A.: Granulomatous aortitis associated with necrotizing angiitis and glomerulonephritis, Acta Pathol. Jpn. 23:129, 1973.
27. Howell, S. B., and Epstein, W. V.: Circulating immunoglobulin complexes in Wegener's granulomatosis, Am. J. Med. 60:259, 1976.
28. Kanfer, A., Sraer, J. D., Feintuch, M. J., Morel-Maroger, L., Beaufils, P., and Richet, G.: Insuffisance rénale aigüe au cours de la périartérite noueuse, Nouv. Presse Med. 5:1883, 1976.
29. Lessana-Leibowitch, M.: Les vascularites allergiques, Nouv. Presse Med. 4:1919, 1975.
30. Levy, M., Broyer, M., Arsana, B., Levy-Bentolila, D., and Habib, R.: Glomérulonephrites du purpura rhumatoïde chez l'enfant. Histoire naturelle et étude immunopathologique, in *Actualités Néphrologique de l'Hôpital Necker* (Paris: Flammarion, 1976), p. 174.
31. McCombs, R. P.: Systemic "allergic" vasculitis, J.A.M.A. 194:157, 1965.
32. Meltzer, M., Franklin, E. C., Elias, K., McCluskey, R. T., and Cooper, N.: Cryoglobulinemia—a clinical and laboratory study. II. Cryoglobulin with rheumatoid factor activity, Am. J. Med. 40:837, 1966.
33. Morel-Maroger, L., and Verroust, P.: Glomerular lesions in dysproteinemias, Kidney Int. 5:249, 1974.
34. O'Neill, W., Hammar, S. P., and Bloomer, H. A.: Giant cell arteritis with visceral angiitis, Arch. Intern. Med. 136:1157, 1976.
35. Paronetto, F.: Systemic nonsuppurative necrotizing angiitis, in Miescher, P. A., and Muller-Eberhard, H. J. (eds.): *Test Book of Immunopathology* (New York: Grune & Stratton, Inc., 1968), vol. 2, p. 722.
36. Razzak, I. A., Bauer, F. W., and Itzel, W.: Hepatitis B antigenemia with panarteritis, diffuse proliferative glomerulonephritis and malignant hypertension, Am. J. Gastroenterol. 68 (6):476, 1975.
37. Richet, G., and Habib, R.: Les localisations rénales de la PAN. J. Urol. Nephrol. (Paris) 65:177, 1959.
38. Rose, G. A., and Spencer, H.: Polyarteritis nodosa, Q. J. Med. 101:43, 1957.
39. Sergent, J. S., Lockshin, M. D., Christian, C. L., and Gocke, D. J.: Vasculitis with hepatitis B antigenemia; Long term observation in nine patients, Medicine 55:1, 1976.
40. Shigematsu, H., Ohtsu, H., and Matsuba, M.: Segmental disorganizing glomerulonephritis in a Wegener's granulomatosis. Virchows Arch. (Pathol. Anat.) 363:359, 1974.
41. Soter, A. N.: Clinical presentations and mechanisms of necrotizing angiitis of the skin, J. Invest. Dermatol. 67:354, 1976.
42. Trepo, C. G., Zuckerman, A. J., and Bird, R. C.: The role of circulating hepatitis B antigen-antibody immune complexes in the pathogenesis of vascular and hepatic manifestations in polyarteritis nodosa, J. Clin. Pathol. 27:863, 1974.
43. Wainwright, J., and Davson, J.: The renal appearances in the microscopic form of periarteritis nodosa, J. Pathol. Bacteriol. 62:189, 1949.
44. Wolff, S. M., Fauci, A. S., Horn, R. G., and Dale, D. C.: Wegener's granulomatosis, Ann. Intern. Med. 81:513, 1974.
45. Zeek, P. M.: Periarteritis nodosa and other forms of necrotizing angiitis, N. Engl. J. Med. 248:764, 1953.

17

Immunologic Alterations in Chronic Renal Insufficiency

J. P. REVILLARD, M.D.

Clinique de Néphrologie et des Maladies Métaboliques et Rénales, Université Claude Bernard, and Hôpital E. Herriot, Lyon, France

With the advent of chronic hemodialysis the prognosis of terminal renal failure was improved dramatically. However, despite this treatment, patients on maintenance hemodialysis (MHD) still suffer from important metabolic disturbances. Furthermore, new manifestations of chronic renal insufficiency are observed with increasing frequency, such as accelerated atherosclerosis with cardiac or cerebral involvement. Among the complications of renal insufficiency, infection remains a predominant cause of morbidity and mortality.[24] Alterations of immune responses can be held responsible for at least some of these infections.

The alteration of nonspecific immunity has been analyzed in a few studies and certainly deserves further investigation. The in vitro phagocytic capacity of monocytes was shown to be reduced in patients with renal insufficiency.[86] In vivo, the inflammatory reaction studied by the skin window test revealed that the migration of polymorphonuclear cells and macrophages was comparable to that in normal controls. However, the phagocytosis of India ink particles was markedly reduced in patients re-

365

0084-5957/79/080365-18 $3.75
© 1979, Year Book Medical Publishers, Inc.

cently started on hemodialysis. This capacity was partially restored after a few months of treatment.[64]

The most frequently encountered infection in hemodialyzed patients is hepatitis B. In contrast to medical personnel, who usually present with an acute hepatitis followed by the immune elimination of the virus, MHD patients often suffer from chronic hepatitis with prolonged antigenemia. This difference in response to the same infectious agent illustrates the consequences of immunologic deficiencies of uremic patients. Despite numerous studies the mechanisms of these changes remain poorly understood.[23]

Antibody Response

There have been few detailed investigations of the antibody response in uremic patients. Balch measured the antibody response to tetanus toxoid in soldiers wounded in battle.[3] He found no difference whether the patient was in acute renal failure or not. Stoloff *et al.* showed that 14 patients with chronic renal insufficiency had positive results on a Schick reaction after vaccination with diphtheria toxoid.[81] However, the exquisite sensitivity of this reaction would not have allowed the authors to observe a possible decreased antibody response in patients. Wilson *et al.* found a depressed response to O and H antigens of *Salmonella typhi*.[89] Boulton-Jones *et al.* immunized their patients with keyhole-limpet hemocyanin, 200 μg intradermally.[10] Antibody titers were measured by passive hemagglutination two weeks later. Antibody titers were markedly depressed both in nondialyzed and uremic patients and, to a lesser extent, in patients on maintenance hemodialysis (MHD). Similar results were obtained by others using influenza vaccine. Patients with creatinine clearances of less than 34 cc/minute had diminished or absent antibody responses to intramuscular and intranasal challenge with vaccine, whereas patients on MHD responded to intramuscular but not to intranasal challenge.[7, 39, 59] In a recent study in hemodialyzed children, antibody responses to toxoid or killed vaccines were normal, whereas responses to live attenuated vaccine were reduced.[46a]

The production of antibodies against HL-A antigens or hepatitis B virus-associated antigens is routinely measured in patients on MHD. However, these data are not informative with respect to possible alterations of antibody response because of the lack of controls. In experimental acute renal failure in rabbits, the primary antibody response to bovine serum albumin was found depressed whereas the anamnestic response remained normal.[29] If similar experiments were performed with experimental models of chronic renal insufficiency, they would help to predict the response of MHD patients to vaccines.

Allograft Rejection

The first study of skin allograft survival in uremic patients was performed by Dammin *et al.* in 1957.[20] Full-thickness skin grafts from different donors were biopsied at intervals from 32 to 115 days. In each of the recipients at least one of the skin allografts was found free of histologic signs of rejection after periods of time much longer than the expected duration of survival in healthy recipients. Similar investigations have not been repeated because of the possible risk of recipient sensitization against transplantation antigens of the prospective donor. In fact this risk may have been overestimated, since Shackman and Castro have recently published their experience with skin grafts from prospective living donors to MHD patients given azathioprine 50 mg daily.[71] In 37 of 43 cases the grafts were accepted without macroscopic alteration after six weeks. Renal transplant survival could be correlated with skin allograft survival though not with stimulation in unidirectional mixed-lymphocyte reaction. Such a selection, according to the authors, could improve the results of renal transplants from haplo-identical donors. However, the survival time of skin grafts from donors sharing zero, one, or two haplotypes with the recipients on MHD was not studied. Despite the lack of control series with azathioprine-treated healthy recipients, the considerable duration of allograft survival is likely to be attributed to renal insufficiency. Other studies have shown a prolonged survival of skin allografts in uremic patients[51] and in rabbits with acute renal failure.[77, 78]

Likewise, the survival of transplanted organs in allogeneic recipients with renal insufficiency is prolonged. Kidneys survive two to three weeks in uremic dogs versus one week in recipients with normal renal function.[46] Similar results were found recently with heart transplants in uremic rats.[80] The first reports of human renal transplants by J. P. Merrill in Boston stressed

the impairment of allograft rejection by uremic patients: in four
of the nine first recipients, survival ranged from 5 to 25 weeks,
whereas survival in allografted dogs seldom exceeded one week.
In addition, the massive cellular infiltration observed in dog
transplants was not found in human allografts.[47] Unfortunately,
initially successful transplantation restores the patient's immunologic responsiveness, thus endowing him with the capacity to
build up a rejection reaction.

Delayed Hypersensitivity Skin Reactions

Delayed-type hypersensitivity in uremic patients was extensively investigated by Kirkpatrick and co-workers in 1964.[43]
Multiple skin tests with various antigens were performed in 28
patients with chronic glomerulonephritis. Each reaction was
recorded as positive or negative. The incidence of positive delayed-type reaction was much lower in uremic (22 of 70) than in
normal subjects (73 of 177). After transplantation, 18 patients
not on steroid treatment developed at least one positive reaction
of the delayed type. The same authors later extended their
studies and showed that the first rejection episode occurred later
in previously anergic patients than in those with positive delayed-type reaction.[88]

In our own studies, we have used four antigens (purified protein derivative, 1 μg; candidin, 1:100; streptokinase, 100 units;
toxoplasmin, 1:100). The chance for a healthy adult to have
negative test results to these four antigens was negligible.
Diameters of erythema and induration were measured 24 and
48 hours after intradermal injection. The results demonstrated
a significant impairment of delayed hypersensitivity in patients with either acute or chronic renal failure. In patients with
mild renal insufficiency (creatinine clearance 8–40 ml/minute),
the reactions were not significantly depressed. MHD treatment
did not improve delayed hypersensitivity.[63] Depressed delayed
hypersensitivity in chronic renal failure patients was also reported by Huber et al.[36] and by Boulton-Jones et al.[10] Finnish
investigators reported a positive correlation between plasma
creatinine levels and the doses of purified protein derivative
(PPD) required to elicit a delayed-type skin reaction.[67] The
seemingly low incidence of anergic patients in Kauffman's series would suggest that MHD results in a partial improvement

of delayed hypersensitivity.[42] However, in the absence of a sequential study of the same patients before and during MHD, no conclusion can be reached. In another study, the percentage of anergic patients was found slightly increased in those who had been on MHD for a long time.[68]

Delayed hypersensitivity skin reactions are more appropriate than any in vitro test to investigate cell-mediated immunity in uremic or MHD patients. However, skin reactions remain difficult to quantitate and can yield variable results when repeated in the same individual. Because of these drawbacks, skin tests have not so far been used for evaluating various methods of MHD or for assaying the effect of nutritional factors. It is not yet known whether the impairment of delayed hypersensitivity reflects a defect of primarily antigen-reaction lymphocytes or mediators of inflammation, or both.

Lymphoid Organs and Populations of Circulating Lymphocytes

Structural alterations of the lymphoid system have not been extensively investigated in patients with renal insufficiency. Kirkpatrick *et al.* noted the presence of atrophic and cystic changes in the thymus that were not found in young adults autopsied after accidental death.[43] Black and de Chabon reported alterations of the lymph nodes with absence of secondary follicles and reduced numbers of plasma cells. In our own studies performed in collaboration with D. Fries and P. A. Bryon, iliac nodes of 27 patients on MHD were examined. The cell density of the deep cortex was reduced in only five patients, whereas in 24 patients germinal centers were sparse or absent and in 17 of them the number of plasma cells was markedly reduced.[63] These structural alterations were not expected in view of the predominant defect of cell-mediated immunity in patients on MHD.

Lymphopenia can be regarded as a typical manifestation of renal insufficiency. It was noted in early reports[62] and confirmed by most authors in cases of acute renal failure,[38, 74, 75, 85] terminal chronic renal insufficiency and patients on MHD.[10, 35, 63, 67, 70, 89] Differential counts of Giemsa-stained smears show that reduced numbers of mononuclear cells can be attributed exclusively to the diminution of small lymphocytes, the numbers of large lymphocytes, monocytes and histiocytes being comparable to those of normal subjects. The selective reduction of small lymphocyte counts that are less than 50% of normal values cannot be attributed to hemodilution. Unlike polymorphs and platelets, lymphocytes do not adhere firmly to artificial membranes and their loss during dialysis remains negligible.[15, 40] Lymphopenia is not reversed by MHD,[10, 63] or is only partially reduced.[35] It is independent of the nature of renal disease and is likely to reflect an overall reduction in the pool of circulating lymphocytes. Hence, the rapidly mobilizable pool of lymphocytes obtained by thoracic duct cannulation patients on MHD ranges from 8 to 110 × 10⁹ cells.[63a] Despite the lack of control values in normal subjects, it is noteworthy that more lymphocytes are collected by thoracic duct drainage in patients with ascitic cirrhosis or rheumatoid arthritis than in patients on MHD.

Differential counts of lymphocyte populations in peripheral blood have not yielded comparable results, perhaps because of insufficient standardization of the techniques and heterogeneity of the patients studied.

We studied the distribution of lymphocyte subpopulations in the peripheral blood in 25 MHD patients free of infection and malnutrition, who were not taking any drugs. The following markers were used: T-lymphocytes were identified by their capacity to form E rosettes with sheep erythrocytes[60] and by the presence of HTLA, a T-cell specific antigen recognized in microlymphocytotoxicity with a specific antiserum prepared from horse antilymphocyte globulin;[14] B cells were identified in microlymphocytotoxicity with an antiserum prepared in rabbits and made specific for B-lymphocytes and monocytes by appropriate absorption;[14] monocytes were characterized by peroxidase staining; lymphocyte suspensions were prepared according to a technique allowing the recovery of more than 70% of the lymphocytes with less than 2.5% contamination by monocytes;[65] receptors for C_3b and C_3d were detected by the EAC rosette technique;[8] receptors for the Fc piece of IgG (Fcγ) were revealed by the EA rosette technique;[13] and receptors for the Fc piece of IgM (Fcμ) by the technique of Moretta et al.[50]

No significant difference was found between patients on MHD and normal controls (Table 17–1) with respect to peripheral blood lymphocyte subpopulations, except for the subset of T-lymphocytes bearing Fcμ receptors, which was lower in patients

TABLE 17-1.—LYMPHOCYTE
POPULATIONS IN PERIPHERAL
BLOOD OF MAINTENANCE
HEMODIALYSIS PATIENTS AND
CONTROLS*

	NORMAL	MHD	p VALUES
HTLA[†]	79.1 + 8.9	72.4 ± 4.3	NS‖
HBLMA[‡]	14.3 ± 6.9	14.4 ± 1.9	NS
"Null"[§]	6.5 ± 1.0	13.3 ± 4.0	NS
E-RFC	74.0 ± 7.8	73.8 ± 2.0	NS
EAC-RFC	16.0 ± 6.4	17.3 ± 2.5	NS
Fcγ	15.2 ± 5.9	15.8 ± 2.2	NS
Fcμ	27.1 ± 3.6	10.4 ± 3.8	0.05

*Results expressed as mean ± standard error. Techniques described in references 8, 13, 14, 25 and 50.

[†]Percent lysed cells in the presence of anti-HTLA serum + complement.

[‡]Percent lysed cells in the presence of anti-HBLMA serum + complement.

[§]Percent lymphocytes not lysed by anti-HTLA + HBLMA.

‖NS = not significant.

on MHD than in controls. These results are in keeping with other reports indicating normal percentages of T cells in patients with chronic renal insufficiency and patients on MHD.[35, 61, 84] Conversely, Sengar and Harris have reported a selective decrease in the number of T cells with a parallel increase in null cells. Incubation with thymosin in vitro was shown to increase the number of E-rosette-forming cells, suggesting that thymosin production might be defective in cases of renal insufficiency. This hypothesis, however, did not rely on measurements of circulating thymic factor.[33] Others have reported decreased relative and absolute counts of B cells[35, 42, 60a] with partial improvement on MHD.[35]

Finally, changes in the relative counts of lymphocyte subsets are restricted within a small range and their biologic significance remains questionable, whereas major lymphopenia is well demonstrated. The use of more discriminative markers of lymphocyte subpopulations (e.g., T-cell subsets) than those presently available may reveal selective defects in patients with renal insufficiency.

In Vitro Lymphocyte Response

The determination of in vitro responses of lymphocytes from uremic patients can be performed using two different approaches. First, peripheral blood lymphocytes can be washed and cultivated in normal serum in the presence of various mitogens, allogeneic cells or antigens to which the patient has been sensitized. Under these conditions, the absence or "paralysis" of a lymphocyte population will result in a defective proliferative response, which might eventually be correlated with changes in the distribution of markers of subpopulations. The second approach analyzes the effects of uremic serum on the responses of normal lymphocytes. If whole uremic serum or its fractions are actually added to normal serum and not used in place of it, then a possible "inhibitory" effect can be demonstrated. Inhibition may or may not be selective; it can be associated with various degrees of toxicity toward lymphocytes with immediate or delayed cell death. However, the possible absence of factor(s) necessary for cell proliferation cannot be detected with such methods. Finally, the in vivo relevance of inhibition by plasma factors cannot be considered unless inhibition is observed in vitro at concentrations found in uremic plasma, and a correlation can be established between the severity of immune deficiency and plasma levels of this factor in individual patients.

Blastogenic Response in Normal Medium

If thymidine incorporation in PHA-stimulated cultures of whole blood was found to be reduced,[45] as expected in lymphopenic patients, lymphocyte proliferative responses in normal medium were reported either normal[10, 41, 52, 63] or diminished.[21a, 36, 49, 53] Methodologic differences, especially in the preparation of lymphocyte suspensions, or sampling heterogeneity might account for the variations among reports. A decreased in vitro survival of uremic lymphocytes might be associated with a low proliferative response.[10, 21]

Antigen-induced lymphocyte proliferation was reported by most investigators to be diminished in uremic and MHD patients,[10, 22, 36, 53] with one exception.[67] Our results indicate a reduced incidence of positive proliferative responses to PPD among patients on MHD (Table 17 – 2). Both stimulation indices

TABLE 17–2.—PHA- AND PPD-INDUCED PROLIFERATIVE
RESPONSES OF PERIPHERAL BLOOD LYMPHOCYTES FROM
NORMAL SUBJECTS AND MHD PATIENTS

STIMULANT	PATIENTS	NO. OF PATIENTS	NATURAL LOGARITHM* (dpm) MEAN ± SD	p VALUES
PHA	Normal	43	11.36 ± 0.74	
	MHD	41	11.55 ± 0.53	NS†
O	Normal	39	6.68 ± 0.85	
	MHD	46	6.85 ± 0.83	NS
PPD	Normal			
	Total	38	10.11 ± 1.29	
	Nonresponder	1	7.80	
	Responders	37‡	10.38 ± 1.07	
	MHD			
	Total	45	9.14 ± 1.66	0.05§
	Nonresponders	12	7.05 ± 0.80	
	Responders	33	9.90 ± 1.15	NS‖

*Normal distribution of the samples is obtained after natural logarithmic transformation.

†Comparison between normal and MHD patients by Student's t test. NS = not significant.

‡Responders are defined as greater than the 90th percentile of response in unstimulated cultures. The difference between numbers of responders in normal and MHD patients was shown to be significant (χ^2 test, $p = 0.05\%$).

§Comparison between whole numbers of normal and MHD patients.

‖Comparison between responders in normal and MHD patients.

and absolute counts of thymidine incorporation show a significant difference between MHD patients and normal controls, with spontaneous thymidine incorporation being similar in both groups. However, the magnitude of the response in positive MHD patients is not lower than that in controls.

Although uremic patients have a reduced response to PPD both in vivo and in vitro, a positive correlation between blastogenic responses and skin reactions could not be demonstrated in individual patients.

PRODUCTION OF LYMPHOKINES

The association of cutaneous anergy with normal lymphocyte proliferative response in some patients suggested that antigen-induced production of lymphokines might be defective.[67] Hence, Boulton-Jones *et al.* reported a diminution of the production of migration-inhibitory factor by lymphocytes stimulated with streptokinase in patients with terminal renal insufficiency or on MHD.[10]

Finally it was reported in an early study on the normal lymphocyte transfer test that lymphocytes taken from uremic patients often failed to elicit an inflammatory reaction when injected intradermally into normal allogeneic recipients.[12]

Cytotoxic Response

With G. Cordier we have studied the cytotoxic capacity of lymphocytes from MHD patients in two in vitro systems: antibody-dependent cell cytotoxicity and PHA-induced cytotoxicity. In the first reaction, the effector cell was shown to be nonadherent, nonphagocytic, and lacking in markers of T- and B-lymphocytes, but to bind erythrocyte-antibody complexes prepared at low antibody concentration ("high-avidity" EA rosettes).[18] This cytotoxic reaction is markedly reduced in patients on MHD (Table 17-3). In PHA-induced cytotoxicity, two populations of effector cells could be identified:[19] one is made of T-lymphocytes bearing Fcγ receptors, and the other of "non-T"-lymphocytes bearing Fcγ but not C_3 receptors. PHA-induced cytotoxicity is defective in MHD patients.[17] These results demonstrate a selective alteration of several cell subsets defined so far by their cytotoxic responses but not yet by surface markers.

TABLE 17-3.—LYMPHOCYTE-MEDIATED
CYTOTOXIC REACTIONS IN NORMAL AND
MHD PATIENTS*

	NORMAL	MHD PATIENTS	p VALUES‡
Antibody-dependent cell cytotoxicity†			
No. of patients	47	22	
Antibody 10^{-4}	65.7 ± 12.5	44.1 ± 19.0	<0.001
Antibody 10^{-5}	47.7 ± 17.0	26.5 ± 19.0	<0.001
PHA-induced cytotoxicity§			
No. of patients	57	22	
PHA	36.3 ± 14.9	21.4 ± 17.0	<0.001

*Results expressed as percent ^{51}Cr release (mean ± SD).
†Rabbit antichicken erythrocytes antiserum at final concentrations of 10^{-4} and 10^{-5}. Details of the technique are described in reference 18.
‡Student's t test.
§Details of the technique are described in reference 19.

Effects of Uremic Serum and Serum Fractions

More than ten years ago it was shown that uremic serum did not support an optimal proliferative response of normal lymphocytes cultivated with PHA or allogeneic cells.[57, 63, 72, 84] Purification of toxic factors from uremic serum was therefore attempted. Though inhibitory, unfractionated uremic serum does not decrease in vitro survival of normal lymphocytes;[76] it does not induce chromium release from ^{51}Cr-labeled normal lymphocytes or cause any ultrastructural alteration.[76]

Serum from patients on MHD taken after hemodialysis was found to be less inhibitory than serum obtained before dialysis.[25, 56, 57] In our own experiments, no clear-cut difference was observed between pre- and postdialysis serum. Furthermore, the effect of in vitro dialysis appeared ambiguous: when normal serum was dialyzed and introduced into lymphocyte cultures, the proliferative response was depressed despite excellent cell variability. A normal response could be restored by the addition of serum dialysate or by a considerable increase of cell concentration.[86a] Hence, in vitro dialysis of uremic serum resulted in the removal of both toxic factors and substances necessary for lymphocyte proliferation.

Several substances present at high concentration in uremic serum can be added to lymphocyte cultures.[63] Unlike phenol, urea (8 mg/ml) and creatinine (300 μg/ml) are not toxic. Methylguanidine decreases the mixed-lymphocyte reaction at 7.5 μg/ml and completely suppresses it at 60 μg/ml.[63] Slightly higher concentrations are required to inhibit the PHA response. Accordingly, Harris *et al.* reported the inhibition of PHA, streptolysine O and streptokinase-induced transformation by methylguanidine.[31, 32, 44] Inhibitory concentrations in vitro are within the range of those measured in uremic serum.[2, 28] In vivo, methylguanidine induces toxic effects comparable to some complications of renal insufficiency.[4, 27] Other derivatives of guanidine were investigated. Despite its effect on platelets,[34] guanidinosuccinic acid is not cytotoxic;[76] its inhibitory effect on lymphocyte proliferative responses has been discussed.[31, 32, 73] Two other guanidine compounds, guanidinopropionic acid and guanidinobutyric acid, cause hemolysis in vitro, but their possible effect on lymphocytes is not known.

Lymphocyte inhibitory factors might be present among nondialyzable substances, especially low-molecular-weight proteins (molecular weight <50,000) that are filtrated through glomeruli and then reabsorbed and catabolized by proximal tubular cells. One typical low-molecular-weight protein is β_2-microglobulin, the plasma levels of which are 8 to 60 times greater in patients on MHD than in normal subjects.[87] Although β_2-microglobulin itself is neither toxic nor inhibitory, other low-molecular-weight proteins might have such effects or might carry toxic or immunoregulatory small molecules. Inhibitory factors were found in the nondialyzable fraction of uremic serum[56] and in the excluded peak after chromatography on Sephadex G-25 fine.[54] Determination of immunoregulatory α-globulins[48] and chalones might provide new insight in the research on uremic immunosuppressive factors.

Considering the efficiency of peritoneal dialysis in the prevention or treatment of complications of chronic renal failure, e.g., neuropathies, Babb *et al.* hypothesized that uremic toxins might be found in the peak of "middle molecules" (molecular weight 500–2000).[1] Such peaks are demonstrable on 254 nm recordings of Sephadex G-25 or G-15 chromatography of uremic serum or urine. Substances recovered from this peak inhibit DNA synthesis by normal lymphocytes stimulated with mitogens or allogeneic cells.[5, 30, 54] In addition, continuous intravenous infusion of middle molecules into the rat delays skin allograft rejection.[55] Incubation of mouse spleen cells in vitro with middle molecules decreases their capacity to induce a graft-versus-host reaction in allogeneic recipients.[55] Comparable preparations of middle molecules inhibit the growth of Wi38 fibroblasts[26] and depress the phagocytic capacity of leukocytes.[58] Bergström and co-workers have attempted to characterize the components of this peak. Many peptidic fractions could be separated, the plasma levels of which vary considerably and independently from patient to patient. One fraction identified as 7c was found to be a potent inhibitor of lymphocyte blastogenesis in vitro.[5, 6]

The evidence that middle molecules may be responsible for the alterations of immune responses in patients on MHD remains circumstantial. No correlation has yet been reported between any clinical manifestation of uremic toxicity and variations in plasma concentrations (estimated by ultraviolet absorption) of this heterogeneous mixture of substances. However, Bergström *et al.* noted that the appearance of a middle molecule peak in plasma was related to episodes of infection, overhydration and malnutrition apparently independent of the dialysis schedule. Furthermore, Hurst *et al.* selectively altered the plasma concentration of "small" and "middle" substances by controlled dialysis procedures.[37] Such alterations did not result in a significant change in the capacity of patient's serum to support a mitogenic response to PHA of lymphocytes from normal subjects. The inhibitory effect of sera from MHD patients was maximal in patients with changes in bone x-rays, although it could not be correlated with parathyroid hormone levels.

Conclusions

Chronic renal insufficiency is associated with important alterations of the lymphoid system and impairment of the immune response. Similar changes are observed in subjects with acute experimental renal failure. The most prominent disturbances are (1) the reduction of the pool of circulating lymphocytes with low numbers of B and T cells, (2) the diminution of primary antibody responses against thymus-dependent antigens and (3) the impairment of delayed hypersensitivity and allograft rejection. These are the consequences on lymphoid cells of multiple metabolic disturbances of renal insufficiency. Although they cannot be accounted for by low protein intake, some of the observed alterations are similar to those of protein-calorie malnutrition,[79] or vitamin deficiency, e.g., pyridoxine.[22] Adaptation of the organism to renal insufficiency implies so many metabolic changes that the immune defect is unlikely to be attributed to a single toxic factor. Several substances may be added to the list of small or "middle" molecular weight factors discussed above. Activators of adenylate cyclase, which depress proliferative and cytotoxic lymphocyte responses,[82] might contribute to the immune defect since plasma levels of cyclic adenosine monophosphate were reported to be increased in patients with renal insufficiency.[66]

The recent discovery by Campbell *et al.* of elevated levels of endogenous serum polyamines in patients in end-stage renal diseases and on MHD introduces a new approach in the search for uremic "toxins."[16] High levels of spermine and spermidine are possibly a consequence of altered monoamine oxidase activity.[83] Some of the effects attributed to middle molecules are similar to certain biologic properties of polyamines. Increased extracellular levels of polyamines may account for dysfunction of membrane-bound Na^+-K-ATPase, decreased tubular reabsorption of sodium, peripheral neuropathies, platelet abnormalities and growth retardation. Radioimmunoassays detecting polyamines in piconanomole quantities will help to evaluate their contribution to uremic toxicity among many other factors.

Acknowledgments

We gratefully acknowledge the communication of unpublished data from Jean Brochier, Geneviève Cordier and Christiane Samarut (INSERM U 80, Hôpital E. Herriot, Lyon).

References

1. Babb, A. L., Popovich, R. P., Christopher, T. C., and Scribner, B. H.: The genesis of the square meter-hour hypothesis, Trans. Am. Soc. Artif. Intern. Organs 17:81, 1971.
2. Baker, I. R. I., and Marshall, R. D.: A reinvestigation of methyl-guanidine concentrations in sera from normal and uraemic subjects, Clin. Sci. 41:563, 1971.
3. Balch, H. H.: The effect of severe battle injury and of posttraumatic renal failure on resistance to infection, Ann. Surg. 142:145, 1955.
4. Barsotti, G., Bevilacqua, G., Morelli, E., Capelli, P., Balesti, P. L., and Giovanetti, S.: Toxicity arising from guanidine compounds: role of methyl guanidine as uremic toxin, Kidney Int. 7:S-299, 1975.
5. Bergström, J., Furst, P., Gordon, A., Asaba, M., Zimmermann, L., and Quadracci, L. J.: Middle molecules in uremia, in *Proc. 6th International Congress on Nephrology* (Basel: Karger, 1975), pp. 600–611.
6. Bergström, J., and Furst, P.: Uremic middle molecules, Clin. Nephrol. 5:143, 1976.
7. Betts, R. F., Douglas, R. G., Roth, F., Pabico, R. C., and Freeman, R. B. Immunoresponsiveness to different influenza vaccines in patients with renal disease (Abstract), American Society of Microbiology, 1974. Interscience Conference on Antimicrobial Agents and Chemotherapy.
8. Bianco, C., Patrik, R., and Nussenzweig, V.: A population of lymphocytes bearing a membrane receptor for antigen-antibody-complement complexes, J. Exp. Med. 132:702, 1970.
9. Black, M. M., and De Chabon, A.: Reactivity of lymph nodes in azotemic patients, Am. J. Clin. Pathol. 41:503, 1964.
10. Boulton-Jones, J. M., Vick, R., Cameron, J. S., and Black, P. H.: Immune responses in uremia, Clin. Nephrol. 1:351, 1973.
11. Bricker, N. S.: On the pathogenesis of the uremic state. An exposition of the "Trade-off Hypothesis," N. Engl. J. Med. 286:1093, 1972.
12. Bridges, J. M.: Evaluation of lymphocyte transfer test in normal and uraemic subjects, Lancet 1:581, 1964.
13. Brochier, J., Samarut, C., and Revillard, J. P.: A rosette technique for identification of human mononuclear cells bearing Fc receptors, Biomedicine 23:206, 1975.
14. Brochier, J., Abou Ahmed, Y. A., Gueho, J. P., and Revillard, J. P.: Study of human T and B lymphocytes with heterologous antisera. I. Preparation, specificity and properties of antisera, Immunology 31:749, 1976.

15. Buscarini, L., and Bassi, F.: Leucocyte loss in hemodialysis, Acta. Haematol. 48: 278, 1972.
16. Campbell, R., Talwalkar, Y., Bartos, F., Musgrave, J., Harner, M., Puri, H., Grettie, D., Dolney, A. M., and Loggan, B.: Polyamines, uremia and hemodialysis, *Advances in Polyamine Research*, in press.
17. Cordier, G., Brochier, J., and Revillard, J. P.: Cytotoxic and proliferative responses of human thoracic duct lymphocytes: effects of thoracic duct drainage in uremic patients, Clin. Immunol. Immunopathol. 5:351, 1976.
18. Cordier, G., Samarut, C., Brochier, J., and Revillard, J. P.: Antibody-dependent cell cytotoxicity (ADCC). Characterization of "killer" cells in human lymphoid organs, Scand. J. Immunol. 5:233, 1976.
19. Cordier, G., Samarut, C., and Revillard, J. P.: Contribution of lymphocytes bearing $Fc\gamma$ receptors in PHA-induced cytotoxicity, Immunology, in press.
20. Dammin, G. J., Couch, N. P., and Murray, J. E.: Prolonged survival of skin homografts in uremic patients, Ann. N.Y. Acad. Sci. 64:967, 1957.
21. Daniels, J. C., Ritzman, S. E., Long, P. A., Gregory, R., and Levin, W. C.: In vitro lymphocyte survival in chronic uremia, Clin. Res. 14:107, 1966.
21a. Daniels, J. C., and Sakia, H., Cobb, E. K., Remmers, A. R., Sarles, H. E., Fish, J. C., Levin, W. R., and Ritzmann, S. E.: Altered nucleic acid synthesis patterns in lymphocytes from patients with chronic uremia, Am. J. Med. Sci. 259:214, 1970.
22. Dobbelstein, H., Korner, W. F., Mempel, W., Grosse-Wilde, H., and Edel, H. H.: Vitamin B_6 deficiency in uremia and its implications for the depression of immune responses, Kidney Int. 5:233, 1974.
23. Dobbelstein, H.: Immune system in uremia, Nephron 17:409, 1976.
24. Drukker, W., Moorhead, J. F., and Cameron, J. S.: Mortality during regular dialysis treatment; an editorial, Lancet 2:968, 1970.
25. Elves, M. W., Israels, M. C. G., and Collinge, M.: An assessment of the mixed leucocyte reaction in renal failure, Lancet 1:682, 1966.
26. Funck-Brentano, J. L., Man, N. K., Sausse, A., Cueille, G., Zingraff, J., Drueke, T., Jungers, P., and Billon, J. P.: Polynévrite urémique et moyennes molécules, Rein Foie 1:317, 1974.
27. Giovanetti, S., Ciorn, L., Balestri, P. L., and Giagini, M.: Evidence that guanidines and some related compounds cause haemolysis in chronic uraemia, Clin. Sci. 34: 141, 1968.
28. Giovanetti, S., Balestri, P. L., and Barsotti, G.: Methylguanidine in uremia, Arch. Intern. Med. 131:709, 1973.
29. Gowland, G., and Smiddy, F. G.: The effect of acute experimental uremia on the immunological responses of the rabbit to bovine serum albumin, Br. J. Urol. 34: 274, 1962.
30. Hanicki, Z., Cichocki, T., Sarnecka-Keller, M., Klein, A., and Komorowska, Z.: Influence of middle-sized molecule aggregates from dialysate of uremic patients on lymphocyte transformation in vitro, Nephron 17:73, 1976.
31. Harris, I., Rashid, A., Copeland, D., Hyslop, D., and Stewart, T.: The effect of methylguanidine (MG) and guanidine succinic acid (GSA) on in vitro lymphocyte responses to mitogenic agents, Clin. Res. 21:1049, 1973.
32. Harris, J. E., Pagé, D., Posen, G., and Stewart, T.: Suppression of in vitro lymphocyte function by uremic toxins, J. Urol. 108:312, 1972.
33. Harris, J., and Sengar, D.: Immunodeficiency in chronic uremia. Preliminary evidence of thymosin deficiency, Transplantation 20:176, 1975.
34. Horowitz, H. I., Stein, I. M., Cohen, B. D., and White, J. G.: Further studies on the platelet inhibitory effect of guanidino-succinic acid and its role in uremic bleeding, Am. J. Med. 49:336, 1970.
35. Hoy, W., Cestero, R. V. M., and Freeman, R. B.: Deficiency of T and B lymphocytes in uremic subjects and partial improvement with maintenance hemodialysis, Nephron, in press.

36. Huber, H., Pastner, D., Dittrich, P., and Braunsteiner, H.: In vitro reactivity of human lymphocytes in uremia. A comparison with the impairment of delayed hypersensitivity, Clin. Exp. Immunol. 5:75, 1969.

37. Hurst, K. S., Saldanha, L. F., Steinberg, S. M., Galen, M. A., Lowrie, E. G., Gagneux, S. A., Lazarus, J. M., Strom, T. B., Carpenter, C. B., and Merrill, J. P.: The effects of varying dialysis regimens on lymphocyte stimulation, Trans. Am. Soc. Artif. Intern. Organs 21:329, 1975.

38. Jensson, O.: Observations on the leucocyte blood picture in acute uremia, Br. J. Haematol. 4:422, 1958.

39. Jordan, M. C., Rousseau, W. E., Tegtmeier, G. E., Noble, G. R., Muth, R. G., and Chin, T. D. Y.: Immunogenicity of inactivated influenza virus vaccine in chronic renal failure, Ann. Intern. Med. 79:790, 1973.

40. Kaplow, L. S., and Gogginet, J. A.: Profound neutropenia during the early phase of hemodialysis, J.A.M.A. 203:1135, 1968.

41. Kasakura, S., and Lowenstein, L.: The effect of uremic blood on mixed leucocyte reactions and on cultures of leucocytes with phytohaemagglutinin, Transplantation 5:283, 1967.

42. Kauffman, C. A., Manzler, A. D., and Phair, J. P.: Cell mediated immunity in patients on long-term hemodialysis, Clin. Exp. Immunol. 22:54, 1975.

43. Kirkpatrick, Ch. H., Wilson, W. E. C., and Talmage, D. W.: Immunologic studies in human organ transplantation, J. Exp. Med. 119:727, 1964.

44. Ku, G., Hird, V. M., Varghese, Z., Ahmed, K. Y., and Moorhead, I. F.: Inhibition of DNA synthesis by guanidine compounds in uraemia, Proc. Eur. Dial. Transplant Assoc. 1974, p. 22.

45. Lopez, C., Simmons, R. L., Touraine, J. L., Park, B. H., Kiskiss, D. F., and Najarian, J. S.: Discrepancy between PHA responsiveness and quantitative estimates of T cell numbers in human peripheral blood during chronic renal failure and immunosuppression after transplantation, Clin. Immunol. Immunopathol. 4:135, 1975.

46. Mannick, J. A., Powers, J. H., Mithoefer, J., and Ferrebee, J. W.: Renal transplantation in azotemic dogs, Surgery 47:340, 1960.

46a. Margolis, A., Kleinknecht, C., Bonnissol, C., Gaiffe, M., Sahyoun, S., and Broyer, M.: Anticorps (Ac) sériques avant et aprés vaccination chez les enfants hémodialysés. Résultats préliminaires, J. Urol. Nephrol. 83:700, 1977.

47. Merrill, J. P.: The immunologic capability of uremic patients, Cancer Res. 28:1449, 1968.

48. Miller, F.: Serum-derived immunosuppressive substances. I. Partial purification and range of action, Transplantation 21:179, 1976.

49. Ming, P. L., Ming, S. C., and Dammin, G. J.: Effect of uremia and azathioprin on lymphocyte response to PHA, Fed. Proc. 27:432, 1968.

50. Moretta, L., Ferrarini, M., Durante, M. L., and Mingari, M. C.: Expression of receptor for IgM by human T cells in vitro, Eur. J. Immunol. 5:565, 1975.

51. Morrison, A. B., Maness, K., and Towes, R.: Skin homograft survival in chronic renal insufficiency, Arch. Pathol. 75:139, 1963.

52. Moynihan, P. C., and Jackson, J. F.: Lymphocyte transformation in acute uraemia, Nature 212:206, 1966.

53. Nakla, L. S., and Goggin, M. J.: Lymphocyte transformation in chronic renal failure, Immunology 24:229, 1973.

54. Navarro, J., Touraine, J. L., Corre, C., and Traeger, J.: Effet in vitro des moyennes molécules sur la prolifération lymphocytaire, Pathol. Biol. 24:189, 1976.

55. Navarro, J., Touraine, J. L., Corre, C., and Traeger, J.: Prolongation of skin allograft survival and inhibition of graft versus host reaction in rodents treated with "middle molecules," Cell. Immunol. 31:349, 1977.

56. Nelson, D. S., and Penrose, J. M.: Effect of hemodialysis and transplantation on inhibition of lymphocyte transformation by sera from uremic patients, Clin. Immunol. Immunopathol. 4:143, 1975.

57. Newberry, M. W., and Sanford, J. P.: Defective cellular immunity in renal failure: depression of reactivity of lymphocytes to phytohemagglutinin by renal failure serum, J. Clin. Invest. 50:1262, 1971.
58. Odeberg, H., Olsson, I., and Thysell, H.: The effect of uremic serum on granulocyte iodination capacity, Trans. Am. Soc. Artif. Intern. Organs 19:484, 1973.
59. Pabico, R. C., Douglas, R. G., Betts, R. F., McKenna, B. A., and Freeman, R. B.: Influenza vaccination of patients with glomerular diseases. Effects on creatinine clearance, urinary protein excretion and antibody response, Ann. Intern. Med. 81: 171, 1974.
60. Pang, G. T. M., Beguley, D. M., and Wilson, J. D.: Spontaneous rosettes as T-lymphocyte marker: a modified method giving consistent results. SRBC rosettes. U, Immunol. Methods. 4:41, 1974.
60a. Quadracci, L. J., Ringden, O., and Drzymanski, M.: The effect of uremia and transplantation on lymphocyte subpopulations, Kidney Int. 10:179, 1976.
61. Reddy, M. M., Goh, K., and Cestero, R. V. M.: T and B lymphocytes in patients with chronic renal disease on hemodialysis, Experientia 31:980, 1975.
62. Reichel, H.: Lymphopenie bei urämie, Klin. Wochenschr. 15:926, 1936.
63. Revillard, J. P., Touraine, J. L., Brochier, J., Manel, A. M., Fries, D., and Traeger, J.: L'immunité cellulaire chez l'urémique, *Actualités Néphrologiques de l'Hôpital Necker* (Paris: Flammarion, 1970), pp. 287–311.
63a. Revillard, J. P., Brochier, J., Samarut, C., and Cordier, G.: Lymphocyte circulation in man, *Transplantation and Clinical Immunology*, vol. 9 (Amsterdam: Elsevier, 1977), in press.
64. Ringoir, S., Van Looy, L., Van de Heyning, P., and Leroux Roels, G.: Impairment of phagocytic activity of macrophages as studied by the skin window test in patients on regular hemodialysis treatment, Clin. Nephrol. 4:234, 1975.
65. Samarut, C., Brochier, J., and Revillard, J. P.: Distribution of cells binding erythrocyte-antibody (EA) complexes in human lymphoid populations, Scand. J. Immunol. 5:221, 1976.
66. Schneider, W., and Jutzler, G. A.: Implications of cyclic adenosine 3',5'-monophosphate in chronic renal failure, N. Engl. J. Med. 291:155, 1974.
67. Sclroos, O., Pasternack, A., and Virolainen, M.: Skin test sensitivity and antigen-induced lymphocyte transformation in uraemia, Clin. Exp. Immunol. 14:365, 1973.
68. Sengar, D. P. S., Rashid, A., and Harris, J. E.: In vitro cellular immunity and in vivo delayed hypersensitivity in uremic patients maintained on hemodialysis, Int. Arch. Allergy Appl. Immunol. 47:829, 1974.
69. Sengar, D. P. S., Hyslop, D. B., Rashid, A., and Harris, J. E.: T rosettes in hemodialysis patients and renal allograft recipients, Cell. Immunol. 20:92, 1975.
70. Sengar, D. P. S., Rashid, A., and Harris, J. E.: Correlation in hemodialysis patients and renal allograft recipients between percent lymphocytes in peripheral blood and in vitro lymphocyte responses to non-specific mitogenic agents, Acta Haematol. 54: 159, 1975.
71. Shackman, R., and Castro, J. E.: Prelusive skin grafts in live-donor kidney transplantation, Lancet 2:521, 1975.
72. Silk, M. R.: The effect of uremic plasma on lymphocyte transformation, Invest. Urol. 5:195, 1967.
73. Slavin, R. G., and Fitch, C. D.: Inhibition of lymphocyte transformation by guanidine succinic acid, a surplus metabolite in uremia, Experientia 27:1340, 1971.
74. Slavin, R. G., Kelly, J. F., and Garrett, J. J.: Lymphocyte response in acute experimental renal failure, J. Immunol. 104:1424, 1970.
75. Slavin, R. G., and Gallagher, N. I.: Lymphocytopenia in acute experimental renal failure, Int. Arch. Allergy Appl. Immunol. 47:80, 1974.
76. Slavin, R. G., Orling, J. F., and Fisher, V. W.: The effect of uremic serum on normal human and guinea pig lymphocytes, Proc. Soc. Exp. Biol. Med. 148:1229, 1975.

77. Smiddy, F. G., Burwell, R. G., and Parsons, F. M.: The effect of acute uraemia upon the survival of skin homografts, Br. J. Surg. 48:328, 1960.
78. Smiddy, F. G., Burwell, R. G., and Parsons, F. M.: Influence of uremia on the survival of skin homografts, Nature 190:732, 1961.
79. Smyth, P. M., Schouland, M., Brereton-Stiles, G. G., Coovadia, H. M., Grace, H. J., Loening, W. E. K., Mafoyane, M., Parent, M. A., and Vos, G. H.: Thymolymphatic deficiency and depression of cell-mediated immunity in protein-malnutrition, Lancet 2:939, 1971.
80. Souhami, R. L., Smith, J., and Bradfield, J. W. B.: The effect of uraemia on organ graft survival in the rat, Br. J. Exp. Pathol. 54:183, 1973.
81. Stoloff, I. L., Stout, R., Myerson, R. M., and Havens, W. P.: Production of antibody in patients with uremia, N. Engl. J. Med. 259:320, 1958.
82. Strom, T. B., Deisseroth, A., Morganroth, J., Carpenter, C. B., and Merrill, J. P.: Alterations of the cytotoxic action of sensitized lymphocytes by cholinergic agents and activators of adenylate cyclase, Proc. Natl. Acad. Sci. USA 69:2995, 1972.
83. Tam, C. F., Kopple, J. D., Wang, M., and Swendseid, M. E.: Alterations of monoamine oxidase activity in uremia, Kidney Int. 7:S-328, 1975.
84. Touraine, J. L., Touraine, F., Revillard, J. P., Brochier, J., and Traeger, J.: T-lymphocytes and serum inhibitors of cell-mediated immunity in renal insufficiency, Nephron 14:195, 1975.
85. Traeger, J., Revillard, J. P., Touraine, J. L., and Brochier, J.: L'immunité cellulaire dans l'insuffisance rénale, Proc. Eur. Dialysis Transplant Assoc. 6:165, 1969.
86. Urbanitz, D., Nolden, H. P., Fechnier, I., Urbanitz, S., Freiberg, J., and Sieberth, H. G.: Zur Monocyten Funktion bei Kranken mit terminaler Niereninsuffizienz, Klin. Wochenschr. 53:59, 1975.
86a. Vincent, C., and Revillard, J. P.: Unpublished data.
87. Vincent, C., Revillard, J. P., Galand, M., and Traeger, J.: Serum B_2 microglobulin in hemodialyzed patients, Nephron, 1977, in press.
88. Wilson, W. E. C., Kirkpatrick, Ch. H., and Talmage, D. W.: Immunologic studies in human organ transplantation. III. The relationship of delayed hypersensitivity to the onset of attempted kidney allograft rejection, J. Clin. Invest. 43:1881, 1964.
89. Wilson, W. E. C., Kirkpatrick, Ch. H., and Talmage, D. W.: Suppression of immunologic responsiveness in uremia, Ann. Intern. Med. 62:1, 1965.

18

Plasma Exchange in Nephritis

C. M. LOCKWOOD, M.B.B.C.H., M.R.C.P.,
B. PUSSELL, F.R.A.C.P., C. B. WILSON, M.D., AND
D. K. PETERS, M.B.B.C.H., F.R.C.P.

Department of Medicine, Royal Postgraduate Medical School, London, England

Since 1974 we have been using a regimen of intensive plasma exchange, cytotoxic drugs and steroids for the treatment of patients with fulminating nephritis. Although initially used to treat diseases associated with antibodies to the glomerular basement membrane (GBM),[10, 11] the regimen was later applied to other forms of nephritis.[12, 13] During the past 3½ years, modifications of the regimen have led to the evolution of a fairly standard approach, which essentially consists of daily 4-L plasma exchange, prednisone in a dosage of 60 mg/day, cyclophosphamide 3 mg/kg/day and azathioprine 1 mg/kg/day. The purpose of this chapter is to describe in detail our experience with this regimen in the treatment of 44 patients — 24 with anti-GBM disease and 20 with putative immune complex (IC) nephritis, six of whom had systemic lupus erythematosus (SLE).

Methods

PLASMA EXCHANGE

Four-liter plasma exchanges were carried out on a cell separator (Haemonetics Model 30). Wherever possible plasma protein

383

fraction (PPF), a semipurified albumin solution (Cohn fraction V) supplied by the National Blood Transfusion Service, was used as plasma replacement. Daily plasma exchange using PPF resulted in depletion of complement and fibrinogen due to the loss of the globulin fraction of plasma, which was not replaced by the PPF. When PPF was not readily available, either reconstituted dried plasma or group-compatible fresh-frozen plasma

TABLE 18–1.–NEPHRITIS: DRUG THERAPY BEFORE TREATMENT REGIMEN

DISEASE	PATIENT	DRUG*	DURATION
Anti-GBM disease	M.D.	Prednisolone, 60–40 mg/day	3 wk
		Cyclophosphamide, 3 mg/kg/day	1 wk
		Heparin, 10,000 IV/6 hourly	1 wk
		Aspirin, 300 mg/day	1 wk
	K.S.	Prednisolone, 30 mg/day	3 wk
		Azathioprine, 1 mg/kg/day	1 wk
	A.W.	Prednisolone, 60 mg/day	2 wk
		Azathioprine, 3 mg/kg/day	2 wk
		Dipyrimadole, 600 mg/day	2 wk
		Heparin, 10,000 IV/8 hourly	2 wk
	R.L.	Prednisolone, 60 mg/day	2 wk
		Cyclophosphamide, 3 mg/kg/day	1 wk
		Azathioprine, 1 mg/kg/day	1 wk
	R.S.	Prednisolone, 60 mg/day	3 wk
		Cyclophosphamide, 3 mg/kg/day	3 wk
IC disease	T.P.	Prednisolone, 45 mg/day	2½ wk
	K.H.	Prednisolone, 60 mg/day	3 wk
		Azathioprine, 2 mg/kg/day	3 wk
	M.B.	Prednisolone, 60 mg/day	10 day
		Cyclophosphamide, 3 mg/kg/day	10 day
		Methylprednisolone, 700 mg/day	3 day
		Heparin, 5000 IV/12 hourly	2 wk
SLE	V.H.	Prednisolone, up to 60 mg/day	6 wk
		Chlorambucil, 10 mg/day	5 wk
	P.F.	Prednisolone, 60 mg/day	3 wk
		Methylprednisolone, 1 gm/day	4 day
	P.D.	Prednisolone, up to 60 mg/day	12 wk
		Azathioprine, up to 150 mg/day	8 wk
		Methylprednisolone, 1 gm/day	4 day
	N.A.	Prednisone, up to 80 mg/day	4 wk

*IV = intravenously.

was used as a substitute (for some patients). In most patients vascular access was by way of an arteriovenous shunt or subcutaneous fistula; in some patients (on shorter-term treatment) a vein-to-vein approach was found satisfactory; and in a few patients direct cannulation of the inferior vena cava by the Seldinger technique was necessary since other access sites were not available. Plasma exchange was continued, usually daily, until clinical and laboratory evidence of control of disease activity was obtained, or until it became evident that no recovery of renal function would occur.

DRUG THERAPY

We attempted to standardize therapy by starting our patients on prednisolone or prednisone 60 mg/day, cyclophosphamide 3 mg/kg/day and azathioprine 1 mg/kg/day. Steroids were generally reduced at weekly intervals, and cytotoxic agents were withdrawn if severe infection occurred or the white blood cell count fell to less than 4,000/cu mm. Cyclophosphamide was withdrawn after eight weeks in most patients. It is now our practice to use a lower dosage (2 mg/kg/day) of cyclophosphamide and to withhold azathioprine in older patients (more than 60 years), whom we have found to be at greater risk from opportunist infection. Some patients had been started on drug therapy before referral (details are provided in Table 18–1.)

HISTOLOGY

Renal tissue was obtained by percutaneous needle biopsy or at autopsy. Specimens were processed for light microscopy and immunofluorescence as described previously.[4]

COMPLEMENT, FIBRINOGEN, IgG AND DNA BINDING

Routine measurements of complement components were carried out by radial immunodiffusion;[15] however, where specific studies of the effect of plasma exchange on concentrations of C3, C5 and factor B were undertaken, "rocket" immunoelectrophoresis techniques were used.[9] Plasma fibrinogen levels were measured by a fibrinogen consumption method,[24] IgG by nephelometry[8] and DNA binding by the Farr ammonium sulfate precipitation technique after decomplementation.[28]

ANTI-GBM ANTIBODY

Assays for circulating anti-GBM antibody were undertaken by Dr. Curtis B. Wilson at the Scripps Clinic and Research Foundation in La Jolla, California. Anti-GBM antibody was measured by a radiolabeled collagenase solubilized human GBM in a double antibody radioimmune assay. The results were expressed as percentage binding of the radiolabeled antigen; this value was less than 1% in patients without other evidence of anti-GBM disease and could be as high as 60% in those with anti-GBM nephritis.[27]

CIRCULATING IMMUNE COMPLEXES

C1Q DEVIATION TEST.[21] — This test is based on the ability of ICs in sera to inhibit the uptake of radiolabeled C1q onto sensitized sheep red blood cells. Results were expressed as the percent of deviation from the radioactivity taken up by normal controls. Deviation of greater than 15% was taken to indicate the presence of C1q binding material such as ICs.

C1Q BINDING ASSAY.[30] — This test depends on the incubation of radiolabeled C1q with polyethylene glycol at a final concentration of 2.8%. The amount precipitated was calibrated by relating it to the precipitation brought about by known quantities of aggregated IgG.

RETICULOENDOTHELIAL FUNCTION

Samples of red blood cells from patients who had group O or A rhesus-positive blood were coated with anti-D non-complement-fixing IgG (as described by Mollison and supplied by him).[16] A standardized quantity was labeled with chromium-51 and reinjected. An initial sample was taken after three minutes and thereafter samples were taken at five-minute intervals for 30 minutes. Samples were counted in a gamma counter and the clearance of the coated cells was calculated by relating the counts per minute in sequential samples to the counts per minute in the initial three-minute sample.

PULMONARY HEMORRHAGE

The presence of fresh lung hemorrhage was measured by changes in the serial measurements of KCO as described by Ewan and Rees.[5] Rises in KCO by more than 30% of the baseline level were taken to indicate the presence of active lung bleeding.

Patients

Details of clinical features and laboratory investigations of the patients are given in Tables 18–2, 18–3 and 18–4.

Results

EFFECTS OF 4-L PLASMA EXCHANGES ON INTRAVASCULAR CONSTITUENTS

ACUTE EFFECTS ON ^{131}I IgG, NATIVE IgG AND EVANS BLUE. — An anuric patient on the therapeutic regimen of cyclophosphamide 3 mg/kg and prednisolone 60 mg/day gave informed consent to the intravenous injection of a trace amount of ^{131}I IgG 48 hours before, and a bolus of Evans Blue immediately before a 4-L plasma exchange. Samples were removed during the course of the exchange in which PPF was substituted for the patient's plasma. The decreases in levels of ^{131}I IgG, native IgG and Evans Blue were determined (^{131}I IgG by gamma counting, native IgG by nephelometry and Evans Blue by optical density techniques). As can be seen from Figure 18–1, a 4-L exchange removed 65% of the ^{131}I IgG and native IgG and 92% of the Evans Blue.

LONG-TERM EFFECTS OF IMMUNOGLOBULIN CONCENTRATIONS. — After a period of intensive plasma exchange, the recovery of native IgG was studied in five immunosuppressed patients. Concentrations of IgG did not return to the normal range for periods ranging from 2½ to 20 weeks (Fig. 18–2). The recoveries of IgA and IgM concentrations are also shown in Figure 18–2.

COMPLEMENT COMPONENTS AND FIBRINOGEN. — The effect of daily 4-L plasma exchange on complement components C3, C5 and factor B and on plasma fibrinogen was studied in two patients. Levels of complement components C3, C5 and factor B were maintained at 20–40% of normal when plasma exchange

TABLE 18-2.—CLINICAL AND LABORATORY FEATURES

PATIENT	AGE (SEX)	PRESENTATION CLINICAL FEATURES	HB (gm/dl)
M.D.	24(M)	Hemopt. (10 wk), microscopic hematuria, deteriorating renal function (August 1974)	7.0
G.W.	54(M)	Minor hemopt. (6 mo), hematuria, renal failure (Feb 1975)	7.5
M.S.	18(M)	Loin pain (3 wk), RPGN, no hemopt. (June 1975)	8.4
C.R.	21(F)	Hemopt., followed 1 mo later by loin pain and RPGN (June 1975)	11.8
D.M.	53(M)	Malaise (6 wk), loin pain, oliguria, hematuria, minor hemopt. (June 1975)	8.9
K.S.	23(M)	Recurrent minor hemopt. (10 wk), hematuria, rising serum creat. clearance (Sept 1975)	14.1
A.W.	20(F)	Hematuria, pyrexia (2 wk); admitted anuric; then severe lung hemorrhage requiring ventilation (Oct 1975)	7.6
M.W.	50(F)	Anemia (19 yr), hemopt. (6 and 12 yr previously), recent hematuria, dyspnea (Dec 1975)	6.5
M.B.	21(F)	Edema (4 wk), loin pain, hematuria, oliguria (Jan 1976)	6.4
F.B.	45(F)	Isolated hemopt. (6 yr before), cough, hemopt., fever (3 wk) (Feb 1976)	10.3
E.M.	56(F)	Dyspnea (2 wk), hematemesis (Feb 1976)	8.0
S.H.	58(M)	Vomiting, headaches (6 wk) (May 1976)	9.7
R.T.	17(M)	Hemopt. (7 mo), malaise, hematuria (3 wk) (Aug 1976)	4.3
D.W.	49(M)	Dyspnea, pleuritic pain (8 days) (Sept 1976)	7.4
M.P.	22(F)	Hemopt. (8 mo), dyspnea, edema, oliguria (Nov 1976)	3.0
P.W.	20(F)	Hemopt. (9 wk), dyspnea, malaise, oliguria (Dec 1976)	4.7
R.L.	61(F)	Headaches, nausea, lethargy, dyspnea (4 mo) (Jan 1977)	6.9
D.D.	66(M)	Hemopt., microscopic hematuria (6 wk) (Feb 1977)	9.9
R.R.	35(M)	Malaise, microscopic hematuria (6 wk) (March 1977)	5.0
R.S.	37(M)	Malaise (4 mo), edema, dyspnea (March 1977)	12.3
R.O.	25(M)	Recurrent hemopt. (1 yr), dyspnea, malaise, microscopic hematuria (May 1977)	8.1
V.S.	29(F)	Recurrent hemopt. (1 yr), dyspnea, ankle edema (4 mo) (Oct 1977)	7.6
C.L.	20(F)	Pleuritic pain, hemopt., arthralgia, headache, hematuria (Oct 1977)	11.0
E.L.	66(F)	Isolated hemopt. (5 yr before), diarrhea, nausea, vomiting (2 mo) (Dec 1977)	10.7

*Abbreviations: Hemopt. = hemoptysis, PD = peritoneal dialysis, HD = hemodialysis,

OF 24 PATIENTS WITH ANTI-GBM DISEASE*

ABNORMAL CXR	CREAT. (μM/L)	ANTI-GBM (LITER %)	EXCHANGES (NO.)	FOLLOW-UP			
				HB (gm/dl)	CREAT. (μM/L)	ANTI-GBM (LITER %)	FOLLOW-UP (MO)
+	460	24	7	14.9	235	−ve	39
+	520	21	16	12.4	200	−ve	30
+	HD	32	7	Died August 75: autopsy showed recurrent lung hemorrhage			
−	PD	28	7		HD	6	24
−	PD	36	7	Died April 1977: one week after transplant			
+	340	26	9	14.0	100	−ve	25
+	HD	42	24		HD	11	20
+	300	25	34	12.9	125	−ve	26
−	PD	34	28		HD	−ve	24
+	480	21	16	12.1	161	−ve	23
+	700	13	3	Died within 72 hours: autopsy showed *Pseudomonas* septicemia and lung hemorrhage			
−	238	6	16	14	104	−ve	16
−	154	36	52	15	101	28	15
+	250	4	16	15.3	112	−ve	16
+	PD	33	27		HD	−ve	12
+	PD	47	9		HD	−ve	12
−	653	24	10		HD	−ve	6
+	528	10	6	Died March 77: autopsy showed presumed vital pneumonitis			
+	180	30	33		HD	31	7
−	260	33	5	11.3	260	−ve	8
+	796	31	37		HD	29	6
+	207	34	7	8.9	221	25	4
+	211	30	29	13.2	76	14	4
−	1000	38	22		PD	30	1

CXR = chest x-ray, Hb = hemoglobin, and Creat. = creatinine.

TABLE 18-3.—CLINICAL AND LABORATORY FEATURES

| | | | PRESENTATION | | |
PATIENT	AGE (SEX)	CLINICAL SYNDROME	CLINICAL FEATURES AND DURATION OF SYMPTOMS (WK)
F.M.	40(M)	MP	Fever, arthralgia, rash, pharyngeal ulceration, weight loss, eosinophilia (12)
P.B.	50(F)	WG	Lethargy, arthralgia, peripheral neuropathy, weight loss (16)
P.R.	53(M)	WG	Fever, ankle edema, cavitating infiltration CXR (4)
W.O.C.	55(M)	MP	Fever, weight loss, cutaneous ulceration, raised IgG level (2)
J.C.	40(M)	WG	Myositis, arthralgia, proximal myopathy, nocturia, weight loss, mononeuritis multiplex eosinophilia (4)
T.P.	66(M)	WG	Lethargy, Wegener's lung lesion excised, fever, rash, jaundice, peripheral neuropathy, eosinophilia (28)
J.R.	42(M)	MP	Otitis media, fever, CVA, arthralgia, jaundice, weight loss, proximal myopathy (2)
K.H.	41(F)	MP	Fever, RUZ opacity, arthralgia, episcleritis, hemoptysis, fits, weight loss (8)
P.P.	59(F)	MP	Fever, diarrhea, microscopic hematuria, arthropathy, hemoptysis, bilateral CXR opacities (20)
D.G.	54(M)	MP	Cough, hemoptysis, nocturia, lethargy (20)
T.D.	56(M)	WG	Deafness, red eyes, cough, pleurisy, dyspnea, peripheral neuropathy, proximal myopathy, dysgraphia, right extensor plantar response, Wegener's lung lesion excised (7)
G.S.	67(M)	WG	Deafness, episcleritis, arthralgia, dyspnea, proximal myopathy, cough, hemoptysis, CXR opacity, fever, eosinophilia, hepatosplenomegaly (60)
M.B.	13(M)	NC	Upper respiratory tract symptoms, hepatosplenomegaly (8)
J.M.	37(F)	WG	Hemoptysis, episcleritis, external otitis, deafness, granuloma, vocal cord, peripheral neuropathy (24)

*Abbreviations: Creat. = creatinine, MP = microscopic polyarteritis, WG = Wegener's x ray, RDT = regular dialysis therapy, CVA = cerebrovascular accident, and NC = not
†Died (see text for details).

OF 14 PATIENTS WITH NONLUPUS RPGN*

| | | FOLLOW-UP | | |
CREAT. (μM/L)	CREAT. CLEARANCE (ml/min)	IMMUNE COMPLEXES	EXCHANGES (NO.)	CREAT. (μM/L)	FOLLOW-UP (MO)
1,100	1	+	7	210	6 (OI)†
Anuric		ND	6	Anuric (RDT)†	
890	3	+	13	230	2½ (OI)†
1,140	1	+	10	221	28
208	28	+	4	122	22
924	ND	−	4	237	2½ (CVA)†
790	6	+	9	146	20
550	2	−	10	HD	20
620	4	−	8	208	16
303	32	−	8	138	14
1,030	ND	+	6	240	2 (OI)†
1,048	2	+	5	300	12
247	11	−	4	131	8
560	ND	−	14	190	4

granulomatosis, OI = opportunistic infection, ND = not detectable, CXR = chest
classified.

TABLE 18-4.—CLINICAL AND LABORATORY FEATURES

PATIENT	AGE (SEX)	CLINICAL FEATURES	CREAT. (μM/L)	ELEVATED DNA BINDING
		PRESENTATION		
V.H.	22(F)	Deteriorating cerebral function, sudden deterioration in renal function despite pred. and chlorambucil for 6 wk	480	+
J.M.	45(F)	Indolent cutaneous vasculitis, sudden-onset cerebral vasculitis, nephritis and pulmonary vasculitis (necessitating ventilation)	260	+
P.F.	21(F)	Onset of edema, rash, thrombocytopenia (70,000/mm) and relentless rise in creatinine clearance occurred in puerperium despite high dose pred. for 3 wk	520	+
J.K.	23(F)	Arthralgia, rash, edema, hematuria, rising creatinine clearance, thrombocytopenia (100,000/mm)	839	+
N.A.	25(F)	Vomiting, anorexia, weight loss, pyrexia, cough, rash, cerebral and pulmonary vasculitis; severe nephritis—anuric at referral; no response to 4 wk pred. (60–80 mg/day)	PD	+
P.D.	21(F)	Rash, arthralgia, edema, nephritis, cerebral and pulmonary vasculitis (ventilated) despite high doses of steroids	800	+

*Abbreviations: Creat. = creatinine, pred. = prednisone, cyclo. = cyclophosphamide,
†Died.

OF SIX PATIENTS WITH LUPUS NEPHRITIS*

IMMUNE COMPLEXES	EXCHANGES (NO.)	FOLLOW-UP		
		OUTCOME	CREAT. (μM/L)	FOLLOW-UP (MO)
ND	8	Elevation of pred. dose (20–40 mg) and PE-induced long remission—disease now controlled with low doses of steroids	105	20
+	11	Introduction of pred. (60 mg), cyclo., aza. and PE followed by resolution of all symptoms—disease controlled by 15 mg pred. daily	95	18
+	15	Started on 60 mg pred. but deteriorated for 3 wk until starting 4×1 gm daily methylpred. and PE simultaneously—then excellent response with fall in creatinine clearance and rise in platelet count to normal range	90	9
+	18	Good remission induced by introduction of combined aza., pred. (60 mg), 3×1 gm daily methylpred. and PE. Relapse when maintenance pred. reduced. Relentless deterioration in renal function despite pred. (60 mg) and 3×1 gm daily methylpred.	See Fig. 18–13	4†
+	2	Cardiac arrest followed cardiac arrhythmia	–	†
+	10	Sudden respiratory arrest caused death after pulmonary vasculitis had cleared radiologically in response to addition of PE, 6×1 gm daily methylpred. and aza., to high dose pred. No response in renal function	–	†

aza. = azathioprine, PE = plasma exchange, and ND = not detectable.

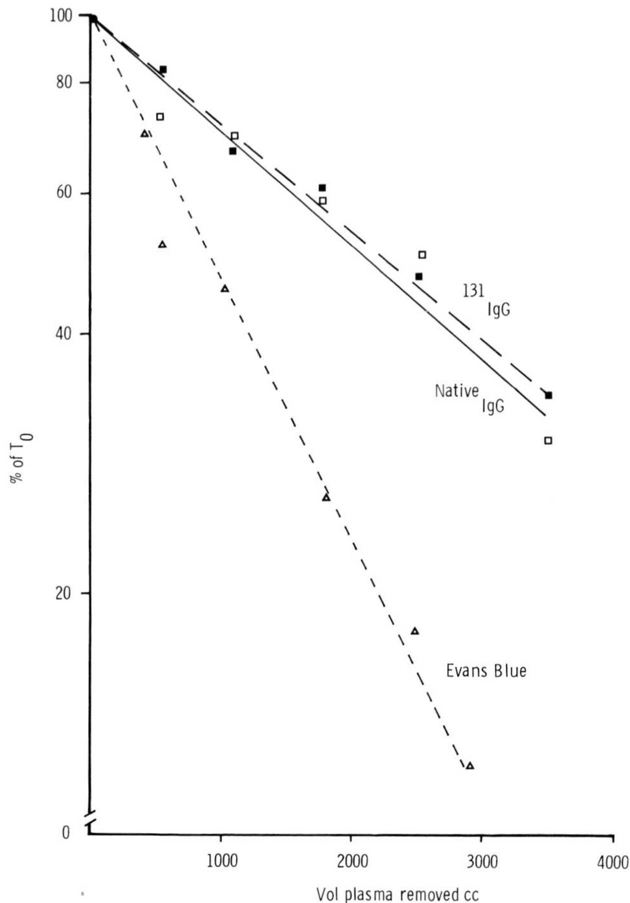

Fig. 18–1.—Effect of one 4-L plasma exchange on levels of [131]I IgG, native IgG and Evans Blue. Sixty-five percent of the ^{131}I and native IgG and 92% of the Evans Blue were removed during the course of one plasma exchange.

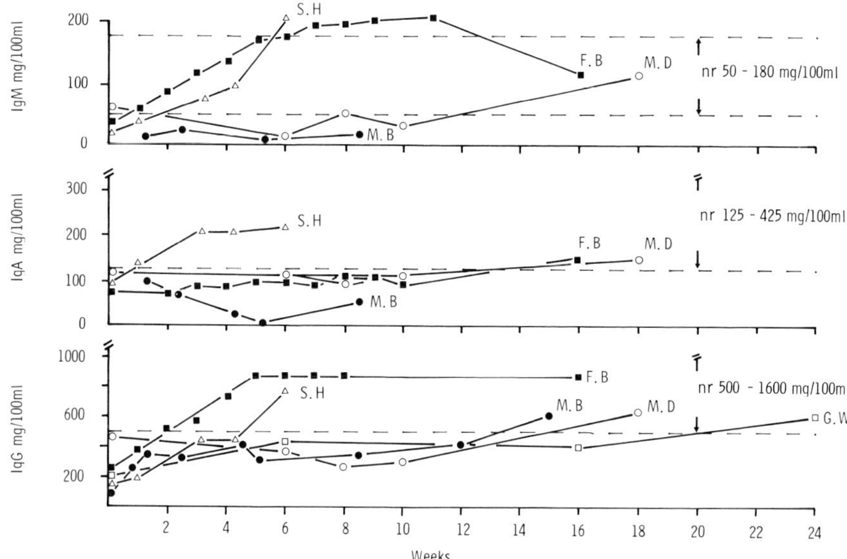

Fig. 18–2. — Recovery of IgG, IgA and IgM levels after intensive plasma exchange in five immunosuppressed patients. Note that the time taken for IgG levels to return to normal ranged from 2½ to 20 weeks, IgA from 1 to 13 weeks, and IgM from 1 to 12 weeks. *nr* = normal range.

was carried out daily; when plasma exchange was discontinued, levels rose to normal within 48 hours with no significant overshoot (Fig. 18 – 3). Daily 4-L plasma exchanges maintained plasma fibrinogen values between 80 and 150 mg/100 ml (Fig. 18 – 3). In other studies (not shown) it was found that an acute phase stimulus, for example, intercurrent infection, prevented this depletion of complement and fibrinogen, presumably because of their increased synthesis rates.

EFFECT OF PLASMA EXCHANGE ON RETICULOENDOTHELIAL FUNCTION

The effect of plasma exchange on the clearance of ^{51}Cr-labeled IgG-coated autologous red blood cells was studied in three patients with nephritis and in one with an immune complex vasculitis affecting the skin but sparing the kidneys. All three patients with nephritis (two with anti-GBM disease and one with Wegener's granulomatosis) had severe renal impairment

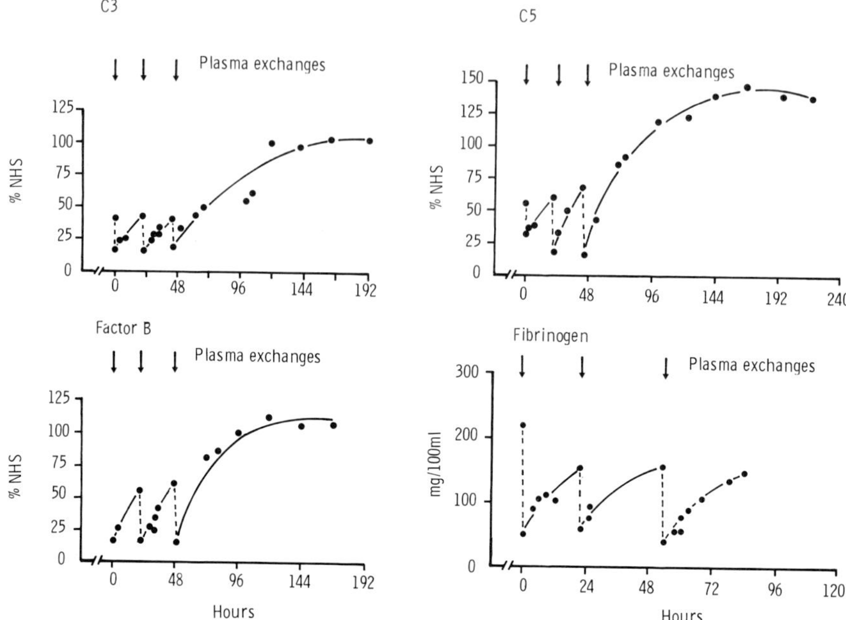

Fig. 18–3.—Effect of daily plasma exchange on complement components C3, C5 and factor B and on plasma fibrinogen. Levels of complement components were maintained at between 20% and 40% of normal during daily plasma exchange and fibrinogen between 80 and 150 mg/100/ml.

(creatinine clearances of $250-1,000$ μM/L) and were treated with plasma exchange, cytotoxic drugs and steroids. The patient with cutaneous vasculitis was treated with plasma exchange without cytotoxic drugs or steroids. In all four patients the red cell clearance times were prolonged before treatment and substantially shortened after (Figs. $18-4$ and $18-5$).

ANTI-GBM NEPHRITIS

Circulating anti-GBM antibodies were detected in all 24 patients in whom a clinical diagnosis of anti-GBM disease had been made, and all 22 patients biopsied showed linear IgG along the GBM by immunofluorescence. Two patients were not biopsied; one (D.W.) had a single kidney and in the other (C.L.) biopsy was deferred for other reasons (see discussion).

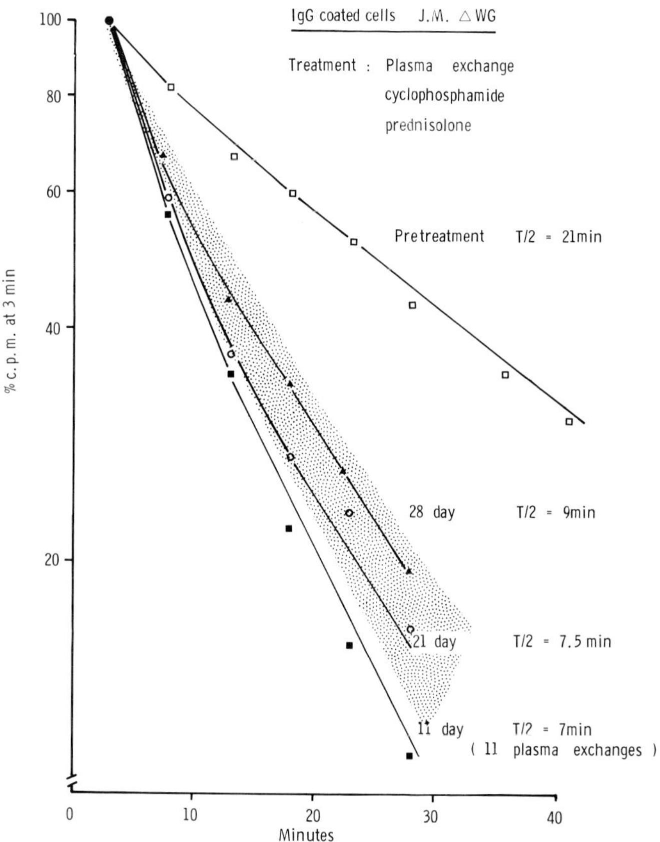

Fig. 18–4.—Clearance of ^{51}Cr-labeled IgG-coated autologous red blood cells in patient J.M. (Wegener's granulomatosis). Note that after treatment with 11 daily plasma exchanges, cyclophosphamide and prednisolone, the 50% clearance time *(T/2)* had fallen from 21 to 7 minutes (normal range, 8–13 minutes). Plasma exchange was discontinued after 14 days: at 21 days and 28 days the 50% clearance times were 7.5 and 9 minutes, respectively. See also Figure 18–12. *c.p.m.* = counts per minute.

                    LOCKWOOD ET AL.

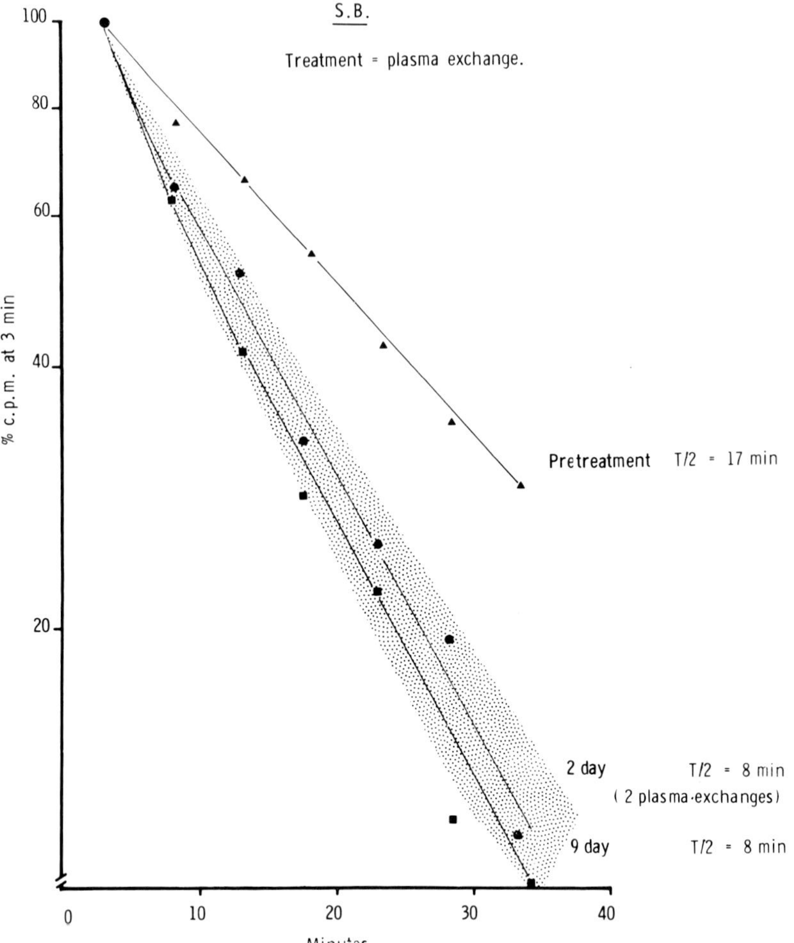

Fig. 18–5.—Clearance of ^{51}Cr-labeled IgG-coated autologous red blood cells in patient S.B. (cutaneous vasculitis — no renal involvement). Before plasma exchange this patient was symptomatic, had detectable levels of circulating complexes by C1q binding assay and had a prolonged 50% clearance time *(T12),* (17 minutes). After two plasma exchanges (each 3 L) she became free from symptoms for four weeks with no detectable complexes: the 50% clearance time after two plasma exchanges was 8 minutes, and one week later (with no further plasma exchange) it was unchanged at 8 minutes. *c.p.m.* = counts per minute.

RENAL FUNCTION. — The overall effects of the treatment regimen on renal function are shown in Table 18 – 2. Seventeen patients had retained some renal function at presentation (M.D., G.W., K.S., M.W., E.M., F.B., D.W., S.H., R.T., D.D., R.L., R.S., R.O., R.R., V.S., C.L., E.L.). One patient (E.M.) died from pulmonary hemorrhage and *Pseudomonas aeruginosa* septicemia within 72 hours of admission. Twelve of the remaining 16 patients (M.D., G.W., K.S., M.W., F.B., D.W., S.H., R.T., D.D., R.S., V.S., C.L.) showed sustained improvement in renal function. However, in four (R.L., R.O., R.R., E.L.), renal function continued to deteriorate. Three of these patients had the most advanced renal failure at referral (E.L., R.O. — creatinine clearances of 1,000 μM/L and 746 μM/L; R.L. — creatinine clearance of 645 μM/L). In the fourth (R.R.), technical problems with vascular access prevented effective early plasma exchange. In five

Fig. 18–6. — Association of intercurrent infection with deterioration in renal function. In all five patients (R.T., M.W., D.D., F.B., R.L.) early improvement in renal function brought about by the treatment regimen was reversed by an intercurrent infection. In all patients, except R.L., there was good response to antibiotic treatment with recovery in renal function. PE = plasma exchange.

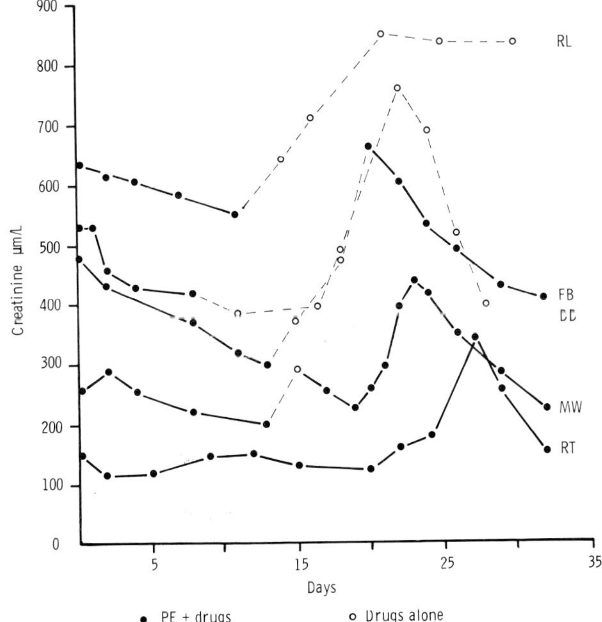

patients (M.W., F.B., R.T., D.D., R.L.), relapse with deterioration of renal function occurred during treatment; in each instance this was associated with intercurrent infection (Fig. 18–6). Appropriate antibiotic treatment was followed by improvement in renal function in four patients, but in the fifth, although deterioration was halted, renal function did not improve (Fig. 18–6). In all seven patients (M.S., C.R., D.M., A.W., M.B., M.P., P.W.) who were anuric at the time of referral, there was no recovery of renal function.

LUNG HEMORRHAGE.—Lung hemorrhage was a clinical feature in 22 of 24 patients, and in two (A.W., E.M.) it was sufficiently severe to require artificial ventilation. Daily measurement of KCO proved a sensitive method of monitoring fresh pulmonary bleeding, which in some instances occurred without radiologic changes or significant hemoptysis (Figs. 18–7 and 18–8). Episodes of lung hemorrhage were usually accompanied

Fig. 18–7.—Serial measurements of serum creatinine clearance and KCO in patient C.L. On day 13 a *Klebsiella* urinary tract infection *(U.T.I.)* developed. Between day 13 and day 14, a 4-gm drop in the hemoglobin level was documented and the KCO rose to its highest level (2.9) on day 15, although there was little change in the chest x-ray (see Fig. 18–8). A convulsion occurred on day 18 (perhaps attributable to central nervous system disease), and microscopic hematuria, which had been heavy since day 13, fell strikingly on day 24. *nr* = normal range.

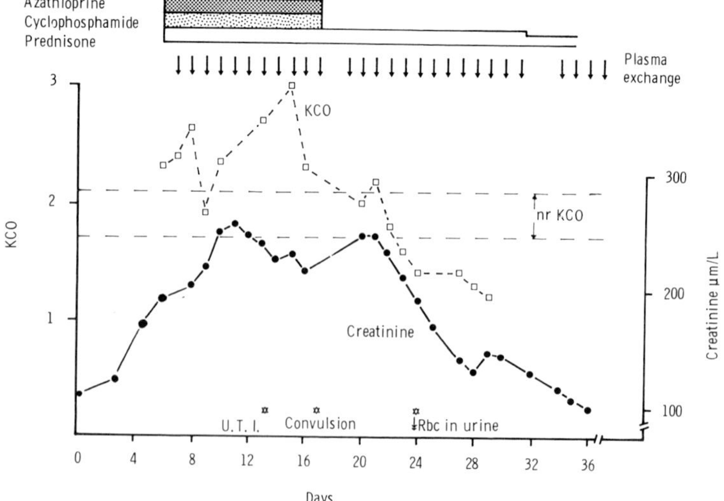

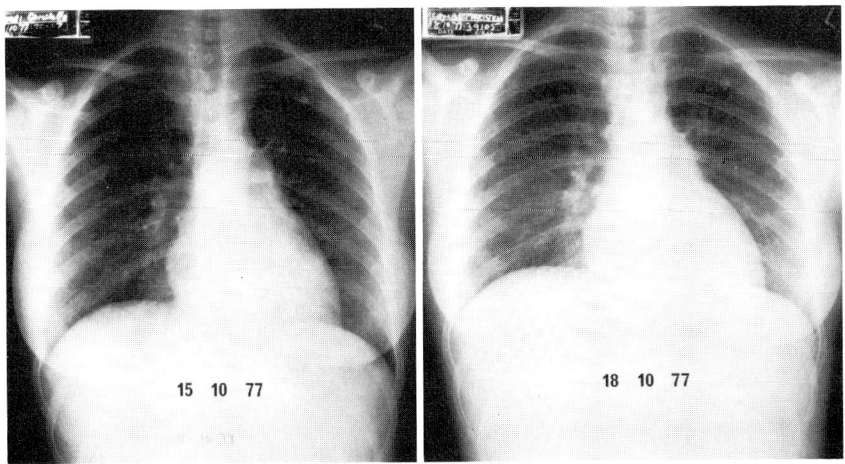

Fig. 18–8.—Chest x-rays taken of patient C.L. on days 11 and 14. The chest x-ray taken on day 16 (not shown) was similar to that taken on day 14.

by deterioration in renal function (Fig. 18–9). With treatment, pulmonary bleeding was controlled in all except one patient (E.M.), who died within 72 hours of referral (see below).

ANTI-GBM ANTIBODY.—The regimen brought about a variable rate of fall in the antibody levels. In certain patients (M.D., K.S., G.W.) a striking decrease was observed and this was always accompanied by rapid improvement; however, in others (R.T., C.L.) sustained improvement occurred despite the persistence of antibody at high titers. In most patients relapse of the disease while on treatment correlated better with other factors such as complicating infection (M.W., F.B., R.T., R.L.),[19] and in respect to pulmonary hemorrhage, fluid overload. In one patient (A.W.), a rise in antibody titers to near pretreatment values (with recurrence of symptoms) occurred after drug therapy and plasma exchange were discontinued. After a short period of plasma exchange, antibody levels seemed to fall spontaneously (Fig. 18–10). In 12 of the 24 patients (M.D., G.W., K.S., M.B., M.W., F.B., R.S., D.D., S.H., D.W., M.P., P.W.), antibody levels eventually fell to within the normal range of the assay after periods ranging from 8 days to 12 months.

RENAL BIOPSIES.—Follow-up renal biopsies were obtained in six patients; in two (M.D., G.W.) who were rebiopsied more than

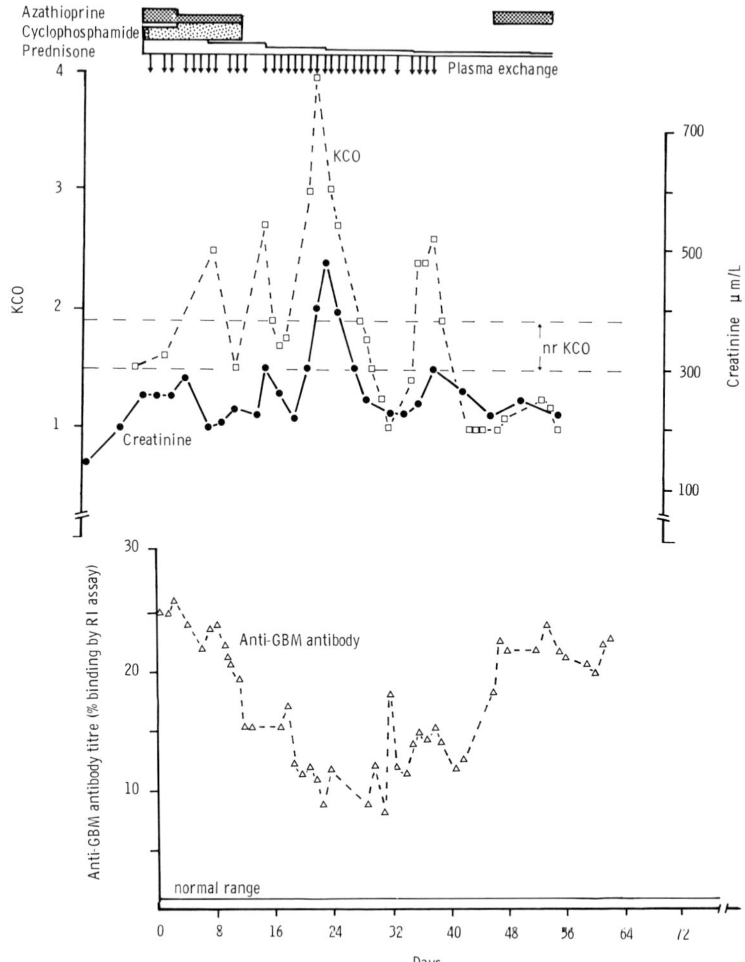

Fig. 18–9.—Serial measurements of serum creatinine clearance and KCO in patient M.W. Note the close correlation between changes in KCO (reflecting active lung bleeding) and serum creatinine clearances. *nr* = normal range. *RI* = radioimmuno.

one year after discharge, decreased intensity of immunofluorescence along the GBM was observed, although this remained strong in the scarred glomeruli. The details of biopsy appearances are shown on Table 18–5.

RECURRENCE OF DISEASE.—Disease recurred in four patients (D.M., D.W., M.S., A.W.) after plasma exchange had been

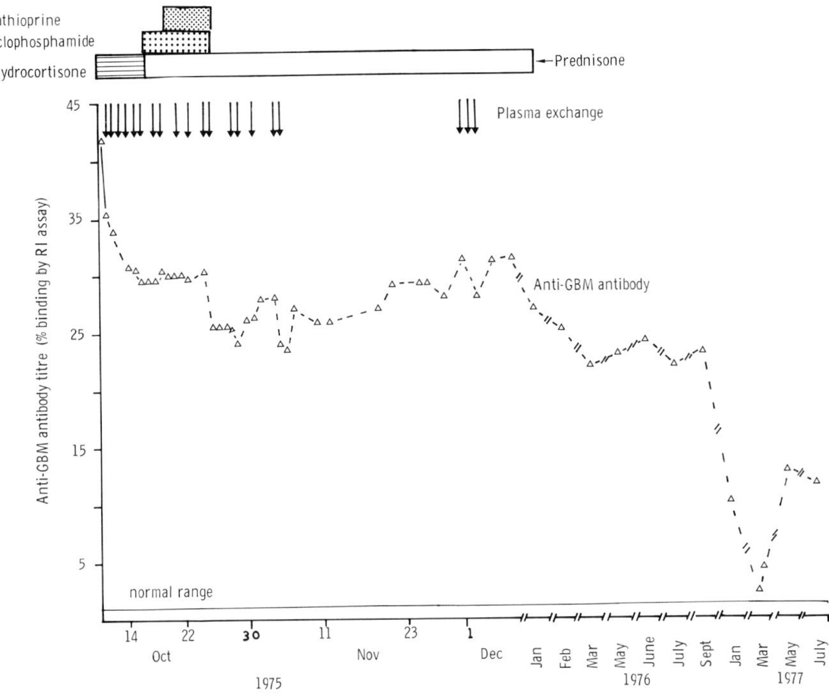

Fig. 18–10.—Serial measurement of anti-GBM antibody in patient A. W. Note the rise in antibody titers when plasma exchange and immunosuppressive drugs were withdrawn. Further hemoptysis occurred in December 1976 and neuropsychiatric disturbances occurred in March 1977 when antibody titers had reached high levels. Improvement in these symptoms occurred after the two related periods of further plasma exchange; thereafter antibody titers seemed to fall spontaneously during 1976. *RI* = radioimmuno.

stopped and drugs were reduced or withdrawn; in all four this was heralded by pulmonary hemorrhage. In only one patient (A.W.) was this deterioration associated with a detectable rise in the level of circulating antibodies; reintroduction of plasma exchange was followed by, and is likely to have been responsible for, resolution of the episode of pulmonary hemorrhage in this patient (Fig. 18–10). In two of the three remaining patients (D.M., D.W.), recurrence was controlled by reintroduction of cytotoxic drugs and/or steroids. However, in the third patient (M.S.), death from pulmonary bleeding occurred despite drug therapy.

TABLE 18–5.—HISTOLOGY: ANTI-GBM DISEASE

PATIENT	BIOPSY DATE	NO. OF GLOMERULI	NO. WITH CRESCENTS	PREDOMINANT FEATURE*
M.D.	July 74	10	2	Segmental proliferation in 6 glomeruli (2 had crescents related to capillary wall breaks); remainder normal
	Sept 74	6	4	Crescent formation with segmental proliferation in 4 glomeruli (2 had extensive obliteration of capillary lumina); remainder normal
	July 75	6	0	2 glomeruli completely sclerosed, 2 partly sclerosed, 2 normal
	April 76	10	0	3 glomeruli completely sclerosed, 2 partly sclerosed, 5 normal
G.W.	March 75	36	9	30 glomeruli sclerosed (3 with crescents); 6 glomeruli compressed by crescents
	April 75	42	6	18 glomeruli sclerosed, 12 showed slight segmental proliferation, 12 normal (6 sclerosed glomeruli had fibrosed crescents)
	April 76	15	4	8 glomeruli sclerosed (4 with fibrosed crescents); 2 partly sclerosed glomeruli; remainder normal
M.S.	May 75	23	22	22 glomeruli obliterated by cellular crescents, 1 normal
	June 75	22	22	All glomeruli surrounded by fibrosed crescents
C.R.	June 75	80	80	All glomeruli occluded by luxuriant crescents
D.M.	June 75	31	31	Extensive necrosis of all glomeruli, 2 completely sclerosed; all compressed by crescents
K.S.	Aug 75	9	0	Early proliferative changes in most glomeruli
	Sept 75	26	0	13 glomeruli showed mesangial hypercellularity; remainder normal
A.W.	Sept 75	19	19	Extensive compression of all glomeruli by crescents
M.W.	Dec 75	8	4	Early focal necrotizing gn with cellular crescents
M.B.	Jan 76	17	16	All glomeruli compressed by cellular crescents
	Feb 76	13	12	Mixture of cellular and fibrosed crescents

F.B.	Feb 76	8	3	Early focal necrotizing gn with cellular crescents
E.M.	Feb 76	12	1	Focal proliferative changes in 6 glomeruli; remainder normal
S.H.	April 76	21	7	Focal proliferative changes in 8 glomeruli, 7 compressed by crescents; remainder normal
R.T.	Aug 76	36	20	Focal proliferative changes in 11 glomeruli; 15 crescents cellular, 5 fibrosed
	Oct 76	9	7	Glomeruli showed focal scarring—areas not scarred were normal, 6 of 7 crescents fibrosed
M.P.	Dec 76	17	17	All glomeruli compressed by luxuriant crescents
P.W.	Jan 77	24	22	Fibrosed crescents obliterated 22 glomeruli, 2 glomeruli sclerosed
R.L.	Feb 77	23	14	All glomeruli showed advanced degree of scarring, crescents fibrosed
D.D.	Feb 77	14	2	Early focal necrotizing gn in 3 glomeruli; 5 partly sclerosed, 2 sclerosed; remainder normal
R.R.	March 77	7	5	Focal proliferative changes in 5 glomeruli progressing to necrosis (prominent crescents); 2 glomeruli showed mesangial proliferation
R.S.	March 77	8	3	3 sclerosed glomeruli, remainder showed focal proliferative changes; crescents mixed fibrous and cellular
R.O.	May 77	32	31	Focal proliferative gn with necrosis; crescent mixed fibrous and cellular
V.S.	Sept 77	20	0	13 sclerosed glomeruli, remainder showed segmental scarring suggestive of late focal proliferative gn
E.L.	Dec 77	10	8	Active cellular crescents compressing most glomeruli, remainder show proliferative changes

Immunofluorescence findings: all patients showed linear deposition of IgG.

*gn = glomerulonephritis.

TRANSPLANTATION. — Transplantation was carried out in three patients (D.M., A.W., C.R.) despite the presence of detectable levels of circulating antibodies. A myocardial infarction caused death one week after transplantation in one patient, hyperacute rejection was responsible for immediate rejection of the graft in the second, and rejection of the graft occurred in the third patient after two months. Recurrence of anti-GBM nephritis was not demonstrated histologically in any of the three patients, although linear GBM fluorescence was present at autopsy of the first patient (D.M.) and in the rejected kidney of the third patient (C.R.).

NONLUPUS CRESCENTIC NEPHRITIS

RENAL FUNCTION. — The overall effects of the treatment regimen on renal function are shown in Table 18–3 and Figure 18–11. Thirteen of the 14 patients were not anuric at presentation: eight of these (F.M., P.R., W.O.C., J.R., T.P., G.S., T.D., J.M.) showed a striking early improvement; of the remaining five (J.C., K.H., P.P., M.B., D.G.), improvement in three (K.H.,

Fig. 18–11.—Measurements of serum creatinine clearance before treatment and at 10, 20 and 30 days after starting the treatment regimen in 13 patients with crescentic (nonlupus) immune complex nephritis.

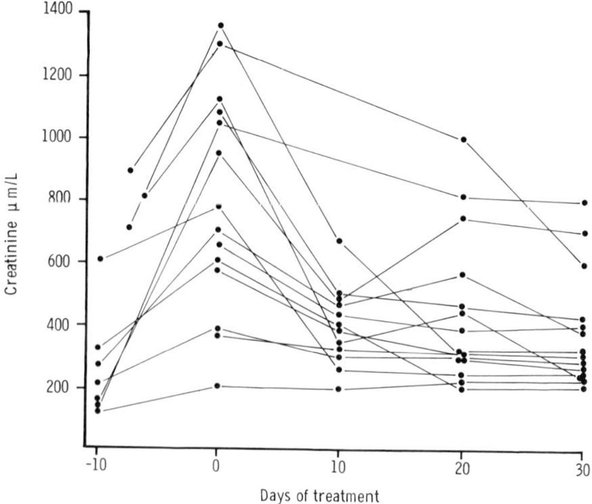

P.P., M.B.) occurred two to three weeks after the start of treatment and could not be confidently attributed to plasma exchange; in the other two patients (D.G., J.C.) an aggressive nephritis (present on biopsy) was arrested and no further deterioration in renal function was observed. Six patients required a short period of dialysis at the start of treatment. No recovery in renal function was observed in the patient (P.B.) who was anuric at the start of therapy. Late deterioration in renal function occurred in one patient (K.H.). In this patient, who had the most severe change on biopsy (22 of 23 glomeruli compressed by crescents) without detectable levels of circulating complexes at the time of deterioration, it was concluded that no useful recovery of renal function could be achieved, and she was not subjected to further plasma exchange.

CIRCULATING IMMUNE COMPLEXES. — Tests for circulating complexes were carried out on sera from 13 patients. C1q assays showed positive results in pretreatment samples taken from six

Fig. 18–12. — Serial measurements of serum creatinine clearance in patient J.M. Complement-dependent assays did not detect immune complexes in this patient, although ^{51}Cr IgG-coated autologous red blood cell clearance titers were prolonged before treatment and normal after starting the therapeutic regimen (see text). $T/2 = 50\%$ clearance time.

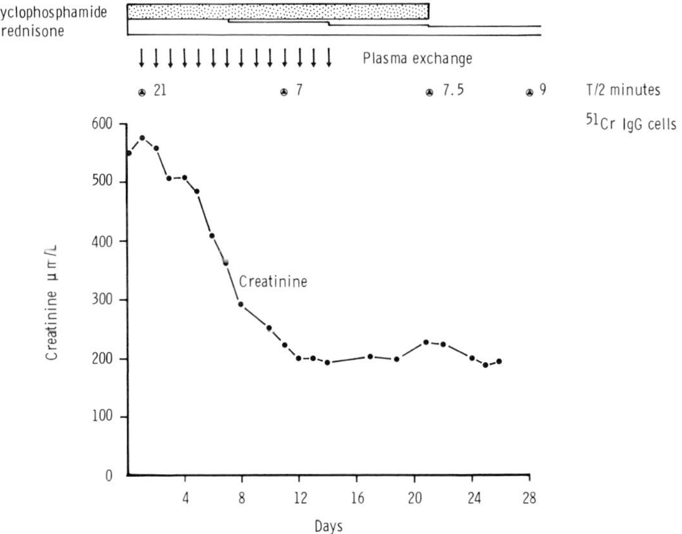

TABLE 18–6.—HISTOLOGY: CRESCENTIC NONLUPUS NEPHRITIS

PATIENT	BIOPSY DATE	NO. OF GLOMERULI	NO. WITH CRESCENTS	PREDOMINANT FEATURES*
F.M.	April 75	13	8	Necrotizing changes in 9 glomeruli, remainder normal; crescents mixed fibrous and cellular
	June 75	13	3	7 sclerosed glomeruli, 3 glomeruli showed focal scarring, 3 normal; crescents fibrosed
	Sept 75	6	1	1 sclerosed glomerulus, 2 partly scarred, 3 normal
	Necrops.	20	3	10 normal glomeruli, 5 partly scarred, 5 sclerosed; crescents fibrosed
P.B.	June 75	25	23	Severe necrotizing glomerulitis affecting 24 glomeruli; crescents all cellular
P.R.	Aug 75	10	7	7 glomeruli showed necrotic changes and were surrounded by cellular crescents, 3 glomeruli normal
	Sept 75	36	7	15 normal glomeruli, 11 showed focal scarring, 10 normal; crescents cellular (2) and fibrous (5)
	Necrops.	20	1	9 normal glomeruli, 5 showed focal scarring, 6 sclerosed
W.O.	Oct 76	20	19	14 glomeruli showed necrotic changes, 5 showed focal scarring; crescents mainly cellular (3)

	Nov 76	9	2	Glomeruli sclerosed (6) or partly scarred (2), 1 normal; both crescents acellular
J.C.	March 76	37	12	Severe necrotizing gn (29); 11 cellular crescents, 1 fibrosed
J.R.	June 76	20	10	Focal necrotizing gn (5) with some glomeruli already hyalinized (8); crescents – mixture of cellular and fibrosed
T.P.	June 76	40	33	Severe necrotizing gn (33) with predominantly cellular crescents (28)
K.H.	June 76	23	22	Advanced necrotic changes in all except one glomerulus with obliteration by cellular crescents
P.F.	Aug 76	27	7	13 glomeruli showed necrosis, 5 sclerosed, 6 focally scarred; remainder normal
D.G.	Oct 76	32	19	9 glomeruli focally scarred, 3 necrotic, 3 normal; most crescents cellular
T.D.	Jan 77	43	27	6 glomeruli showed necrosis, 27 compressed by cellular crescents (11 showed focal proliferation), crescents cellular
G.S.	Dec 76	12	9	Most glomeruli compressed by crescents, one sclerosed and two partly scarred
M.B.	Jan 77	14	5	Hypercellular glomeruli with occasional sclerotic areas within mesangium

Immunofluorescence findings: Fibrin was present in all crescents examined. No immunoglobulins or complement were found in patients FM and WOC; IgG and C3 were deposited segmentally in mesangium of patients PR and JC; granular IgG, IgM and C3 in capillary loops in patient PB; granular deposition IgG, IgA and C3 in capillary loops and mesangium in patient KH; granular deposition IgG and C3 in capillary loops and granular C3 in crescents in patient TD; granular C3 in glomeruli, Bowman's capsule and capillary walls in patient GS.

*gn = glomerulonephritis.

patients (F.M., P.R., W.O.C., J.R., J.C., T.D.) and in one patient (G.S.) early in treatment (ten days after referral); with therapy, levels of complexes fell to within the normal range in all cases. Six of the seven patients with detectable levels of circulating complexes showed a striking early response to therapy (Fig. 18–11). However, good clinical responses were also seen in two patients (T.P., J.M.) in whom C1q binding tests were negative. In one patient (T.P.), treatment with steroids and cytotoxic drugs had been started 2½ weeks before referral. In another patient (J.M.), impaired reticuloendothelial clearance was shown by the ^{51}Cr-labeled IgG-coated red blood cell technique (Fig. 18–12).

RENAL BIOPSIES.—Six of the eight patients from whom tissue was available (P.B., P.R., J.R., K.H., T.D., G.S.) showed granular deposits of immunoglobulin or complement within the glomeruli. Four of these six (P.R., J.R., T.D., G.S.) also had detectable levels of circulating complexes. However, circulating complexes were found in two patients (F.M., W.O.C.) in whom biopsy immunofluorescence results were negative. Follow-up renal biopsies (carried out on three patients—F.M., P.R., W.O.C.) showed a striking cessation of disease activity; glomeruli were either normal or scarred to a variable extent, and crescents had become fibrosed and acellular. The details of renal biopsies are given in Table 18–6.

LUPUS NEPHRITIS

Six patients with SLE were treated with high doses of steroids, cytotoxic drugs and plasma exchange (Table 18–4). Five of the six (V.H., P.F., J.K., P.D., N.A.) were known to have lupus nephritis before referral and had entered a fulminating phase of the disease requiring increasing doses of steroids and cytotoxic drugs; the sixth patient (J.M.) presented undiagnosed, with life-threatening pulmonary vasculitis necessitating artificial ventilation. Circulating ICs were detected in five patients (J.M., P.F., J.K., P.D., N.A.) at the time of referral. Plasma exchange was used as a final stage in the escalation of treatment, which had already involved a rapid increase in steroid therapy (prednisolone 40–100 mg/day in all six patients) and culminated in "pulse" dosage with 1-gm doses of methyl prednisolone in three patients (P.F., J.K., P.D.).

RENAL FUNCTION. — Four of the six patients (V.H., J.M., P.F., J.K.) showed an initial good response to treatment. However, no improvement in renal function occurred in two patients (P.D., N.A.) and both required dialysis. One (J.K.) had a relapse after four months and the presence of severe infection and lack of vascular access precluded plasma exchange. Although steroids (including "pulse" dosage of methyl prednisone) and high doses of cytotoxic drugs were used, renal function continued to deteriorate until the patient died (Fig. 18 – 13).

Fig. 18–13.—Serial measurements of immune complex levels, DNA binding and serum creatinine *(S. Creat.)* clearance in patient J.K. Note the rise in complex levels and the arrest in improvement of renal function that occurred when plasma exchange was interrupted. A relapse at 16 weeks was associated with rising levels of complexes despite increased drug therapy. *Aza* = azathioprine.

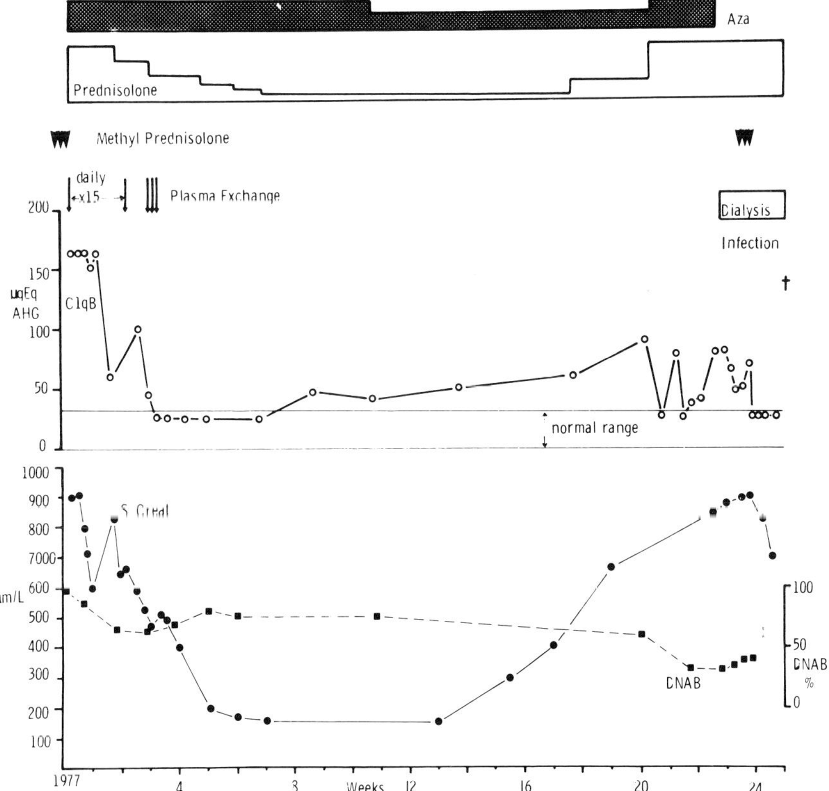

OTHER MANIFESTATIONS OF LUPUS. — Cerebral involvement was a feature of two patients (V.H., J.M.); thrombocytopenia (platelet count less than 50,000/cu mm) was present in two patients (P.F., J.K.); and severe pulmonary vasculitis necessitating ventilation was present in two patients (J.M., P.D.). Improvement eventually occurred in all patients following treatment with the regimen.

CIRCULATING IMMUNE COMPLEXES. — In four patients, samples were available to study the serial levels of ICs. In three patients (J.M., J.K., P.F.), levels fell to within normal limits after plasma exchange was started and as recovery of renal function occurred. In the fourth patient (P.D.) there was no clear response in terms of levels of complexes and there had been no recovery of renal function by the time of her death, which occurred unexpectedly ten days after the start of plasma exchange.

PLASMA EXCHANGE. — Because of the complicated therapeutic regimen involving stepwise increases in drug therapy and eventual introduction of plasma exchange, the beneficial effect of treatment could not always be confidently attributed to plasma exchange. However, in one patient (J.K.), more data are available (Fig. 18–13): cessation of daily exchange was accompanied by a rise in the levels of circulating complexes and an arrest in the recovery of renal function; reintroduction of plasma exchange brought about further improvement in renal function and disappearance of ICs.

DEATHS

ANTI-GBM DISEASE. — Four patients with anti-GBM disease died; death was due principally to lung complications in three patients and to myocardial infarction in the fourth. One patient (E.M.) had lung hemorrhage and *Pseudomonas aeruginosa* septicemia with lung abscesses, which caused death 72 hours after referral. One patient (M.S.) died from lung hemorrhage two months after stopping plasma exchange despite a falling anti-GBM titer. Another patient (D.D.) died from a presumed viral pneumonitis one month after discharge, when other signs of disease activity had been resolved. In one patient (D.M.) death was due to myocardial infarction occurring one week after renal transplantation.

NONLUPUS IC NEPHRITIS. — Five patients died. Three died from opportunistic infection when other signs of disease activity had regressed: the first (T.D.) died four weeks after admission from *Pneumocystis carinii* infection, the second (P.R.) died ten weeks after admission from *Pseudomonas* septicemia, and the third (F.M.) died two months after discharge from *Pneumocystis carinii* infection. One patient (T.P.) died from a cerebrovascular accident ten weeks after discharge. One patient (P.B.) who was anuric did not recover renal function and died on renal dialysis therapy following return to her local hospital.

LUPUS NEPHRITIS. — Death due principally to disease activity occurred in three patients. One patient (N.A.) died within 48 hours of starting plasma exchange after an arrhythmia caused cardiac arrest. The second patient (P.D.) died suddenly from a respiratory arrest ten days after plasma exchange and drug therapy had produced radiologic resolution of a pulmonary vasculitis which had required ventilation. The third patient (J.K.) had a relapse of her disease after a two-month remission had been produced by the treatment regimen. Plasma exchange could not be reintroduced because of severe infection and, although high-dosage steroid therapy and cytotoxic agents were used, disease activity progressed. Death was due to uncontrollable bleeding from ulceration of the stomach associated with *Candida albicans* infection.

Discussion

We have outlined our experience in using plasma exchange, cytotoxic drugs and steroids in the treatment of 44 patients with potentially fulminating nephritis. It is useful to evaluate separately our experience with patients in the three broad groups of diseases to which we have applied this treatment.

ANTI-GBM DISEASE

We believe our regimen represents a considerable advance in the management of patients with anti-GBM antibody-mediated nephritis. As recently as 1970 it was reported that anti-GBM disease was almost uniformly fatal; half the victims died from renal disease and half from lung hemorrhage in one series of 50 patients.[18] In 1973 only four of 32 patients in another series retained their own renal function at follow-up.[26] In our series, 12 of 24 patients showed improvement of renal function. Such improvement was seen only when the patients were not anuric at referral (as was the case in 17 of our 24 patients). Only four of 16 patients failed to respond; in one, technical difficulties with vascular access precluded effective plasma exchange, and the remaining three had the most advanced renal disease in this group at the time of presentation. Our treatment thus appears to have produced a radical improvement in the prognosis of anti-GBM nephritis. Although our experience is uncontrolled, we cannot accept that such improvement is not attributed to the regimen.

Turning to the question of lung hemorrhage, our results suggest that this aspect of anti-GBM disease is also better controlled by our approach. We again believe that the regimen is superior to previously available treatment. Only one of our patients died from lung hemorrhage while receiving the plasma-exchange regimen, and in this case the clinical problem was complicated by severe infection. However, it must be admitted that response to drugs alone and spontaneous remission of lung hemorrhage may occur in patients with Goodpasture's syndrome, and that other factors are important, such as control of fluid and electrolyte balance and prompt and efficient eradication of infection, which precipitates and exacerbates lung injury in patients with anti-GBM disease.[19]

The question of which component of the regimen is responsible for the apparent benefit cannot be resolved with certainty. Study of individual case charts has provided clear examples in which withdrawal of the plasma-exchange component (for technical reasons) was followed by relapse, and reinstitution of plasma exchange was followed by response. We feel that in patients with life-threatening anti-GBM disease, it is not now justifiable to study the effect of plasma exchange alone. On theoretical grounds, removal of antibody is likely to be followed by a rebound in synthesis if not accompanied by treatment with immunosuppressive drugs.[3] However, in another antibody-mediated autoallergic disease—myasthenia gravis—we have been able to demonstrate that plasma exchange per se leads to remission, and that response correlates with the removal of specific antibody.[17] Some support for our reservation about using plasma exchange without cytotoxic drugs has lately been provided by the experience of Swainson and his colleagues in Edinburgh:[23]

therapy by plasma exchange alone for a patient with Goodpasture's syndrome was followed by remission of lung hemorrhage, but also by progression of nephritis; following transplantation, the same patient developed nephritis (while on standard immunosuppressive therapy) and this time plasma exchange led to remission of both lung and kidney disease.

As already indicated, the best response occurred in patients referred at an apparently early phase in the disease, as judged by clinical and histologic criteria. The need for early institution of therapy has been emphasized by our experience: certain patients have shown dramatic loss of renal function, with one patient's condition deteriorating from near normal glomerular function to anuria in less than two weeks. Clearly no regimen, however effective it may be at removing antibody or controlling its synthesis, can be expected to reverse gross derangement and scarring of glomeruli.

We have been interested in whether glomerular necrosis, through the release of GBM antigen, might contribute to the accelerated synthesis of anti-GBM antibody. Although there is no direct evidence for this, recent experimental work in guinea pigs has suggested that antibody-mediated damage in the case of tubular basement membrane (TBM) can, in susceptible animals, lead to secondary auto-anti-TBM antibody production.[6] If a similar process occurs in humans, this would be another reason for early plasma exchange — to interrupt this postulated vicious circle.

At a practical level we regard the prompt institution of therapy as sufficiently important to justify making the diagnosis of anti-GBM disease on clinical grounds, and not allowing investigative procedures such as renal biopsy to delay therapy. When control of the disease is established, biopsy can be undertaken electively at a later stage.

Nonlupus Crescentic Nephritis

Analysis of the contribution of plasma exchange is more difficult. Cytotoxic drugs and steroids have been the drugs most commonly used in treatment[1, 22] and a number of centers have claimed benefit from the additional use of anticoagulants and antiplatelet agents.[2, 7] A major difficulty is that this type of nephritis may be a manifestation of a heterogeneous group of diseases, such as Wegener's granulomatosis, polyarteritis and Henoch-Schönlein purpura, or it may occur without evidence of other specific system involvement. These diseases are rare and attempts at controlled trials of treatment have presented great difficulty. Uncontrolled experience certainly suggests that some drugs are beneficial under certain circumstances: for example, there is a measure of agreement that cyclophosphamide alone is of value in treating Wegener's granulomatosis.[29]

In considering our results, we have, in addition to using standard methods of assessing organ damage, examined the effects of therapy on circulating ICs. From first principles, plasma exchange, if it were to have any place in treating this group of diseases, might be expected to have its greatest value in those patients with high levels of circulating ICs. Overall, this has been our experience: of the nine patients showing the best response to therapy, seven had complexes that were easily detectable. We hope that more selective use of plasma exchange may become possible when better tests for ICs become available. In this connection, improvement in the clearance of antibody-coated erythrocytes following plasma exchange was sometimes observed in patients who did not have detectable levels of ICs. We are in the process of evaluating further the relationships between circulating IC, clearance of labeled erythrocytes and response to treatment.

Lupus Nephritis

In SLE, although much publicity has been given to plasma exchange[20, 25] and our own experience suggests that it has some role, evaluation and definition of criteria for its use present great difficulty. There are a number of reasons for this; they include the well-known spontaneous variation in disease activity, the undeniable value of steroid therapy and the difficulty in standardizing the doses of other drugs, such as cytotoxic agents, in patients with the severe and life-threatening disease who are likely to be referred for plasma exchange.

General Considerations

In all conditions, as well as with the removal of the primary nephrotoxic agents, depletion of mediators, such as complement and coagulation factors brought about by the substitution of albumin (PPF) for plasma, may also contribute to the effect of the regimen. As well as having direct effects on the inflammatory response, perturbation of complement function may alter the disposal of IC by the reticuloendothelial system. Whether or not this would be of therapeutic value remains unclear. In any event, plasma exchange provides the first effective method of altering the internal macromolecular environment and provides opportunities for studying its function in health and disease.

References

1. Bacani, R. A., Velasquez, F., Kanter, A., Pirani, C. L., and Pollak, V. E.: Rapidly progressive (non-streptococcal) glomerulonephritis, Ann. Intern. Med. 69:463, 1968.
2. Brown, C. B., Wilson, D., Turner, D., Cameron, J. S., Ogg, C. S., Chantler, C., and Gill, D.: Combined immunosuppression and anticoagulation in rapidly progressive nephritis, Lancet 2:1166, 1974.
3. Bystryn, J. C., Schenken, I., and Uhr, J. W.: A model for the regulation of antibody synthesis by serum antibody, in Amos, B. (ed.): *Progress in Immunology* (London: Medical Press, 1971), p. 630.
4. Evans, D. J., Gwyn-Williams, D., Peters, D. K., Sissons, J. G. P., Boulton-Jones, J. M., Ogg, C. S., Cameron, J. S., and Hoffbrand, B. I.: Glomerular deposition of properdin in Henoch-Schönlein syndrome and idiopathic focal nephritis, Br. Med. J. 3:326, 1973.
5. Ewan, P. W., Jones, H. A., Rhodes, C. G., and Hughes, J. M. B.: Detection of intrapulmonary hemorrhage with carbon monoxide uptake: application in Goodpasture's syndrome, N. Engl. J. Med. 295:1391, 1976.
6. Hall, C. L., Calvin, R. B., Carey, K., and McCluskey, R. T.: Passive transfer of autoimmune disease with isologous IgG_1 and IgG_2 antibodies to the tubular basement membrane in strain XIII guinea pigs. Loss of self tolerance induced by auto antibodies, J. Exp. Med., 146:1246, 1977.
7. Kincaid-Smith, P., Laver, M. C., Fairley, K. F., and Mathews, D. C.: Dipyrimadole and anticoagulants in renal disease due to glomerular and vascular lesions, Med. J. Aust. 1:145, 1970.
8. Larson, C., Gorman, J. M., and Becket, A.: Advances in automated analysis, Technicon International Congress, vol. 4, 1972.
9. Laurell, C. B.: Quantitative estimation of proteins by electrophoresis in agarose gel containing antibodies, Anal. Biochem. 10:358, 1966.
10. Lockwood, C. M., Boulton-Jones, J. M., Lowenthal, R. M., Simpson, I. J., Peters, D. K., and Wilson, D. B.: Recovery from Goodpasture's syndrome after immunosuppressive treatment and plasmapheresis, Br. Med. J. 2:252, 1975.
11. Lockwood, C. M., Rees, A. J., Pearson, T. A., Evans, D. J., Peters, D. K., and Wilson, D. B.: Immunosuppression and plasma-exchange in the treatment of Goodpasture's syndrome, Lancet 1:711, 1976.
12. Lockwood, C. M., Rees, A. J., Pinching, A. J., Pussell, B., Sweny, P., Uff, J., and Peters, D. K.: Plasma-exchange and immunosuppression in the treatment of fulminating immune complex crescentic nephritis, Lancet 1:63, 1977.
13. Lockwood, C. M., Rees, A. J., Pussell, B., and Peters, D. K.: Experience of the use of plasma-exchange in the management of potentially fulminating glomerulonephritis and SLE, Exp. Hematol. 5(S):117, 1977.

14. Lockwood, C. M., Worlledge, S., and Peters, D. K.: Effect of plasma-exchange on reticulo-endothelial function: a study of clearance of ^{51}Cr-labelled Ig-G coated autologous red cells, in preparation.
15. Mancini, G., Carbonara, A. O., and Heremans, J. F.: Immunochemical quantitation of antigens by single radial immunodiffusion, Int. J. Immunochem. 2:235, 1965.
16. Mollison, P. L.: *Blood Transfusion in Clinical Medicine* (Oxford: Blackwell, 1974), p. 462.
17. Pinching, A. J., Peters, D. K., and Newsome-Davis, J.: Remission of myaesthenia-gravis following plasma-exchange, Lancet 2:1373, 1976.
18. Proskey, A. J., Wetherbee, L., Easterling, R. E., Greene, J. A., and Weller, J. M.: Goodpasture's syndrome, Am. J. Med. 48:162, 1970.
19. Rees, A. J., Lockwood, C. M., and Peters, D. K.: Enhanced allergic tissue injury in Goodpasture's syndrome by intercurrent bacterial infection, Br. Med. J. 2:723, 1977.
20. Rossen, R. D., Hersh, E. M., Sharp, J. T., McCredie, K. B., Gyorkey, F., Suki, W. N., Eknoyan, G., and Reisberg, M. A.: Effect of plasma-exchange on circulating immune complexes and antibody formation in patients treated with cyclophosphamide and prednisone, Am. J. Med. 63:674, 1977.
21. Sobel, A. T., Bokisch, V. A., and Muller-Eberhard, H. J.: C1q deviation test for the detection of immune complexes, aggregates of IgG and bacterial products in human serum, J. Exp. Med. 142:139, 1975.
22. Sonsino, E., Nabarra, B., Kazatchkine, M., Hinglais, N., and Kreis, H.: Extracapillary proliferative glomerulonephritis so-called malignant glomerulonephritis, Adv. Nephrol. 2:121, 1972.
23. Swainson, C. P., Robson, J. S., Urbaniak, S. J., Keller, A. J., and Kay, A. B.: Treatment of Goodpasture's disease by plasma exchange and immunosuppression, Clin. Exp. Immunol. 32:233, 1978.
24. Vermylen, D., DeVreker, R. A., and Verstraete, M.: A rapid enzymatic method for assay of fibrinogen-fibrin polymerisation time (FPT test), Clin. Chim. Acta 10:418, 1963.
25. Verrier-Jones, J., Cumming, R. J., Bucknall, R. C., Asplin, C. M., Fraser, I. D., Bothamley, J., Davis, P., and Hamblin, T.: Plasmapheresis in the management of acute systemic lupus erythematosus? Lancet 1:709, 1976.
26. Wilson, C. B., and Dixon, F. J.: Anti-glomerular basement membrane antibody-induced glomerulonephritis, Kidney Int. 3:74, 1973.
27. Wilson, C. B., Marquardt, H., and Dixon, F. H.: Radioimmune assay for circulating antiglomerular basement membrane antibody, Kidney Int. 6:114A, 1974 (Abstract).
28. Wold, R. T., Young, F. E., Tan, E. M., and Farr, R. S.: Deoxyribonucleic acid antibody: a method to detect its primary interaction with deoxyribonucleic acid, Science 161:806, 1968.
29. Wolff, S. M., Fauci, A. S., Horn, R. G., and Dale, D. C.: Wegener's granulomatosis, Ann. Intern. Med. 81:513, 1974.
30. Zubler, R. H., Nydegger, U., Perrin, L. H., Fehr, K., McCormick, J., Lambert, P. H., and Miescher, P. A.: Circulating and intra-articular complexes in patients with rheumatoid arthritis. Correlation of ^{125}I-C1q binding activity with clinical and biological features of the disease, J. Clin. Invest. 57:1308, 1976.

Index